Drug Therapy pocket 2006–2007

Hematology	3
Respiratory System	4
Rheumatology	5
Metabolic, Endocrine	6
Gastroenterology	7
Nephrology, Urology	8
Infections	9
Neurology	10
Psychiatry	11
Ophtalmology	12
ENT	13
Dermatology	14
Oncology	15
Toxicology	16

www.media4u.com

MW00682900

Contributing Authors:
Albrecht, Carter, Casper, Cheung, Daley, D'Souza, Endres, Freytes, Gilkeson, Jazieh, Kaliszky, Krystal, Levine, Lien, Mukherjee, Pritchard, Smolinske, Tyor, Ur, Walker, Walsh, Woodson

Cover Illustration: Lucy Mikyna
Production: Sylvia Engel
Publisher: Börm Bruckmeier Publishing LLC, www.media4u.com

© 2003–2006, by **Börm Bruckmeier Publishing LLC**
63 16th Street, Hermosa Beach, CA 90254
www.media4u.com
Second Edition

Published in the Middle East by GMG Diagnostics Ltd. by arrangement with Börm Bruckmeier LLC

IMPORTANT NOTICE – PLEASE READ!
This book is based on information from sources believed to be reliable, and every effort has been made to make the book as complete and accurate as possible and to describe generally accepted practices based on information available as of the printing date, but its accuracy and completeness cannot be guaranteed. Despite the best efforts of authors, editors and publisher, the book may contain errors, and the reader should use the book only as a general guide and not as the ultimate source of information about the subject matter.
This book is not intended to reprint all of the information available to the author or publisher on the subject, but rather to simplify, complement and supplement other available sources. The reader is encouraged to read all available material and to consult the package insert and other references to learn as much as possible about the subject.
This book is sold without warranties of any kind, expressed or implied, and the publisher and author disclaim any liability, loss or damage caused by the content of this book.
IF YOU DO NOT WISH TO BE BOUND BY THE FOREGOING CAUTIONS AND CONDITIONS , YOU MAY RETURN THIS BOOK TO THE PUBLISHER FOR A FULL REFUND.

Printed in al-ahram commercial press
ISBN 1-59103-227-X

Preface

Readers have been writing regularly to tell us that they'd like to have drug therapy diagrams. Dr. Karsten Junge kindly compiled a preliminary set of diagrams for us, but it turned out to be so extensive that we decided to recruit additional experts and publish this material in its own booklet, the **Drug Therapy pocket**. As the name implies, it is conceived and designed as a supplement to our familiar **Drug pocket**.

For the **Drug Therapy pocket**, we have chosen a compact 4-column layout for much of the book (see inside front cover).

For the individual diseases or diagnoses, you will find the appropriate class of active substance (e.g. loop diuretics) with the mechanism of action indicated (e.g. volume reduction). In the third column you will find an example of an existing drug, i.e. an active substance with its trade names (e.g. furosemide: Lasix.....). Of course, other equally appropriate pharmaceuticals can be selected from the **Drug pocket**. In the fourth column, you will find facts about dosage and, if applicable, duration of therapy. The first column simply lists qualifying remarks, for example whether a particular drug can be used generally or only in special cases.

When using these therapy tables, please note that they cover drug therapies only. You will not find other therapeutic measures (e.g. surgery) in this book, although they may be more appropriate to the case in question. We have also omitted details about adverse effects and contraindications of medical drugs, even though these considerations are an integral part of drug therapy. Our goal in this volume was to condense a huge amount of information into a single, fundamental drug therapy diagram in the interest of clarity and validity. Each of our expert authors has selected this essential material from the numerous possible drug therapies. This is the main focus of the **Drug Therapy pocket**. Please consult other sources for supplementary information or alternate therapy plans.

We hope you enjoy using the **Drug Therapy pocket**. Please write (service@media4u.com) to tell us what we can do to make it even better.

From the authors and the publisher   February 2006

Contributing Authors

Helmut Albrecht, MD
(Infections)

Assistant Professor, Director, Emory Healthcare Infectious Diseases Clinic, Emory University, Atlanta, GA

Timothy D. Carter, MD
(Neurology)

Associate Professor, Department of Neurology, Medical University of South Carolina, Charleston, SC

Daniel S. Casper, MD
(Ophthalmology)

Assistant Professor, Director of Ophthalmology, Naomi Berrie Diabetes Center, Columbia University Medical Center, New York, NY

Pamela Cheung, MD
(Ophthalmology)

Assistant Professor, Department of Ophthalmology, College of Physicians and Surgeons of Comlumbia University, New York, NY

Charles L. Daley, MD
(Respiratory System)

Professor of Medicine, Division of Mycobacterial and Respiratory Infections, National Jewish Medical and Research Center, Denver, CO

D. Cyril D'Souza, MD
(Psychiatry)

Associate Professor, Department of Psychiatry, Yale University School of Medicine, New Haven, CT

Stefan Endres, MD
(Gastroenterology)

Professor, Chief, Division of Clinical Pharmacology, University of Munich, Munich, Germany

Cesar O. Freytes, MD
(Hematology)

Associate Professor, FACP, Director, Adult Bone Marrow Transplant Program, University of Texas Health Science Center at San Antonio, TX

Gary Gilkeson, MD
(Rheumatology)

Professor, Division of Rheumatology and Immunology, Department of Medicine, Medical University of South Carolina, Charleston, SC

Abdul-Rahman Jazieh, MD
(Oncology)

Professor, M.P.H., Acting Division Director, Hematology/Medical Oncology, Department of Internal Medicine, University of Cincinnati, Cincinnati, OH

Zoltan Kaliszky, MD
(Neurology)

Department of Neurology, Medical University of South Carolina, Charleston, SC

John H. Krystal, MD
(Psychiatry)

Professor, Department of Psychiatry,
Yale University School of Medicine, New Haven, CT

Norman Levine, MD
(Dermatology)

Professor of Medicine (Dermatology), Department of
Medicine, Arizona Health Sciences Center, University
of Arizona, Tucson, AZ

Y. Howard Lien, MD
(Fluids, Electrolytes,
Urology, Nephrology)

Professor, Chief, Section of Nephrology,
Department of Medicine, College of Medicine,
University of Arizona, Tucson, AZ

Debabrata Mukherjee, MD
(Cardiovascular System)

Tyler Gill Professor, Gill Heart Institute,
University of Kentucky, Lexington, KY

Paul B. Pritchard, III, MD
(Neurology)

Professor, Department of Neurology,
Medical University of South Carolina, Charleston, SC

Susan Smolinske, Ph.D.
(Toxicology)

Managing Director, Regional Poison Control Center,
Children's Hospital of Michigan, Wayne State
University, Detroit, MI

William R. Tyor, MD
(Neurology)

Professor, Department of Neurology,
Medical University of South Carolina, Charleston, SC

Ehud Ur, MB, FRCP
(Metabolic, Endocrine)

Head, Division of Endocrinology & Metabolism,
Dalhousie University, Halifax, Nova Scotia, Canada

Aljoeson Walker, MD
(Neurology)

Assistant Professor, Department of Neurology,
Medical University of South Carolina, Charleston, SC

Tracey Walsh, Pharm.D.
(Hematology)

Pharm.D., BCOP,
Department of Pharmacy, Tripler Army Medical Center,
Honolulu, HI

Gayle Ellen Woodson, MD
(ENT)

Professor, Division of Otolaryngology,
Southern Illinois University, Springfield, IL

Additional titles in this series:
Anatomy pocket
Differential Diagnosis pocket
Drug pocket 2006
Drug pocket plus 2006–2007
Canadian Drug pocket 2006–2007
ECG pocket
ECG Cases pocket
EMS pocket
Homeopathy pocket
Medical Abbreviations pocket
Medical Classifications pocket
Medical Spanish pocket
Medical Spanish Dictionary pocket
Medical Spanish pocket plus
Normal Values pocket
Respiratory pocket

Börm Bruckmeier Publishing LLC on the Internet:
www.media4u.com

Contents

8   Contents

10 Contents

How to use the Drug Therapy pocket

6.11 Hyperthyroidism
6.11.1 Grave's Disease, Thyrostatic

Antithyroid (peroxidase inhibition ⇒ hormone synthesis ↓)	**Methimazole** (Tapazole, Gens)	*Ini 10-20mg PO qd, maint dose 10mg/d PO qd; euthyroid usually after 2-8wk, try to discontinue after 12-18mo; Caution: check blood count due to AE (agranulocytosis 0.1-1%)*
or sos **Antithyroid** (conversion T4 → T3 ↓, peroxidase inhibition ⇒ hormone synthesis ↓)	**Propylthiouracil** (Gens)	*ini 150-400mg div into bid, maint dose 50-150mg qd*

Disease group
Subgroup
Dosage

Generic drug name
Brand name
Qualifying remark
Drug category
Mechanism of action
Sources

98. Leech NJ, Controversies in the management of Graves' disease, Clinical Endocrinology, 1998, 49, 273-80
99. Reinwein D, A prospective randomized trial of antithyroid drug dose in Grave' disease therapy, J Clin Endocrinol Metabol, 1993, 76, 1516-21
100. Weetman AP: Graves' disease. N Engl J Med 2000 Oct 26; 343(17): 1236-48

- Fundamental drug therapy diagramms
- 4-column layout:
    + 1st column: qualifying remarks
    + 2nd column: drug class, mechanism of action
    + 3rd column: active agent, brand name
    + 4th column: dosage, route of administration, duration of therapy
- Covering most medical specialties
- Also available as PDA software

1. Cardiovascular System

Debabrata Mukherjee, MD, FACC
Tyler Gill Professor, Gill Heart Institute
University of Kentucky, Lexington, KY

1.1 Hypertension

1.1.1 JNC VII Hypertension Guideline

Classification and management of blood pressure for adults*

BP Classification	SBP* (mmHg)	DBP* (mmHg)	Lifestyle Modification	Initial Drug Therapy Without Compelling Indications	With Compelling Indications (see Table 5)
Normal	< 120	and < 80	Encourage	No antihypertensive drug indicated.	Drug(s) for compelling indications***
Prehypertension	120 - 139	or 80 - 89	Yes		
Stage 1 Hypertension	140 - 159	or 90 - 99	Yes	Thiazide-type diuretics for most. May consider ACEI, ARB, BB, CCB, or combination	Drug(s) for the compelling indications. Other antihypertensive drugs (diuretics, ACEI, ARB, BB, CCB) as needed.
Stage 2 Hypertension	≥ 160	or ≥ 100	Yes	Two-drug combination for most** (usually thiazide-type diuretic and ACEI or ARB or BB or CCB).	

DBP: diastolic blood pressure; SBP: systolic blood pressure; ACEI: angiotensin converting enzyme inhibitor; ARB: angiotensin receptor blocker; BB: beta-blocker; CCB: calcium channel blocker.

*   Treatment determined by highest BP category.
** Initial combined therapy should be used cautiously in those at risk for orthostatic hypotension.
*** Treat patients with chronic kidney disease or diabetes to BP goal of < 130/80 mmHg.

Identifiable causes of hypertension

- Sleep apnea
- Drug-induced or related causes
- Chronic kidney disease
- Primary aldosteronism
- Renovascular disease
- Chronic steroid therapy and Cushing's syndrome
- Pheochromocytoma
- Coarctation of the aorta
- Thyroid or parathyroid disease

Cardiovasular risk factors

Major Risk Factors	Target Organ Damage

• Hypertension*
 • Cigarette smoking
 • Obesity* (body mass index ≥ 30 kg/m^2)
 • Physical inactivity
 • Dyslipidemia*
 • Diabetes mellitus*
 • Microalbuminuria GFR < 60 mL/min
 • Age (> 55 years for men, > 65 years for woman)
 • Family history of premature cardiovascular
    disease (men < 55 years or woman < 65 years)
	• Heart
	    - Left ventricular hypertrophy
	    - Angina or prior myocardial infarction
	    - Prior coronary revascularization
	    - Heart failure
	 • Brain
	    - Stroke or transient ischemic attack
	 • Chronic kidney disease
	 • Peripheral arterial disease
	 • Retinopathy

GFR: glomerular filtration rate., * components of the metabolic syndrome.

Lifestyle modifications to manage hypertension

Modification	Recommendation*, **	Approximate SBP Reduction (Range)
Weight reduction	Maintain normal body weight (body mass index 18.5 - 24.9 kg/m^2)	5 - 20 mmHg/ 10 kg weight loss
Adopt DASH eating plan	Consume a diet rich in fruits, vegetables, and lowfat dairy products with a reduced content of saturated and total fat	8 - 14 mmHg
Dietary sodium reduction	Reduce dietary sodium intake to no more than 100 mmol per day (2.4 g sodium or 6 g sodium chloride)	2 - 8 mmHg
Physical activity	Engage in regular aerobic physical activity such as brisk walking (at least 30 min per day, most days of the week)	4 - 9 mmHg
Moderation of alcohol consumption	Limit consumption to no more than 2 drinks (1 oz or 30 mL ethanol; e.g., 24 oz of beer, 10 oz wine, or 3 oz 80-proof whiskey) per day in most men and to no more than 1 drink per day in woman and lighter weight persons	2 - 4 mmHg

DASH: Dietary Approaches to Stop Hypertension
* For overall cardiovascular risk reduction, stop smoking.
** The effects of implementing these modifications are dose and time dependent, and could be greater for some individuals.

Clinical trial and guideline basis for compelling indications for individual drug classes

Compelling Indication*	Recommended Drugs**						Clinical Trial Basis***
	Diuretic	BB	ACEI	ARB	CCB	Aldo ANT	
Heart failure	x	x	x	x		x	ACC/AHA Heart Failure Guideline, MERIT-HF, COPERNICUS, CIBIS, SOLVD, AIRE, TRACE, ValHEFT, RALES
Postmyocardial infarction		x	x			x	ACC/AHA Post-MI Guideline, BHAT, SAVE, Capricorn, EPHESUS
High coronary disease risk	x	x	x		x		ALLHAT, HOPE, ANBP$_2$, LIFE, CONVINCE

Diabetes	x	x	x	x	x	NKF-ADA Guideline, UKPDS, ALLHAT
Chronic kidney disease			x	x		NKF Guideline, Captopril Trial, RENAAL, IDNT, REIN, AASK
Recurrent stroke prevention	x		x			PROGRESS

* Compelling indications for antihypertensive drugs are based on benefits from outcome studies or existing clinical guidelines; the compelling indication is managed in parallel with the BP.
** Drug abbreviations: ACEI, angiotensin converting enzyme inhibitor; ARB, angiotensin receptor blocker; Aldo ANT, aldosterone antagonist; BB, beta-blocker; CCB, calcium channel blocker.
*** Conditions for which clinical trials demonstrate benefit of specific classes of antihypertensive drugs.

Determine Blood Pressure Stage (JNC VI)

Category	Systolic	Diastolic
Optimal	< 120	< 80 (mmHg)
Normal	< 130	< 85
High-normal	130-139	85-89
Stage I	140-159	90-99
Stage II	160-179	100-109
Stage III	≥ 180	≥ 110
Isol. syst. hypertension	≥ 140	< 90

Major Risk Factors:
- Smoking
- Dyslipidemia
- Diabetes mellitus
- Gender:
  - Men
  - Postmenopausal women
- Age > 60 years
- Family history of cardiovascular disease:
  - Women < age 65
  - Men < age 55

Determine Risk Group

Risk Group	
A	No major risk factors, no TOD/CCD
B	At least one major risk factor, not including diabetes; no TOD/CCD
C	TOD/CCD and/or diabetes, with or without other risk factors

Target Organ Damage (=TOD), Clinical Cardiovascular Disease (=CCD)
- Left ventr. hypertrophy
- Angina/prior myocardial infarction
- Prior coronary artery bypass graft
- Heart failure
- Stroke or TIA
- Nephropathy
- Peripheral arterial disease
- Hypertensive retinopathy

Choose Therapy Concept

HT Treatment	Risk Group		
	A	B	C
High-normal	*	**	***
I	*	**	
II and III			

Example: 66 year old patient with diabetes mellitus, BP 145/95 mmHg
➡ Hypertension Stage I; Risk Group C
➡ immediate initiation of lifestyle modification and drug therapy
* up to 1 year, ** up to 6 months
*** in patients with diabetes mellitus, heart failure or renal failure

JNC VII, Joint National Committee on High BLood Pressure, May 2003

1.1.2   Monotherapy

Diuretic

	Thiazide diuretic (renal H_2O/Na^+Cl^- loss, endogen vasoconstrictive stimuli ↓)	**Hydrochlorothiazide** (Esidrix, Hydrodiuril, Microside, Oretic, Gens)	*12.5-50mg PO qd*
poss	**Potassium-saving diuretic** (renal H_2O/Na^+Cl^- loss, K^+ secretion ↓)	**Triamterene** (Dyrenium)	*50mg PO bid (1-1-0)*
		Amiloride (Midamor, Gens)	*5mg PO qd*
		Spironolactone (Aldactone, Gens)	*25-100mg PO qd*
		Eplerenone (Inspra)	*50mg qd-bid*

Renal Na^+Cl^- mobilization, Caution: only effective if creatinine < 2mg/dl

Beta blocker

	Beta-1-selective blocker (CO↓, neg. chronotropic, neg. inotropic, renin secretion↓, central sympathetic activity↓)	**Metoprolol** (Lopressor, Toprol-xl, Gens)	*50-100mg PO qd-bid*
		Atenolol (Tenormin, Gens)	*25-100mg PO qd*
		Bisoprolol (Zebeta, Gen)	*2.5-10mg PO qd*
		Carvedilol (Coreg)	*6.25-25mg PO bid*

Caution: Uncontrolled heart failure, high grade AV-block, bronchial asthma

Calcium channel blocker (CCB)

	CCB – non-dihydropyridine (chrono-, dromo-, inotropic↓, afterload↓)	**Diltiazem** (Cardizem, Cartia XT, Tiamate, Tiazac, Gens)	*60-90mg PO tid, 90-180mg SR PO qd, 240mg SR PO qd*
or		**Verapamil** (Calan, Covera-HS, Isoptin, Verelan, Gens)	*80-120mg PO tid, 120-240mg SR PO bid*
or	**CCB – dihydropyridine** (chrono-, dromo-, inotropic↓, afterload↓)	**Nifedipine** (Adalat, Adalat cc, Procardia, Procardia XL, Gens)	*20mg SR PO bid, 10mg PO tid*
or		**Amlodipine** (Norvasc)	*5-10mg PO qd*

ACE inhibitor

	ACE inhibitor (vasodilation↑, renal perfus.↑, aldosterone↓, catecholamine↓)	Captopril (Capoten, Gens)	*Incr slowly to 12.5–50mg PO bid-tid*
or		Enalapril (Lexxel, Vaseretic, Vasotec, Gens)	*Incr slowly to 5–20mg PO qd*
or		Lisinopril (Prinivil, Zestril)	*Incr slowly to 2.5–40mg PO qd*
or		Ramipril (Altace)	*Incr slowly to 2.5–10mg PO qd-bid*

Angiotensin receptor blocker (ARB)

	ARB (specific blockade of angiotensin-II type 1 receptor ⇒ angiotensin effects↓)	Losartan (Cozaar)	*50mg PO qd, max 100mg/d*
or		Candesartan (Atacand)	*8–32mg PO qd*
or		Valsartan (Diovan)	*80–320mg PO qd*
or		Irbesartan (Avapro)	*150–300mg PO qd*
or		Telmisartan (Micardis)	*40–80mg PO bid*

Alpha-1-blocker

	Alpha-1-Blocker (vasodilation↑, afterload↓, preload↓)	Prazosin (Minipress, Minipress XL, Gens)	*1–5mg PO bid-tid, 4–6mg SR PO qd*
or		Doxazosin (Cardura, Gens)	*2–8mg PO qd, max 16mg PO qd*

1.1.3 Double Therapy (Two Drug Combination)

Diuretic + Beta blocker or + CCB or + ACE inhibitor or + ARB	**CCB** + Beta blocker or + ACE inhibitor	**ACE-inhibitor** + ARB

1.1.4 Triple Therapy (Three Drug Combination)

Diuretic + Beta blocker + Vasodilator	**Diuretic** + ACE inhibitor + CCB	**Diuretic** + Antisympathotonic + Vasodilator

Vasodilator: CCB, ACE inhibitor, alpha-1 blocker, hydralazine

1.2 Hypertensive Emergency
1.2.1 In General

First measures

	Nitrate (pre-/afterload ↓, venous pooling)	Nitroglycerin (Nitrolingual, Nitrostat)	0.4mg SL, rep prn q5min up to 3 doses in 15min

If persistent

	Central Alpha-2-Agonist (norepinephrine release ↓, periph. sympathetic tone ↓, renin ↓)	Clonidine (Catapres, Catapres-TTS, Gens)	Ini 0.1-0.2mg PO, then 0.05-0.2mg qh until total dose of 0.5-0.7mg
or	ACE inhibitor (vasodilation ↑, renal perfus. ↑, aldosterone ↓, catecholamine ↓)	Captopril (Capoten, Gens)	12.5-25mg PO
or	Beta blocker (neg. ino-, chronotropic ⇒ cardiac output ↓)	Labetalol (Normodyne, Trandate, Gens)	0.5-2mg/min slowly IV up to total of 50-200mg
		Esmolol (Brevibloc)	Loading dose 250-500µg/kg IV over 1min, then 50-100µg/kg/min for 4min, sos rep prn
or	Direct vasodilator (peripheral resistance ↓, afterload ↓)	Hydralazine (Apresoline, Gens)	5-10mg IV (range: 5-20mg) q20-30min prn

In pulmonary edema additionally

	Loop diuretic (excretion of H_2O, Na^+, Cl^-, K^+, Ca^+, Mg^+ ↑)	Furosemide (Lasix, Gens)	20-40mg IV, poss rep after 30min
plus	Opioid (analgesic, sedative)	Morphine sulfate (Astramorph, Avinza, Duramorph, Infumorph, Kadian, Numorphan, Roxanol, Gens)	5-10mg IV (diluted 1:10)
plus	Gas (blood oxygenation)	Oxygen	2-4l/min nasal cannula

If therapy fails			
poss	**Direct vasodilator** (peripheral resistance↓, afterload↓)	Diazoxide (Hyperstat, Proglycem)	*50-150mg IV, rep q5-15min, or 15-30mg/min IV Inf to max 600mg*
poss	**Direct vasodilator** (pre-/afterload↓)	Nitroprusside sodium (Nipride, Nitropress)	*0.25-10mg/kg/min IV*

1.2.2	In Pheochromocytoma		
	Alpha blocker (vasodilation↑, afterload↓, preload↓)	Phentolamine (Regitine, Rogitine, Gens)	*5-10mg IV, then 0.25-1mg/min Inf*
or		Phenoxybenzamine (Dibenzyline)	*1mg/kg over 2-4h in 200ml NS*
poss plus	**Beta blocker**: use only after primary treatment with alpha blocker. **Caution: serious blood pressure elevation without concomitant alpha-blockade!**		
	(CO↓, neg. chronotropic, neg. inotropic, renin secretion↓, central sympathetic activity↓)	Propranolol (Inderide LA, Gens)	*1mg slowly IV, rep prn, 40-80mg PO bid-tid*
		Metoprolol (Lopressor, Toprol, Gens)	*5mg IV, rep prn, 50-200mg XL PO qd*

1.3   Hypotension and Syncope

In neurally mediated syncope			
poss	**Methylxanthine** (Phosphodiesterase inhibition ⇒ cAMP↑⇒ central stimulation of respiration, positive inotropic/chronotropic, vasodilation)	Theophylline (Aerolate, Elixophyllin, Slo-bid, Slo-Phyllin, Theo-24, Theo-DurUni-Dur, Uniphyl, Gens)	*6-12mg/kg/d*
poss	**Beta-1-selective blocker** (CO↓, neg. chronotropic, neg. inotropic, renin secretion↓, central sympathetic activity↓)	Metoprolol (Lopressor, Toprol)	*50-200mg PO qd*
		Atenolol (Tenormin, Gens)	*25-200mg PO qd*

In decreased sympathetic tone

poss	**Alpha-beta-adrenergic agonist** (vasoconstriction, CO↑ ⇒ BP↑)	**Pseudoephedrine** (Sudafed, Afrin)	60mg q4–6h
		Ephedrine (Gens)	25mg PO qd–qid

Consider atrioventricular pacing in refractory cases

In hypocortisolism, diabetic autonomic neuropathy

Drug therapy should be used only after nondrug therapies e.g., support hose, increased sodium intake, lifestyle modifications and fluid expansion have failed.

poss	**Mineralocorticoid** (H_2O and Na^+ resorption ⇒ circulating volume↑)	**Fludrocortisone** (Florinef)	0.1–1.0mg PO qd
poss	**Vasopressor** (alpha-adrenergic agonist ⇒ vasoconstriction)	**Midodrine** (ProAmatine)	2.5mg PO bid–tid

1.4   Coronary Artery Disease

1.4.1   Acute Angina Pectoris

	Nitrate (pre-/afterload↓, venous pooling)	**Nitroglycerin** (Nitrolingual, Nitrostat)	0.4mg SL, rep prn q5min up to 3 doses in 15min
plus	**Gas** (blood oxygenation)	**Oxygen**	2–4l/min nasal cannula
plus	**Antiplatelet drug** (phosphodiesterase/ platelet aggregation-adhesion inhibition)	**Aspirin – ASA** (Ascriptin, Aspergum, Asprimox, Bayer Aspirin, Bufferin, Easprin, Ecotrin, Empirin, Genprin, Halfprin, St. Joseph Pain Reliever, Zorprin, Gens)	81–325mg PO chewed
plus	**Antiplatelet agent** (blockage of platelet ADP-receptors)	**Clopidogrel** (Plavix)	300–600mg loading dose followed by 75mg PO qd

plus	**Opioid** (analgesic, sedative)	**Morphine sulfate** (Astramorph, Avinza, Duramorph, Infumorph, Kadian, Numorphan, Roxanol, Gens)	*5–10mg IV (diluted 1:10)*
plus	**Beta-1-selective blocker** (CO↓, neg. chronotropic, neg. inotropic, O_2 consumption↓, central sympathetic activity↓)	**Metoprolol** (Lopressor, Toprol-xl, Gens)	*5–10mg slowly IV, titrate to HR and BP*
		Atenolol (Tenormin, Gens)	*5mg IV, rep prn*
		Bisoprolol (Ziac, Gens)	*2.5–10mg PO qd*

Under relative contraindication: calcium channel blockers, digitalis glycosides

1.4.2 Chronic Stable Angina Pectoris

In general

	Antiplatelet drug (phosphodiesterase/ platelet aggregation-adhesion inhibition)	**Aspirin – ASA** (Ascriptin, Asprimox, Bayer Aspirin, Bufferin, Easprin, Ecotrin, Empirin, Genprin, Halfprin, St. Joseph Pain Reliever, Zorprin, Gens)	*81–325mg PO qd*
or	**Antiplatelet drug** (blockage of platelet ADP-receptors)	**Clopidogrel** (Plavix)	*75mg PO qd*
plus	**Nitrate** (pre-/afterload↓, venous pooling, coronary spasmolysis, O_2-consumption↓)	**Isosorbide mononitrate** (Imdur, ISMO, Monoket, Gens)	*20–40mg PO bid (1-1-0), 40–100mg SR PO qd*
or / poss plus	**Beta-1-selective blocker** (CO↓, neg. chronotropic, neg. inotropic, O_2 consumption↓, central sympathetic activity↓)	**Metoprolol** (Lopressor, Toprol-xl, Gens)	*50–100mg PO qd-bid*
		Atenolol (Tenormin, Gens)	*25–100mg PO qd*
		Bisoprolol (Ziac, Gens)	*1 x 2.5–10mg PO*

Prinzmetal's angina

	Nitrate (pre-/afterload↓, venous pooling, coronary spasmolysis, O_2-consumption↓)	**Isosorbide mononitrate** (Imdur, ISMO, Monoket, Gens)	20-40mg PO bid (1-1-0), 40-100mg SR PO qd
plus	**Calcium channel blocker (CCB)** (chrono-, dromo-, inotropic↓, afterload↓, O_2-consumption↓)	**Diltiazem** (Cardizem, Cartia XT, Tiamate, Tiazac, Gens)	60-90mg PO tid, 90-180mg SR PO bid, 240mg SR PO qd
		Amlodipine (Norvasc)	5-10mg PO qd
poss	**Beta-1-selective blocker** (CO↓, neg. chronotropic, neg. inotropic, O_2 consumption↓, central sympathetic activity↓)	**Metoprolol** (Lopressor, Toprol-xl, Gens)	50-100mg PO qd-bid
		Atenolol (Tenormin, Gens)	25-100mg PO qd

Poss antihypertensive therapy in CAD

	Beta-1-selective blocker (CO↓, neg. chronotropic, neg. inotropic, O_2-consumption↓)	**Metoprolol** (Lopressor, Toprol-xl, Gens)	50-100mg PO qd-bid
		Atenolol (Tenormin, Gens)	25-100mg PO qd
or	**ACE inhibitor** (vasodilation↑, renal perfusion↑, aldosterone release↓, catecholamine release↓)	**Captopril** (Capoten, Gens)	Incr slowly to 12.5-25mg PO bid
		Enalapril (Lexxel, Vaseretic, Vasotec, Gens)	2.5-20mg PO qd, max 40mg qd; IV ini 1.25mg, then 1.25-2.5mg IV qid
		Lisinopril (Prinivil, Zestril)	2.5-40mg PO qd
		Ramipril (Altace)	1.25-5mg PO qd-bid max 20mg qd
or	**Calcium channel blocker (CCB)** (O_2-consumption↓, inotropic↓, afterload↓)	**Amlodipine** (Norvasc)	5-10mg PO qd

Acute coronary syndrome without ST-elevation			
	Heparin, unfractionated (coagulation factor inhibition ↑, embolism prophylaxis)	Heparin (Gens)	*5000 U IV bolus, then 1000 U/h; aim for aPTT ratio of 1.5–2.5*
or	**Heparin – low-molecular-weight** (LMWH)	Enoxaparin (Lovenox)	*30mg IV bolus, then 1mg/kg SC bid*
plus	**Antiplatelet drug** (phosphodiesterase/ platelet aggregation-adhesion inhibition)	Aspirin – ASA (Ascriptin, Asprimox, Bayer Aspirin, Bufferin, Easprin, Ecotrin, Empirin, Genprin, Halfprin, St. Joseph Pain Reliever, Zorprin, Gens)	*325mg PO chewed*
plus	**Antiplatelet drug** (blockage of platelet ADP-receptors)	Clopidogrel (Plavix)	*300-600mg loading dose then 75mg PO qd*
plus	**Nitrate** (pre-/afterload↓, venous pooling, scientifically disputed)	Nitroglycerin (Nitrolingual, Nitrostat)	*0.4mg SL, rep prn q5min up to 3 doses in 15min*
plus	**Opioid** (analgesic, sedative)	Morphine sulfate (Astramorph, Avinza, Duramorph, Infumorph, Kadian, Numorphan, Roxanol, Gens)	*5-10mg IV (diluted 1:10)*
plus	**Beta-1-selective blocker** (CO↓, neg. chronotropic, neg. inotropic, O_2 consumption↓, central sympathetic activity↓)	Metoprolol (Lopressor, Toprol-xl, Gens)	*5mg IV x 3; Caution: BP↓, HR↓*
		Atenolol (Tenormin, Gens)	*5mg IV, rep prn*
plus	**Statins** (intracell. cholesterol synthesis↓, LDL↓, HDL↑)	Atorvastatin (Lipitor)	*10-80mg PO qd*
		Pravastatin (Pravachol)	*10-20 mg PO qd*
		Simvastatin (Zocor)	*10-40mg PO qd*

1.5 Myocardial Infarction
1.5.1 First Measures

	Antiplatelet drug (phosphodiesterase/ platelet aggregation- adhesion inhibition)	**Aspirin – ASA** (Ascriptin, Asprimox, Bayer Aspirin, Bufferin, Easprin, Ecotrin, Empirin, Genprin, Halfprin, St. Joseph Pain Reliever, Zorprin, Gens)	*325mg PO chewed*
plus	**Nitrate** (pre-/afterload ↓, venous pooling, scientifically disputed)	**Nitroglycerin** (Nitrolingual, Nitrostat)	*0.4mg SL, rep prn q5min up to 3 doses in 15min*
poss	**Opioid** (analgesic, sedative)	**Morphine sulfate** (Astramorph, Avinza, Duramorph, Infumorph, Kadian, Numorphan, Roxanol, Gens)	*5-10mg IV (diluted 1:10)*
plus	**Heparin, unfractionated** (coagulation factor inhibition ↑, embolism prophylaxis)	**Heparin** (Gens)	*5000-10000 U IV*
plus	**Gas** (blood oxygenation)	**Oxygen**	*2-6l/min nasal cannula*
poss	**Benzodiazepine** (sedative, anxiolytic, muscle relaxing)	**Diazepam** (Diazepam Intensol, Valium, Gens)	*5-10mg IV sos*
poss	**ACE inhibitor** (vasodilation ↑, renal perfus. ↑, aldosterone ↓, catecholamine ↓)	**Captopril** (Capoten)	*6.25–25mg PO tid*
		Enalapril (Vasotec)	*2.5–20mg PO qd*
		Lisinopril (Zestril)	*2.5–10mg PO qd*
		Ramipril (Altace)	*2.5–5mg PO bid*
poss only if CV-stable	**Beta-1-selective blocker** (CO ↓, neg. chronotropic, neg. inotropic, O$_2$ consumption ↓, central sympathetic activity ↓)	**Metoprolol** (Lopressor, Toprol-xl, Gens)	*5mg IV; Caution: BP↓, HR↓*
		Atenolol (Tenormin, Gens)	*5mg IV, rep prn*

1.5.2   Revascularization Therapy

Primary percutaneous intervention (PCI)

or	**Thrombolytic** (plasminogen activation ⇒ fibrin proteolysis, recanalization, limitation of myocard necrosis, mortality↓)	**Streptokinase** (Streptase)	*1.5 M IU over 1h IV*
or		**rt-PA** (Alteplase)	*15mg IV as bolus, then 0.75mg/kg (max 50mg) over 30min, then 0.5mg/kg (max 35mg) over 1h*
or		**Reteplase** (Retevase)	*10 U as bolus IV, rep after 30min*
or		**Tenecteplase** (TNKase)	*30–50mg IV over 5sec, dose based on body weight*
plus	**Heparin, unfractionated** (coagulation factor inhibition ↑, embolism prophylaxis)	**Heparin** (Gens)	*Concomitant heparin: 5000 U IV bolus, then 1000 U/h (no heparin with streptokinase)*

If possible: primary angioplasty, ICU admission. IV Heparin not necessary with Streptokinase. SC heparin may be used in these patients for thromboprophylaxis.
CI of thrombolytics: severe HTN, aortic aneurysm, endocarditis, GI ulcers, pancreatitis, advanced malignant tumors, pathologic hemostasis, head trauma, internal bleeding, operation or puncture < 10d, IM injection < 7d, esophageal varices; CI of anistreplase/streptokinase: hypersensitivity to these products

1.5.3   Therapy of Complication

Ventricular tachyarrhythmias

poss	**Antiarrhythmic, class Ib**	**Lidocaine** (Xylocaine)	*Ini 50-100mg IV, then Inf at 2-4mg/min*
	Antiarrhythmic, class Ia	**Procainamide** (Pronestyl)	*17mg/kg bolus, then Inf at 1-4mg/min*
or poss	**Antiarrhythmic, class III** (blockage of K+ channels ⇒ action potential length ↑, refractory time↑)	**Amiodarone** (Cordarone, Pacerone, Gens)	*IV 150mg over 30min, then 1mg/min for 6h Inf, then 0.5mg/min for 18h, or d1-10: 1000mg PO div in 5 doses, then 200mg/d*

Atrial fibrillation

	Beta-1-select. blocker (CO↓, neg. chronotropic, neg. inotropic, renin secretion↓, central sympathetic activity↓)	**Metoprolol** (Lopressor, Toprol-xl, Gens)	*50–100mg PO qd-bid*
		Atenolol (Tenormin, Gens)	*25–100mg PO qd*
plus	**Antiarrhythmic, class III** (blockage of K⁺ channels ⇒ action potential length ↑, refractory time↑)	**Amiodarone** (Cordarone, Pacerone, Gens)	*d1-10: 1000mg PO div in 5 doses, then 200mg qd*

Sos cardioversion!

or	**Calcium channel blockers (CCB) – non-dihydropyridine** (chrono-, dromo-, inotropic↓, afterload↓, O₂-consumption↓)	**Diltiazem** (Cardizem, Cartia XT, Tiamate, Tiazac, Gens)	*15–25mg IV bolus, then 10mg/h Inf*
		Verapamil (Calan, Covera-HS, Isoptin, Verelan, Gens)	*5mg slowly IV, then 5–10mg/h, max 100mg/d*

Bradycardia

	Antiarrhythmic (parasympatholytic, chronotropic↑)	**Atropine** (Atropen)	*0.5–1mg IV*

Sos pacemaker!

Heart Failure

poss	**Loop diuretic** (excretion of H₂O, Na⁺, Cl⁻, K⁺, Ca⁺, Mg⁺↑)	**Furosemide** (Lasix, Gens)	*20–40mg IV*
plus	**Nitrate** (pre-/afterload↓, venous pooling)	**Nitroglycerin** (Nitro-Bid, Nitrolingual, Nitrostat, Tridil, Gens)	*0.4mg SL, rep prn q5min up to 3 doses in 15min; IV Inf 5–200µg/min*
plus	**Gas** (blood oxygenation)	**Oxygen**	*2-4l/min nasal cannula*
plus	**ACE inhibitor** (vasodilation↑, renal perfus.↑, aldosterone↓, catecholamine↓)	**Captopril** (Capoten)	*Incr slowly to 12.5–25mg PO bid*
		Enalapril (Vasotec)	*2.5–20mg PO qd*
		Lisinopril (Zestril)	*2.5–40mg PO qd*

Cardiogenic shock

Primary therapy goal: placement of intra-aortic balloon pump, revascularization with angioplasty or surgery.

	Gas (blood oxygenation)	**Oxygen**	*2-4l/min nasal cannula*
plus	**Loop diuretic** (excretion of H_2O, Na^+, Cl^-, K^+, Ca^+, $Mg^+\uparrow$)	**Furosemide** (Lasix, Gens)	*20-80mg IV qd*
poss	**Vasopressor** (dose-dependent dopamine-, beta-alpha-adrenergic agonism $\Rightarrow$ inotropia$\uparrow$, CO$\downarrow$, renal vasodilation, vasoconstriction)	**Dopamine** (Intropin, Gens)	*Ini 2-5µg/kg/min, incr by 1-4µg/kg/min q10-30min, max 50µg/kg/min; Renal dose: 0.5-5µg/kg/min, beta-stim. at 5-10µg/kg/min, alpha stimulation at 10-20µg/kg/min*
poss	**Phosphodiesterase inhibitor** (intracell. cAMP$\uparrow$ $\Rightarrow$ $Ca^{++}\uparrow$ $\Rightarrow$ chrono-/inotropia$\uparrow$, CO$\uparrow$, vasodilation)	**Milrinone** (Primacor)	*50µg/kg IV over 10 min, maint 0.5µg/kg/min Inf*
poss	**Vasopressor** (primarily beta-adrenergic agonist, inotropia$\uparrow$, no vasoconstriction)	**Dobutamine** (Dobutrex, Gens)	*Ini 0.5-1µg/kg/min IV, incr to 2.5-20µg/kg/min*

1.5.4   Secondary Prophylaxis after Infarction

	Antiplatelet drug (phosphodiesterase/platelet aggregation-adhesion inhibition)	**Aspirin – ASA** (Ascriptin, Asprimox, Bayer Aspirin, Bufferin, Easprin, Ecotrin, Empirin, Genprin, Halfprin, St. Joseph Pain Reliever, Zorprin, Gens)	*81-325mg PO qd*
or	**Antiplatelet drug** (blockage of platelet ADP-receptors)	**Clopidogrel** (Plavix)	*75mg PO qd*

plus	Beta-1-selective blocker (CO↓, neg. chronotropic, neg. inotropic, renin secretion↓, central sympathetic activity↓)	Metoprolol (Lopressor, Toprol-xl, Gens)	*50-100mg PO qd-bid*
		Atenolol (Tenormin, Gens)	*25-100mg PO qd*
		Bisoprolol (Ziac, Gens)	*2.5-10mg PO qd*
plus	ACE inhibitor (vasodilation↑, renal perfusion↑, aldosterone↓, catecholamine↓)	Captopril (Capoten, Gens)	*Incr slowly to 12.5-25mg PO bid*
		Lisinopril (Zestril)	*2.5-40mg PO qd*
		Enalapril (Lexxel, Vaseretic, Vasotec, Gens)	*2.5-20mg PO qd, max 40mg qd; IV ini 1.25mg, then 1.25-2.5mg IV qid*
		Ramipril (Altace)	*1.25-5mg PO qd max 10mg qd*
plus	HMG-CoA-reductase inhibitor (intracell. cholesterol synthesis↓, LDL↓, HDL↑)	Atorvastatin (Lipitor)	*10-20mg PO qd*
		Pravastatin (Pravachol)	*10-20 mg PO qd*
		Simvastatin (Zocor)	*10-40mg PO qd*

1.6 Heart Failure

1.6.1 Determine Heart Failure Stage

ACC/AHA

Stage	A	B	C	D
Definition	At high risk for heart failure but without structural heart disease or symptoms of HF	Structural heart disease but without symptoms of HF	Structural heart disease with prior or current symptoms of HF	Refractory HF requiring specialized interventions
e.g. Patients with	- Hypertension - CAD - Diabetes mell. - FHx CM or Patients using cardiotoxins	- Previous MI - LV systolic dysfunction - Asymptomatic valvular disease	- Known struct. heart disease - Shortness of breath, fatigue, reduced exercise tolerance	- Marked symptoms at rest despite max. medical Tx; frequently hospitalized (1)

ACC: American College of Cardiology; AHA: American Heart Association

New York Heart Association (NYHA)

Stage	NYHA I	NYHA II	NYHA III	NYHA IV
Symptoms	no symptoms	during ordinary physical strain	during slight physical strain	symptoms during rest
CO	normal	normal	during physical strain ↓	at rest ↓
LVEDP	during physical strain ↑	at rest ↑	at rest ↑	at rest ↑

Classification after NYHA (= New York Heart Association)
CO = Cardiac output, LVEDP = Left ventricular end-diastolic pressure

1.6.2 Evaluation of Heart Failure + Concomitant Disorders

Concomitant DOs	Evaluation
Cardiovascular Hypertension Hyperlipidemia Diabetes mellitus CAD Supraventr. arrhythmias Ventr. arrhythmias Prevention of sudden death Prev. of thrombotic events **Noncardiovascular** Renal insufficiency Pulmonary disease Cancer Thyroid disease (1)	Thorough **H + P** (identify cardiac and noncardiac DO)
	Assess patient's ability to perform routine and desired **activities of daily living** (initial, ongoing)
	Volume status (initial, ongoing)
	Initial laboratory: CBC, UA, serum electrolytes (incl Ca⁺⁺, Mg⁺), BUN, serum creatinine, blood glucose, LFTs, TSH (initial)
	Serial laboratory: serum electrolytes, renal function
	Initial 12-lead **ECG** and chest **X-ray**
	Initial 2-dimensional **echocardiography** with **Doppler** or **radionuclide ventriculography** (assess left ventr. syst. function)
	Cardiac catheterization with **coronary arteriography** in patients with angina who are candidates for revascularization (1)

1.6.3   Start Therapy

	A	B	C	D
Therapy: **General Measures** + **Pharmacologic Treatment of Heart Failure** + **Treatment of Concomitant Disorders**	- Encourage smoking cessation and regular exercise - Discourage alcohol intake, illicit drug use - Treat **hypertension** - Treat **lipid DO** - ACE inhibitors in appropriate patients[a] - Control HR in supraventricular tachyarrhythmias - Treat **thyroid DO** - Evaluate periodically for heart failure	**All measures under stage A +** - ACE inhibitors in appropriate patients[b] - Beta-blockers in appropriate patients[c] - Valve replacement or repair for patients with significant valvular stenosis or regurgitation - Evaluate regularly for heart failure	**All measures under stage A +** - Dietary salt restriction - Diuretics in patients with fluid retention - ACE inhibitors in all patients unless CI - Beta-blockers in all stable patients unless CI - Digitalis for TX of symptoms of HF unless CI - Withdrawal of drugs known to adversely affect HF (e.g. CCBs)	**All measures under stages A, B and C +** - Control of fluid retention - Mechanical assist devices - Referral for cardiac transplantation in eligible patients - Continous IV inotropic infusion for palliation - Hospice care

a) with a Hx of atherosclerotic valvular disease, diabetes mellitus, or hypotension and associated cardiovascular risk factors

b) with a recent or remote Hx of myocardial infarct. regardless of ejection fraction OR in patients with a reduced ejection fraction, whether or not they have experienced a myocardial infarction

c) with a recent myocardial infarction regardless of ejection fraction OR in patients with a reduced ejection fraction whether or not they have experienced a myocardial infarction   (1)

1.6.4   Therapy Goals

Decrease mortality   **Improve symptoms (quality of life)**
Stop progression   **Decrease hospitalization rate**

Drug Class	Decrease in Mortality	Inhibition of Progression	Symptom Improvement	Decrease in Hospitaliz. Rate	Improved Hemodyn. Parameters
ACE Inhib.	A	A	A	A	A
Beta Blocker	A	A	A	A	A
Diuretic Loop	C	C	B	B	B
Aldost. Antag.	B	B	B	B	B
Glycoside	C	C	B	B	B
ARB	B	B	A	B	B

A: Several randomized controlled clinical studies
B: One randomized controlled clinical study or good evidence through clinical experience
C: No sure study results that prove beneficial or damaging effects
D: Negative results based on one or more studies   (1)

1.6.5   Pharmacological Treatment of Heart Failure

DrugClass	Drug	Initial Dose	Max. Dose
ACE Inhib	Captopril	6.25-12.5mg tid	450mg/d
		Monitor blood pressure. Increase gradually depending on patient's response.	
	Enalapril	2.5mg qd	20 mg bid
		Monitor blood pressure, renal function. Uptitrate as tolerated over a few days or weeks.	
	Lisinopril	5mg qd	40 mg qd
		Monitor blood pressure. Increase by no greater than 10mg, at intervals of at least 2 weeks to the highest tolerated dose up to max. 40mg/d.	
	Quinapril	5 mg bid	20 mg bid
		If well tolerated titrate weekly intervals until effective dose is reached	
Beta Blocker	Carvedilol	3.125mg bid	25mg bid; >85kg: 50mg bid
		Individualize dosage and monitor closely during up-titration! If well tolerated increase to 6.25, 12.5 and 25mg over successive intervals of at least two weeks to the highest tolerated dose. Carvedilol has demonstrated improved survival compared to metoprolol in one randomized trial (COMET).	
	Metoprolol succinate	12.5-25mg qd	200mg qd
		Monitor closely during up-titration. Double dose every 2 weeks to the highest dosage level tolerated by the patient or up to max 200mg/d.	
Diuretic (loop)	Bumetanide	0.5-2mg qd	10mg qd
		Uptitrate by giving 2nd or 3rd dose at 4-5h intervals up to max. 10mg/d	
	Ethacrynic acid	50 mg qd	100-200mg bid
		After diuresis has been achieved give minimally effective dose.	
	Furosemide	20-80mg as single dose	600mg qd
		If needed repeat same dose after 6-8h or increase. Raise by increments of 20-40mg and administer not sooner than 6-8h after prvios dose. Give individually determined single dose qd or bid. Titrate up to max 600mg/d.	
	Torsemide	10-20mg qd	200 mg qd
		Uptitrate by approx. doubling until desired diuretic response is obtained.	

Diuretic (thiazide)	Hydrochloro-thiazide	25mg qd	25-100mg qd
		Many patients respond to intermittent therapy e.g. on alternate days.	
	Metolazone	5mg qd	20mg qd
		Titrate to gain an initial therapeutic response and to determine the minmal dose possible to maintain the desired therapeutic response.	
Diuretic (aldost. antag.)	Spironolactone	25mg qd (100mg qd)	200mg qd
		If an adequate diuretic effect has not occurred after five days, add second diuretic that acts more proximally in the renal tubule.	
	Eplerenone	25mg qd	50mg qd
		Monitor serum K^+! Titrate to target dose of 50mg/d within 4 wks as tolerated.	
Glycoside	Digoxin	Digitalization, e.g.: ini **0.4-0.6mg IV**, then 0.1-0.3mg q6-8h until adequate effect; maint 0.125(0.0625)-0.5mg qd	
		Titrate according to the patient's age, lean body weight and renal function.	
ARB (angio-tensin rec. blocker)	Valsartan	40mg bid	160mg bid
		Uptitrate to the highest dose (to 80mg bid and 160mg bid), as tolerated by the patient.	

(1)Hunt SA, Baker DW, Chin MH, Cinquegrani MP, Feldmann AM, Francis GS, Ganiat TG, Goldstein S, Gregoratos G, Jessup ML, Noble RJ, Packer M, Silver MA, Stevenson LW. ACC/AHA guidelines for the evaluation and management of chronic heart failure in the adult. 2001. American College of Cardiology

ACE inhibitor (vasodilation ↑, renal perfus. ↑, aldosterone ↓, catecholamines ↓)	**Captopril** (Capoten, Gens)	*Incr slowly to 12.5-25mg PO bid*
	Lisinopril (Zestril)	*2.5-40mg PO qd*
	Enalapril (Lexxel, Vaseretic, Vasotec, Gens)	*2.5-20mg PO qd, max 40mg qd; IV ini 1.25mg, then 1.25-2.5mg IV qid*
	Ramipril (Altace)	*1.25-10mg PO qd-bid, max 20mg qd*
ARB (specific blockade of angiotensin-II type 1 receptor ⇒ angiotensin effects ↓)	**Losartan** (Cozaar)	*50mg PO qd max 100mg/d*
	Candesartan (Atacand)	*8-32mg PO qd*
	Valsartan (Diovan)	*80-320mg PO qd*
	Irbesartan (Avapro)	*150-300mg PO qd*
	Telmisartan (Micardis)	*40-80mg PO qd*
Beta-1-selective blocker (CO ↓, neg. chronotropic, neg. inotropic, renin secretion ↓, central sympathetic activity ↓)	**Metoprolol** (Lopressor, Toprol-xl, Gens)	*50-100mg PO qd-bid, ini with very small doses, then slowly incr*
	Atenolol (Tenormin, Gens)	*25-100mg PO qd*
	Bisoprolol (Ziac, Gens)	*2.5-10mg PO qd*
Beta-adrenergic blocker, nonselective	**Carvedilol** (Coreg)	*3.125-50mg PO bid*
Thiazide diuretic (renal H_2O/Na^+Cl^- loss, endog. vasoconstrictive stimuli ↓)	**Hydrochlorothiazide** (Esidrix, Hydrodiuril, Microside, Oretic, Gens)	*12.5-50mg PO qd (caution: only effective if creatinine < 2mg/dl, then furosemide)*
Loop diuretic (excretion of H_2O, Na^+, Cl^-, K^+, Ca^+, Mg^+ ↑)	**Furosemide** (Lasix)	*20-80mg IV qd*
	Torasemide (Demadex)	*2.5-10mg PO qd-bid, 10-20mg IV qd-tid, max 200mg PO/IV qd*
or **Aldosterone antagonist** (renal H_2O/Na^+Cl^- loss, K^+ secretion ↓)	**Spironolactone** (Aldactone, Gens)	*d1-5: 50-100mg bid-qid, then 50-100mg PO qd-bid*
	Eplerenone (Inspra)	*25-50mg PO qd*

| **Cardiac glycoside** (chrono-, dromo-↓, inotropic↑, AV node refract. time↑, economy of coronary work↑) | **Digoxin** (Digoxin pediatric, Lanoxi Cap, Lanoxin, Lanoxin pediatric, Gens) | *Ini 0.5mg IV, then 0.25mg q6h for 2 doses, (total 1mg), then 0.25mg PO qd* |
| **Nitrate** (pre-/afterload↓, venous pooling, coronary spasmolysis, O_2-consumption↓) | **Isosorbide mononitrate** (Imdur, ISMO, Monoket, Gens) | *20-40mg PO bid (1-1-0), 30-120mg SR PO qd* |

1.7   Arrhythmias
1.7.1   Sinus Tachycardia

Find cause i.e hypovolemia, anxiety

| **Beta-1-selective blocker** (CO↓, neg. chronotropic, neg. inotropic, renin secretion↓, central sympathetic activity↓) | **Metoprolol** (Lopressor, Toprol-xl, Gens) | *50-100mg PO qd-bid* |
| | **Atenolol** (Tenormin, Gens) | *25-100mg PO qd* |

1.7.2   Atrial Flutter

Heart rate control

poss	**Cardiac glycoside** (chrono-, dromo-↓, inotropic↑, AV node refract. time↑, economy of coronary work↑)	**Digoxin** (Digoxin pediatric, LanoxiCap, Lanoxin, Lanoxin pediatric, Gens)	*Ini 0.5mg IV, then 0.25mg q6h for 2 doses, (total 1mg), then 0.25mg PO qd*
plus	**Beta-1-selective blocker** (CO↓, neg. chronotropic, neg. inotropic, renin secretion↓, central sympathetic activity↓)	**Metoprolol** (Lopressor, Toprol-xl, Gens)	*50-100mg PO qd-bid*
		Atenolol (Tenormin, Gens)	*25-100mg PO qd*

or	CCB – non-dihydropyridine (chrono-, dromo-, inotropic↓, afterload↓, O_2-consumption↓)	Verapamil (Calan, Covera-HS, Isoptin, Verelan, Gens)	5mg slowly IV, then 5-10mg/h, max 100mg/d
		Diltiazem (Cardizem, Cartia XT, Tiamate, Tiazac, Gens)	IV 15-25mg bolus, then 10mg/h Inf; 60-90mg PO tid, 90-180mg SR PO bid, 240mg SR PO qd

Catheter ablation

1.7.3 Atrial Fibrillation

Embolism prophylaxis

poss	Heparin, unfractionated (coagulation factor inhibition↑, embolism prophylaxis)	Heparin (Gens)	5000 U IV bolus, then 1000 U/h; aim for a PTT ratio of 1.5-2.5
plus	Antiplatelet drug (phosphodiesterase/ platelet aggregation-adhesion inhibition)	Aspirin – ASA (Ascriptin, Asprimox, Bayer Aspirin, Bufferin, Easprin, Ecotrin, Empirin, Genprin, Halfprin, St. Joseph Pain Reliever, Zorprin, Gens)	81-325mg PO qd
or	Oral anticoagulant (vit. K antagonism ⇒ clotting factors II, VII, IX, X↓ ⇒ longterm anticoag.)	Warfarin (Coumadin, Gens)	2-10mg PO qd to keep INR 2-2.5 times normal

Heart rate control

poss	Cardiac glycoside (chrono-, dromo-↓, inotropic↑, AV node refract. time↑, economy of coronary work↑)	Digoxin (Digoxin pediatric, LanoxiCap, Lanoxin, Lanoxin pediatric, Gens)	Ini 0.5mg IV, then 0.25mg q6h for 2 doses, (total 1mg), then 0.25mg PO qd
plus	Beta-1-selective blocker (CO↓, neg. chronotropic, neg. inotropic, renin secretion↓, central sympathetic activity↓)	Metoprolol (Lopressor, Toprol-xl, Gens)	50-100mg PO qd-bid
		Atenolol (Tenormin, Gens)	25-100mg PO qd

| or | **CCB – non-dihydropyridine** (chrono-, dromo-, inotropic↓, afterload↓, O_2-consumption↓) | **Verapamil** (Calan, Covera-HS, Isoptin, Verelan, Gens) | 5mg slowly IV, then 5-10mg/h, max 100mg/d; 80-120mg PO tid-qid |
| | | **Diltiazem** (Cardizem, Cartia XT, Tiamate, Tiazac, Gens) | IV 15-25mg bolus, then 10mg/h Inf; 60-90mg SR PO tid, 90-180mg SR PO bid, 240mg SR PO qd |

Restoration of sinus rhythm

Primary method: DC cardioversion

poss	**Antiarrhythmic, class III** (blockage of K^+ channels ⇒ action potential length ↑, refractory time↑)	**Amiodarone** (Cordarone, Pacerone, Gens)	150mg IV over 30min, then 1mg/min Inf for 6h, then 0.5mg/min for 18h
		Ibutilide (Corvert)	1mg IV, rep once prn
or	**Antiarrhythmic, class III** (blockage of K^+ channels + beta-receptor blocker ⇒ refractory time↑)	**Sotalol** (Betapace, Betapace AF, Gens)	80-160mg PO bid; Caution: contraindicated in CAD

Urgent restoration of normal sinus rhythm only indicated in patients with hypotension, shock, heart failure

1.7.4	Relapse Prophylaxis		
poss	**Antiarrhythmic, class III** (blockage of K^+ channels ⇒ action potential length ↑, refractory time↑)	**Amiodarone** (Cordarone, Pacerone, Gens)	d1-10: 1000mg PO div in 5 doses, then 200mg qd
or	**Antiarrhythmic, class III** (blockage of K^+ channels + beta-receptor blockage ⇒ refractory time↑)	**Sotalol** (Betapace, Betapace AF, Gens)	80-160mg PO qd-bid; Caution: proarrhythmic
or	**Antiarrhythmic, class IC** (Na^+ influx block ⇒ conduction↑, refractory time↑)	**Propafenone** (Rythmol, Gens)	150mg tid or 300mg bid PO; Caution: proarrhythmic

Ablation is possible in selected cases

1.7.5	Supraventricular Tachycardia in WPW Syndrome, AV Node Tachycardia		
Attack			
If appl. radiofrequeny ablation (frequently first choice)			
poss	**Antiarrhythmic** (short-term blockade of AV node)	Adenosine (Adenocard)	6mg IV bolus, then 12-18mg IV prn
poss	**CCB – non-dihydropyridine** (chrono-, dromo-, inotropic↓, afterload↓, O₂-consumption↓)	Diltiazem (Cardizem, Cartia XT, Tiamate, Tiazac, Gens)	15-25mg IV bolus, then 10mg/h Inf; Not in atrial fibrillation!
		Verapamil (Calan, Covera-HS, Isoptin, Verelan, Gens)	5mg slowly IV, then 5-10mg/h, max 100mg/d; Not in atrial fibrillation!
Prophylaxis			
poss	**Antiarrhythmic, class III** (blockage of K⁺ channels + beta-receptor blocker ⇒ refractory time↑)	Sotalol (Betapace, Betapace AF, Gens	80-160mg PO bid-tid; Caution: proarrhythmic
or	**Antiarrhythmic, class Ic** (Na⁺ influx block ⇒ conduct.↑, refrac. time↑)	Flecainide (Tambocor)	100-200mg PO bid Caution: proarrhythmic
or	**Antiarrhythmic, class III** (block. of K⁺ channels ⇒ action potent. length↑, refractory time↑)	Amiodarone (Cordarone, Pacerone, Gens)	d1-10: 1000mg PO div in 5 doses, then 200mg qd; Caution: proarrhythmic

Radiofrequency ablation is curative!

1.7.6	Ventricular Tachycardia		
Attack			
	Antiarrhythmic, class Ib (conduction, refr. time↑)	Lidocaine (Gens)	Ini 50-100mg IV, then 2-4mg/min Inf
or poss	**Antiarrhythmic, class III** (blockage of K⁺ channels ⇒ action potential length↑, refractory time↑)	Amiodarone (Cordarone, Pacerone, Gens)	150mg IV over 30min, then 1mg/min for 6h Inf, then 0.5mg/min for 18h, or d1-10: 1000mg PO div in 5 doses, then 200mg/d

DC cardioversion if evidence of hemodynamic compromise.

Prophylaxis

	Antiarrhythmic, class III (block. of K^+ channels $\Rightarrow$ action potent. length $\uparrow$, refractory time $\uparrow$)	**Amiodarone** (Cordarone, Pacerone, Gens)	*d1-10: 1000mg PO div in 5 doses, then 200mg qd*
or	**Antiarrhythmic, class III** (blockage of K^+ channels + beta-receptor blocker $\Rightarrow$ refractory time $\uparrow$)	**Sotalol** (Betapace, Betapace AF, Gens	*80-160mg PO qd-bid*
poss plus	**Beta-1-selective blocker** (CO$\downarrow$, neg. chronotropic, neg. inotropic, renin secretion $\downarrow$, central sympathetic activity $\downarrow$)	**Metoprolol** (Lopressor, Toprol-xl, Gens)	*25-200mg PO qd-bid; Caution: not with Sotalol*
		Atenolol (Tenormin, Gens)	*25-100mg PO qd; Caution: not with Sotalol*

Sos consider implantable defibrillator, especially if LVEF < 35%

1.7.7 Torsades De Pointes

Usually **sign of proarrhythmic effects** of other antiarrhythmics - discontinue.
Consider pacemaker to increase heart rate and decrease QTc.

Attack

	Magnesium (antiarrhytmic)	**Magnesium Sulfate** (Gens)	*1-6g IV over several min, then 3-20mg/min IV for 5-48h*
poss plus	**Beta-adrenergic agonist** (chronotropic $\uparrow$, inotropic $\uparrow$, HR $\uparrow$, CO $\uparrow$, peripheral vasodilatation)	**Isoproterenol** (Isuprel, Gens)	*Ini 0.02-0.06mg IV bolus, then Inf at 2-10µg/min*

Prophylaxis

1. Choice: discontinue antiarrhythmics
2. Sos stimulation
3. Poss pacemaker

1.7.8 Extrasystoles

Supraventricular Extrasystoles

	Beta-1-selective blocker (CO↓, neg. chronotropic, neg. inotropic, O$_2$ consumption↓, central sympathetic activity↓)	**Metoprolol** (Lopressor, Toprol-xl, Gens)	5-10mg slowly IV, max 20mg IV; 25-100mg PO qd-bid, 100-200mg SR PO qd
		Atenolol (Tenormin, Gens)	25-100mg PO qd

Mg^{2+}, K$^+$ replacement, treat cause, e.g. hyperthyroidism

Ventricular Extrasystoles

	Beta-1-selective blocker (CO↓, neg. chronotropic, neg. inotropic, O$_2$ consumption↓, central sympathetic activity↓)	**Metoprolol** (Lopressor, Toprol-xl, Gens)	25-100mg PO qd-bid, 100-200mg SR PO qd, 5-10mg slowly IV, max 20mg IV
		Atenolol (Tenormin, Gens)	25-100mg PO qd
	Electrolytes (symptomatic)	**Mg$^+$-K$^+$ supplement** (Mag-ox, Gens)	400mg PO bid-tid

Mg^{2+}, K$^+$ replacement, treat cause. Antiarrhythmics NOT indicated!

1.7.9 Bradycard Arrhythmias

poss	**Parasympatholytic** (chronotropic↑)	**Atropine** (Atropine sulfate)	0.5-1mg IV

Usually pacemaker

1.8 Infective Endocarditis
1.8.1 Rheumatic Fever

Acute Rheumatic Fever

	Penicillin (antibiotic)	**Benzathine Penicillin** (Bicillin L-A, Permapen)	1.2 M U IM as single dose
or		**Penicillin V** (Betapen-VK, Ledercillin-VK, Pen-vee K, Uticillin VK, V-cillin VK, Gens)	250-500mg PO tid for 10d

plus	**NSAID – salicylate** (anti-inflammatory, antipyretic)	**Aspirin – ASA** (Ascriptin, Asprimox, Bayer Aspirin, Bufferin, Easprin, Ecotrin, Empirin, Genprin, Halfprin, St. Joseph Pain Reliever, Zorprin, Gens)	*2-3g qd PO (until infection signs ↓)*
plus	**Glucocorticoid** (anti-inflammatory, immunosuppressive)	**Prednisone** (Deltasone, Meticorten, Prednisone Intensol, Gens)	*1-2mg/kg PO qd slowly decreasing (until infection signs ↓)*

Relapse prophylaxis

	Penicillin (antibiotic)	**Benzathine Penicillin** (Bicillin L-A, Permapen)	*1.2 M U IM q3wk (until 25years of age)*
or	In penicillin allergic patients:		
	Macrolide	**Erythromycin** (E-Base, E-Mycin, Eryc, Ery-Tab, Ilosone, Ilotycin, PCE, Gens)	*250mg PO bid (until 25years of age)*

1.8.2   Bacterial Endocarditis

Streptococci

	Benzylpenicillin (antibiotic)	**Penicillin G** (Penicillin, Penicillin G Potassium, Pfizerpen, Gens)	*12–18 M U IV per 24h*
or	In penicillin allergic patients:		
	Glycopeptide (antibiotic)	**Vancomycin** (Vancocin HCT, Vancoled, Gens)	*30mg/kg IV q24h, div in 2 doses*
plus	**Aminoglycoside** (antibiotic)	**Gentamicin** (Garamycin, U-gencin, Gens)	*1mg/kg IV tid or 3mg/kg qd for 2wk*

Staphylococci

	Isoxazylpenicillin (antibiotic)	**Oxacillin** (Bactocill)	*2g q4h for 6wk*
or	**Glycopeptide** (antibiotic)	**Vancomycin** (Vancocin HCT, Vancoled, Gens)	*30mg/kg IV q24h div in 2 doses*
plus	**Aminoglycoside** (antibiotic)	**Gentamicin** (Garamycin, U-gencin, Gens)	*1mg/kg tid or 3mg/kg qd for 6wk*

Enterococci			
	Aminopenicillin (antibiotic)	**Ampicillin** (Omnipen, Omnipen-N, Principen, Totacillin, Totacillin-N)	*12g cont IV over 24h or in six divided doses for 4-6wk*
or	Glycopeptide (antibiotic)	**Vancomycin** (Vancocin HCT, Vancoled, Gens)	*30mg/kg IV q24h in two divided doses for 4-6wk*
plus	Aminoglycoside (antibiotic)	**Gentamicin** (Garamycin, U-gencin, Gens)	*1mg/kg IV tid or 3mg/kg IV qd for 4-6wk*
Pneumococci			
	Benzylpenicillin (antibiotic)	**Penicillin G** (Penicillin, Penicillin G Potassium, Pfizerpen, Gens)	*12-18 M U/24h cont IV or div in 6 doses*

1.9   Endocarditis Prophylaxis

1.9.1   No Penicillin Allergy - Normal risk (e.g. rheumatic. valve defect, HOCM)

Oropharynx, GI, Urogenital			
	Aminopenicillin (antibiotic)	**Amoxicillin** (Amoxil, Larotid, Trimox, Wymox, Gens)	*2g PO 1h before procedure*

1.9.2   No Penicillin Allergy - Higher risk (e.g. artificial heart valve, after bact. endocarditis)

Oropharynx, GI, Urogenital			
	Aminopenicillin (antibiotic)	**Amoxicillin** (Amoxil, Larotid, Trimox, Wymox, Gens)	*2g PO (or 2g IV) 1h before, and 1g PO each 8 + 16h after procedure*
plus	Aminoglycoside (antibiotic)	**Gentamicin** (Garamycin, U-gencin, Gens)	*1.5mg/kg IV 1h before, and 1mg/kg IV each 8 + 16h after procedure*
Skin			
	Isoxazylpenicillin (antibiotic)	**Cloxacillin** (Cloxacillin sodium)	*2g PO 1h before, and 500mg PO each 8 + 16h after procedure*
		Cefazolin (Ancef)	*1g IV before, and 1g IV each 8 + 16 h after procedure*

1.9.3   In Penicillin Allergy – Normal Risk (e.g. rheumatic. valve defect, HOCM)

Oropharynx, Skin

Lincosamide (antibiotic)	**Clindamycin** (Cleocin, Gens)	*600mg PO 1h before procedure*

GI, Urogenital

Glycopeptide (antibiotic)	**Vancomycin** (Vancocin HCT, Vancoled, Gens)	*1g IV 1h before procedure*

1.9.4   In Penicillin Allergy – Higher Risk (e.g. artificial heart valve, after bact. endocarditis)

Oropharynx

Lincosamide (antibiotic)	**Clindamycin** (Cleocin, Gens)	*600mg PO 1h before, and 300mg PO each 8 + 16h after procedure*

GI, Urogenital, Skin

Glycopeptide (antibiotic)	**Vancomycin** (Vancocin HCT, Vancoled, Gens)	*1g IV 1h before, and 1g IV each 8 + 16h after procedure*

1.10   Pericarditis

1.10.1   Bacterial

Antibiotics only after testing, think of tuberculosis!

1.10.2   Dressler's Syndrome (after myocardial infarctions, cardiac operations)

poss	**NSAID acid derivative** (NSAID; anti-inflammatory, analgesic)	**Diclofenac** (Voltaren, Voltaren-XR, Gens)	*50mg PO qd-tid, 100mg SR PO qd, 75mg IM qd*
		Ibuprofen (Advil, Ibu, Motrin, Gens)	*600–800mg PO tid*
poss	**Glucocorticoid** (anti-inflammatory, antiallergic, immuno-suppressive)	**Prednisone** (Deltasone, Meticorten, Prednisone Intensol, Gens)	*Depending on clinical signs 5–20mg PO qd*

1.11 Intermittent Claudication
1.11.1 Stage II: Walking Regimen

More important is prevention of cardiovascular morbidity and mortality with appropriate use of statins, antiplatelet drugs and beta blockers

	Antiplatelet drug (phosphodiesterase/ platelet aggregation-adhesion inhibition)	**Aspirin – ASA** (Ascriptin, Asprimox, Bayer Aspirin, Bufferin, Easprin, Ecotrin, Empirin, Genprin, Halfprin, St. Joseph Pain Reliever, Zorprin, Gens)	*81–325mg PO qd*
poss plus	**Antiplatelet drug** (blockage of platelet ADP-receptors)	**Clopidogrel** (Plavix)	*75mg PO qd*
or / poss plus	**Hemorheologic** (erythrocyte flexibility↑, rheology↑)	**Pentoxifylline** (Pentoxil, Trental, Gens)	*400mg PO tid*
		Cilostazol (Pletal)	*100mg PO bid*
plus	**Statins** (intracellular cholesterol synthesis↓, LDL↓, HDL↑)	**Atorvastatin** (Lipitor)	*10-80mg PO qd*
		Pravastatin (Pravachol)	*40-80mg PO qd*

1.11.2 Stage III/IV in Inoperability, Buerger's Disease

	Angiogenic growth factors (experimental protocols)	**Vascular endothelial growth factor** (VEGF$_{165}$)	*Gene therapy*

1.12 Superficial Vein Thrombosis
1.12.1 In General

poss	**Antiplatelet drug** (phosphodiesterase/ platelet aggregation-adhesion inhibition)	**Aspirin – ASA** (Ascriptin, Asprimox, Bayer Aspirin, Bufferin, Easprin, Ecotrin, Empirin, Genprin, Halfprin, St. Joseph Pain Reliever, Zorprin, Gens)	*325-1950mg PO bid-tid*

1.12.2   In Great Saphenous Vein Thrombosis

| poss | **Heparin – low-molecular-weight** (LMWH, coagulation factor inhibition↑) | **Dalteparin** (Fragmin) | *2850 U SC qd* |
| | | **Enoxaparin** (Lovenox) | *30mg SC bid* |

1.13   Deep Vein Thrombosis

1.13.1   In Popliteal Vein Thrombosis

| | **Heparin, unfractionated** (coagulation factor inhibition↑, embolism prophylaxis) | **Heparin** (Gens) | *5000 U IV bolus, then 1000 U/h; aim for a PTT ratio of 1.5–2.5* |
| then | **Oral anticoagulant** (vit. K antagonism ⇒ clotting factors II, VII, IX, X↓ ⇒ longterm anticoag.) | **Warfarin** (Coumadin, Gens) | *2–10mg PO qd to achieve INR of 2–2.5* |

1.13.2   In Extensive Cases

	Thrombolytic (plasminogen activation ⇒ fibrin proteolysis)	**Streptokinase** (Streptase, Kabikinase)	*250,000 U over 30min, then 100,000 U/h x 24h*
or		**Urokinase** (Abbokinase)	*4400 U/kg IV over 10min, then 4400 U/kg/h IV for 12h*
or		**rt-PA** (Alteplase)	*100mg IV Inf over 2h*
then	**Oral anticoagulant** (vit. K antagonism ⇒ clotting factors II, VII, IX, X↓ ⇒ longterm anticoag.)	**Warfarin** (Coumadin, Gens)	*2–10mg PO qd to achieve INR of 2–2.5 for 6mo*

1.14   Thrombosis Prophylaxis
1.14.1   Thrombosis Risk Factor Assessment

Each Risk Factor Represents 1 Point

- Age 41 to 60 years
- Minor surgery planned
- History of prior major surgery (<1mo)
- Varicose veins
- Inflammatory Bowel Disease
- Swollen legs (current)
- Obesity (BMI > 25)

Each Risk Factor Represents 3 Points

- Age over 75 years
- History of DVT/PE
- Family history of thrombosis
- Major surgery with additional risk factors such as myocardial infarction, congestive heart failure, sepsis, serious lung disease, or abnormal pulmonary function, such as COPD
- Medical patient with additional risk factors, such as stroke, myocardial infarction, etc.
- Factor V Leiden
- Prothrombin 20210A
- Serum homocysteine
- Lupus anticoagulant
- Anticardiolipin antibodies
- Other congenital or acquired thrombophilia; If yes: Type: ....
- Other risk factors ....

Each Risk Factor Represents 2 Points

- Age 60-74 years
- Malignancy (present or previous)
- Major surgery (>45 min)
- Laparoscopic surgery (>45 min)
- Patient confined to bed (>72h)
- Immobilizing plaster cast (<1mo)
- Central venous access

Each Risk Factor Represents 5 Points

- Elective major lower extremity arthroplasty
- Hip, pelvis or leg fracture (<1mo)
- Stroke (<1mo)
- Multiple trauma (<1mo)
- Acute spinal cord injury (paralysis, <1mo)

For Women Only (Each Represents 1 Point)

- Oral contraceptives or hormone replacement therapy
- Pregnancy or postpartum (<1mo)
- History of stillborn infant, spontaneous abortion, premature birth with toxemia or placental insufficiency

Total Risk Factor Score

1.14.2 Prophylaxis Regimen

Total Risk Factor Score	Incidence of DVT	Risk Level	Prophylaxis Regimen
0-1	<10%	Low Risk	No specific measures, early ambulation
2	10-20%	Moderate Risk	**ES** or **IPC** or **LDUH** or **LMWH**
3-4	20-40%	High Risk	**IPC** or **LDUH** or **LMWH**
5 or more	40-80%	Highest Risk	Pharmacological: **LDUH, LMWH, Warfarin,** or **Fac X*** alone or in combination with **ES** or **IPC**

ES - Elastic Stockings; **IPC** - Intermittent Pneumatic Compression; **LDUH** - Low Dose Unfractionated Heparin; **LMWH** - Low Molecular Weigth Heparin; **Fac X** - Factor X Inhibitor
*For use with total hip replacement, total knee replacement and hip fracture

© Evanston Northwestern Healthcare, JA Caprini, www.venousdisease.com;
Based on:
1. Geerts WH et al: Prevention of Venous Thromboembolism. Chest 2001; 119:132S-175S;
2. Nicolaides AN et al: 2001 International Consensus Statement: Prevention of Venous Thromboembolism, Guidelines According to Scientific Evidence;
3. Caprini JA, Arcelus JI et al: State-of-the-Art Venous Thromboembolism Prophylaxis. Scope 2001; 8: 228-240;
4. Oger E: Incidence of Venous Thromboembolism: A Community-based Study in Western France. Thromb Haemost 2000; 657-660; and
5. Turpie AG, Bauer KA, Ericsson BI, et al. Fondaparinux vs. Enoxaparin for the Prevention of Venous Thromboembolism in Major Orthopedic Surgery: a Meta-analysis of 4 Randomized Double-blind Studies. Arch Intern Med 2002; 162(16):1833-40.

1.15 Acute Aortic Dissection

Opioid (analgesic, sedative)	**Morphine sulfate** (Astramorph, Avinza, Duramorph, Infumorph, Kadian, Numorphan, Roxanol, Gens)	*5-10mg IV prn (diluted 1:10)*
Beta blocker (to reduce sheer stress, negative inotrope, negative chronotrope)	**Labetalol** (Normodyne, Trandate, Gens)	*0.5-2mg/min IV Inf, total dose 50-200mg*
	Esmolol (Brevibloc)	*Ini IV loading dose 250-500µg/kg over 1min, then 50-100µg/kg/min for 4min, sos rep prn*

If beta blockers are contraindicated, consider negative chronotrope CCBs

	CCB – non-dihydropyridine (chrono-, dromo-, inotropic↓, afterload↓)	**Diltiazem** (Cardizem, Cartia XT, Tiamate, Tiazac, Gens)	*15–25mg IV bolus, then 10mg/h Inf*
		Verapamil (Calan, Covera-HS, Isoptin, Verelan, Gens)	*5mg slowly IV, then 5-10mg/h, max 100mg/d*
then	**Direct vasodilator** (pre-/afterload↓)	**Nitroprusside sodium** (Nipride, Nitropress)	*0.25-10mg/kg/min; Caution: use after beta blocker admin*

Emergent surgical repair is indicated for Type A dissection

2. Fluids, Electrolytes

Y. Howard Lien, MD
Professor, Section of Nephrology, College of Medicine,
University of Arizona, Tucson, AZ

2.1 Volume Depletion

2.1.1 Isotonic Volume Depletion

Mild

Saline solution (volume expansion + electrolyte replacement)	Saline or sugar-electrolyte solutions (sport drinks)	10g Na^+Cl^- in 2-3l PO Recommendation of WHO for **diarrhea**: 3.5g Na^+Cl^- + 2.5g $Na^+H^+CO_3^-$ + 1.5g K^+Cl^- + 20g glucose in 1000ml water PO

Severe

	Isotonic saline solution (volume expansion + electrolyte replacement)	Normal Saline 0.9% (154meq/l)	IV according to CVP and urine output
If low K^+	Crystalloid plasma expander (volume expansion + electrolyte replacement)	Ringer's solution	IV according to CVP and urine output

In oliguria/anuria or renal failure

Isotonic saline solution (potassium free volume + electrolyte replacement)	Normal Saline 0.9% (154meq/l)	IV according to CVP and urine output

In profound circulatory failure

plus	Colloid plasma expander (volume expansion)	Albumin 5% (Albuminar, Buminate, Plasbumin)	250-500ml IV

Only as acute therapy, later replace with saline or Ringer's solution

2.1.2 Hypotonic Volume Depletion

Mild

	Saline solution (volume expansion + electrolyte replacement)	Saline or sugar-electrolyte solutions (sport drinks)	10g Na⁺Cl⁻ in 2-3l PO Recommendation of WHO for diarrhea: 3.5g Na⁺Cl⁻ + 2.5g NaHCO₃ + 1.5g K⁺Cl⁻ + 20g glucose in 1000ml water PO

where the chemical formulas read: $10g\ Na^+Cl^-$ in 2-3l PO; $3.5g\ Na^+Cl^-$ + $2.5g\ NaHCO_3$ + $1.5g\ K^+Cl^-$ + 20g glucose in 1000ml water PO

Severe

	Isotonic saline solution (volume expansion + electrolyte replacement)	Normal Saline 0.9% (154meq/l)	IV according to CVP Keep Na⁺ increase <10meq/l/d
(1:1) plus	Crystalloid plasma expander (volume expansion + electrolyte replacement)	Ringer's solution	IV according to CVP Keep Na⁺ increase <10meq/l/d

2.1.3 Hypertonic Volume Depletion

Mild

	Free water replacement (volume expansion)	Water, tea	2-3l PO

Severe

first	Isotonic saline solution (volume expansion)	Normal Saline 0.9% (154meq/l)	1-2l IV according to CVP
then	Hypotonic saline solution (free water replacement)	Half Saline 0.45% (77meq/l)	Slowly IV. Caution: cerebral edema
or	Glucose solution (free water replacement)	Glucose 5% (D5W)	Slowly IV. Caution: cerebral edema

Water deficit (l) = [(Na/140)−1] x 0.5 x kg (man, for woman use 0.4)
Correction rate <0.5meq/h
Caution: rapid correction may cause cerebral edema

2.2   Volume Overload

2.2.1   Isotonic Volume Overload

sos	Loop diuretic	Furosemide (Lasix, Gens)	20mg IV, sos↑ dose

Poss. + fluid/Na⁺ restriction

2.2.2   Hypotonic Volume Overload

	Fluid restriction	Reduce free water	<1.5 l/d
	Loop diuretic	Furosemide (Lasix, Gens)	20mg IV, sos↑ dose

Water excess (l) = $(1-Na/140) \times 0.6 \times kg$ (man, for woman use 0.5)

2.2.3   Hypertonic Volume Overload

	Na⁺ restriction	Reduce Na⁺ intake	Remove iatrogenic causes
	Loop diuretics	Furosemide (Lasix, Gens)	20mg IV with D5W

Hypertonic volume overload due to primary aldosteronism

	Aldosterone antagonist	Spironolactone (Aldactone, Gens)	25-100mg q 8h

2.3   Generalized Edema

	Low-dose heparinization (DVT prophylaxis)	Enoxaparin (Lovenox)	40mg SC qd
	Loop diuretic	Furosemide (Lasix, Gens)	20-40mg PO or IV
plus sos	Thiazide diuretic	Metolazone (Zaroxolyn)	2.5-5mg PO given same time as PO Lasix or IV 30min earlier than Furosemide. Watch K⁺ deficit
Cirrhosis	Aldosterone antagonist	Spironolactone (Aldactone, Gens)	25-100mg bid-qid

2.4   Hyponatremia
2.4.1   Hypovolemic Hyponatremia

Mild

Saline solution (volume expansion + electrolyte replacement)	Saline or sugar-electrolyte solutions (sport drinks)	10g Na^+Cl^- in 2-3l PO Recommendation of WHO for diarrhea: 3.5g Na^+Cl^- + 2.5g $NaHCO_3$ + 1.5g K^+Cl^- + 20g glucose in 1000ml water PO

Severe (Na^+ < 125 mmol/l or symptomatic)

Isotonic saline solution (volume expansion + electrolyte replacement)	Normal Saline 0,9% (154 meq/l)	IV according to CVP Keep Na^+ increase <10 meq/l/d

Emergency (severe CNS symptoms, i.e. seizure and coma)

Hypertonic saline solution (volume expansion + electrolyte replacement)	Hypertonic Saline 3% (513 meq/l)	Correct Na^+ 1.5-2 meq/l for 3-4h and keep Na^+ increase < 10 meq/l/d

2.4.2   Hypervolemic Hyponatremia (Cirrhosis, Congestive Heart Failure and Nephrotic Syndrome)

Fluid restriction (reduce free water intake)	Fluid restriction	Limit fluid intake <1000-1500ml/d

Severe CNS symptoms due to hyponatremia

	Hypertonic saline solution (electrolyte replacement)	Hypertonic Saline 3% (513meq/l)	Correct Na^+ 1.5-2 meq/l for 3-4h and keep Na^+ increase < 10 meq/l/d
plus	Loop diuretic	Furosemide (Lasix, Gens)	40-100mg IV q6-8hS

2.4.3   Isovolemic Hyponatremia (SIADH)

Without severe CNS symptoms

Fluid restriction (reduce free water intake)	Fluid restriction	Limit fluid intake <1000-1500ml/d

Severe CNS symptoms due to hyponatremia

	Hypertonic saline solution (electrolyte replacement)	Hypertonic Saline 3% (513meq/l)	*Correct Na$^+$ 1.5-2 meq/l for 3-4h and keep Na$^+$increase <10 meq/l/d*
plus	Loop diuretics	Furosemide (Lasix, Gens)	*40-100mg IV q6-8h*

Chronic treatment

	Tetracycline (induce nephrogenic DI)	Demeclocycline (Declomycin)	*300-600mg PO bid* **Caution:** *renal failure*

2.4.4   Hyponatremia due to Water Intoxication

Without severe CNS symptoms

Fluid restriction (reduce free water intake)	Fluid restriction	*Limit fluid intake <1000-1500ml/d*

Severe CNS symptoms due to hyponatremia

Hypertonic saline solution (electrolyte replacement)	Hypertonic Saline 3% (513meq/l)	*Correct Na$^+$ 1.5-2 meq/l for 3-4h and keep Na$^+$ increase < 10 meq/l/d*

Caution: central pontine myelinolysis if hyponatremia corrected too quickly. Rapid correction can be applied when hyponatremia develops within 24h.

Na$^+$ deficit for initial therapy (meq): 10 x 0.6 x kg (man, for woman use 0.5)

2.5   Hypernatremia
2.5.1   Hypernatremia due to Volume Depletion

first	Isotonic saline solution	Normal Saline 0.9% (154meq/l)	*1-2l IV according to CVP*
then	Hypotonic saline solution (free water replacement)	Half Saline 0.45% (77meq)	*Slowly IV* **Caution:** *cerebral edema*
or	Glucose solution (free water replacement)	Glucose 5% (D5W)	*Slowly IV* **Caution:** *cerebral edema*

2.5.2	Hypernatremia due to Excessive Salt (Primary Aldosteronism, Cushing's Syndrome, Acute Salt Loads)		
	Hypotonic saline solution (free water replacement)	Half Saline 0.45% (77meq)	*Slowly IV* **Caution:** *cerebral edema*
or	Glucose solution (free water replacement)	Glucose 5% (D5W)	*Slowly IV* **Caution:** *cerebral edema*
plus	Loop diuretic	Furosemide (Lasix, Gens)	*20-40mg PO bid*
or	Aldosterone antagonist	Spironolactone (Aldactone, Gens)	*25-100mg q8h*

2.5.3	Hypernatremia due to Diabetes Insipidus (DI)		
Mild (Na$^+$ <160mmol/l or symptomatic)			
	Free water replacement (volume expansion)	Water, tea	*Several liters PO driven by thirst*
Severe (Na$^+$ >160mmol/l)			
	Glucose solution (free water replacement)	Glucose 5% (D5W)	*Slowly IV* **Caution:** *cerebral edema*
Specific treatment for central DI			
	Vasopressin (replacement)	Desmopressin (DDAVP)	*0.05-0.5mg PO bid or 0.1-0.2ml (10-20µg) intranasally bid*
Specific treatment for nephrogenic DI			
	Thiazide diuretic	HCTZ	*25-50mgPO qd*
plus	K$^+$ sparing diuretic	Amiloride	*5-10mg PO qd*

Water deficit (l) = ((Na$^+$/140) − 1) x 0.5 x kg (man, for woman use 0.4)
Correction rate <0.5meq/h **Caution:** *rapid correction may cause cerebral edema*

2.6 Hypokalemia
2.6.1 Mild Hypokalemia

sos	Potassium preparation (replacement)	K$^+$Cl$^-$ (K-Dur, K-Lor, Micro-K, Ram-K, Slow-K)	*20-80meq PO qd (40meq ⇒ approx. K$^+$ 0.3meq/l↑)*

2.6.2	Severe Hypokalemia (K⁺ deficit: 200meq, if K⁺<3meq/l, and no intracellular K⁺ shift)		
	Potassium preparation (replacement)	K⁺Cl⁻ solution (injectable, 1.5 or 2meq/ml)	*Peripheral line: 20-40meq in 1 l NS IV over 2-4h. Central line: 10-20meq in 50ml NS IV over 1h. ECG monitor*

2.7 Hyperkalemia
2.7.1 Mild Hyperkalemia

	K⁺ restriction	Low K⁺ diet	*<2g/d*

2.7.2	Severe Hyperkalemia (> 6meq/l or ECG changes)		
	Loop diuretic (K⁺ excretion)	Furosemide (Lasix, Gens)	*40-80mg IV*
sos	Cation exchangers (remove K⁺ from GI)	Sodium polystyrene sulfonate (Kayexalate)	*20g in 100ml 20% sorbitol every 4-6h prn* **Contraindication:** *Bowel obstruction*
	Redistribution (intracellular shift of K⁺)	Glucose 50% + Regular insulin	*50ml + 10units IV over 20min*
plus sos	Redistribution (intracellular shift of K⁺)	Sodium bicarbonate 8.4% (1meq/ml)	*50ml IV over 5min*
plus sos	Membrane antagonism (inhib. of depolarization)	Calcium gluconate 10% (4.5meq/ml, Gens)	*10ml IV over 2-3min* **Caution:** *digitalis toxicity*
or	Redistribution (intracellular shift of K⁺)	Albuterol (Proventil, Ventolin, Gens)	*0.5mg IV slowly in 15min or 10-20mg in 4ml saline nasal inhal. over 10min*
sos	Hemodialysis (removal of K⁺)	Hemodialysis	*Use 1meq/l K⁺ bath and ECG monitoring*

2.8 Hypocalcemia
2.8.1 Mild Hypocalcemia

	Calcium preparation (replacement)	Ca⁺⁺ carbonate (Mylanta, Titralac, Tums)	*1-2g PO qd*

	Vitamin D (increase Ca+ absorption)	**Ergocalciferol** (Drisdol, Gens)	*50,000 IU PO qd*
sos	**1,25OH Vitamin D** (increase Ca+ absorption)	**Calcitriol** (Rocaltrol)	*0.25µg PO tiw*

2.8.2	Acute Hypocalcemic Crisis		
	Calcium preparation (replacement)	**Ca++ gluconate 10%** (4.5meq/ml)	*Ini: 1g slowly IV, then: 1mg/kg/h in D5W* **Caution:** *digitalis toxicity*
If low Mg+	**Magnesium preparation** (replacement)	**Mg++ sulfate 50%** (4meq/ml)	*2g in 100ml D5W IV over 1h*

2.9	**Hypercalcemia**		
2.9.1	Mild Hypercalcemia		
sos	**Isotonic saline solution** (volume expansion)	**Normal Saline 0.9%** (154meq/l)	*1-2l IV*
sos	**Loop diuretic** (Ca excretion)	**Furosemide** (Lasix, Gens)	*20-40mg IV*

2.9.2	Hypercalcemic Crisis		
	Isotonic saline solution (volume expansion)	**Normal Saline 0.9%** (154meq/l)	*1-2l IV, max. 10l/24h*
sos	**Loop diuretic** (Ca++ excretion)	**Furosemide** (Lasix, Gens)	*Only after volume repletion, 20-40mg IV q4-6h*
sos	**Bisphosphonate** (osteoclast inhibition)	**Pamidronate** (Aredia)	*60 or 90mg IV over 4 or 24h*
sos	**Calcitonin** (osteoclast inhibition)	**Calcitonin** (Calcimar, Miacalcin)	*4IU/kg SC q 12h (only works for a few d)*
sos malig-nancy	**Cytotoxic** (osteoclast inhibition)	**Mithramycin** (Mithracin)	*25µg/kg over 6h.* **Caution:** *bone marrow toxicity*
sos malig-nancy	**Glucocorticoid** (inhibition of Vitamin D synthesis)	**Prednisone** (Deltasone, Meticorten, Prednisone Intensol, Gens)	*0.5-1mg/kg qd*

2.10 Hypomagnesemia

2.10.1 Chronic Hypomagnesemia

Magnesium preparation (replacement)	Mg^+Cl^- (Slow Mg) Mg^+ lactate (Mg-Tab) Mg^+ oxide (Mag-ox)	1-2 PO bid

2.10.2 Acute Symptomatic Hypomagnesemia

Magnesium preparation (replacement)	Mg^+ sulfate 50% (4meq/ml)	2g in 100ml D5W IV over 1h

2.11 Hypermagnesemia

	Loop diuretic (Mg^+ excretion)	Furosemide (Lasix, Gens)	20-40mg IV
sos	Membrane antagonism (inhibit depolarization)	Ca^{++} gluconate 10% (4.5meq/ml)	10ml slowly IV
plus sos	Isotonic saline solution (volume expansion)	Normal Saline 0.9% (154meq/l)	IV according to CVP

Require hemodialysis if renal failure

2.12 Metabolic Acidosis

2.12.1 Chronic Metabolic Acidosis

	Alkaline preparation (bicarbonate replacement)	Na^+ citrate and citric acid (Shohl's solution)	15-30ml PO bid
or	Alkaline preparation (bicarbonate replacement)	Sodium bicarbonate 8.4% (1meq/ml)	30-100meq PO qd

2.12.2 Acute Non-Anion Gap Acidosis Due to Bicarbonate Loss

Alkaline preparation (bicarbonate replacement)	Sodium bicarbonate 8.4% (1meq/ml)	Ini Tx (meq) = (desired bicarb - observed bicarb) x 0.5 x kg IV over 24h

2.12.3   Acute High Anion Gap Acidosis due to Intoxication

Methanol or ethylene glycol overdose

	Alcohol dehydrogenase inhibitor (reduce toxic metabolites of methanol or ethylene glycol)	Fomepizole (Antizol)	15mg/kg loading, then 10mg/kg IV q12h, follow toxin levels **Contraindication**: renal failure
plus	Loop diuretics (force diuresis)	Furosemid (Lasix, Gens)	40-80mg IV q6h
sos	Hemodialysis (removal of methanol or ethylene glycol)	Hemodialysis	Monitor methanol or ethylene glycol level **Caution**: increase fomepizole to q4h

Salicylate overdose

	Forced alkaline diuresis (increase renal excretion of salicylate)	Sodium Bicarbonate 8.4% (1meq/ml)	50-100mmol to 1l of 0.45% saline IV at 250-500ml/h. Keep urine pH >7.5 **Caution**: potassium depletion
sos	Hemodialysis or hemoperfusion (removal of salicylate)	Hemodialysis or hemoperfusion	Monitor salicylate level

2.12.4   Lactic Acidosis

Typ A due to tissue hypoxia

	Buffer (pH neutralization)	Sodium Bicarbonate 8.4% (1meq/ml)	Ini Tx (meq) = (12 - bicarb) x 0.5 x kg IV over 4-8h **Caution**: intracellular acidosis, worsening respiratory acidosis
	Dialysis (removal of lactate)	Continous venous-venous hemofiltration/ dialysis or hemodialysis	Daily

First: stabilize hemodynamics and establish ventilation. Bicarbonate indicated for pH<7.5

Typ B Not due to tissue hypoxia			
	Thiamine (replace thiamine)	**Thiamine**	*100mg IV qd x 1, then 50mg qd*

First: treat underlying disease. Thiamine indicated for thiamine deficiency

2.12.5 Diabetic Ketoacidosis (DKA)			
	Saline solution (volume expansion and increase renal excretion of ketones)	**Normal saline 0.9%** (154meq/l) or **Half saline 0.45%** (77meq/l)	*Ini Tx: 0.9% NaCl IV over 0.5-1h then 0.9% or 0.45% NaCl 200-1000 ml/h according to BP and urine output*
plus	**Insulin** (reduce ketones and glucose)	**Human insulin**	*Ini Tx: 0.1-0.15U/kg IV bolus, then 0.1U/kg/h. Monitor glucose and ketone levels*
plus	**Glucose solution** (avoid insulin-induced hypoglycemia)	**Glucose 5%** (D5W) or **Glucose 10%** (D10W)	*Add to IV fluid and maintain glucose level 150-250 mg/dl*
plus	**Potassium preparation** (replacement)	K+Cl- or **Potassium phosphate**	*Add 20-40 meq/l to IV fluid when K+<5.5. Use KCl/KPi 2:1 if phosphate depletion*

2.12.6 Alcoholic Ketoacidosis			
	Glucose and saline solution (Volume expansion and carbohydrate repletion)	**Glucose 5%/ normal saline 0.9%** (154meq/l) (D5NS)	*Ini Tx: 1l IV over 0.5-1h, then 200-1000ml/h according to BP and urine output*
	Thiamine (replace thiamine)	**Thiamine**	*100mg IV qd x 1 then 50mg qd*
	Potassium preparation (replacement)	K+Cl- or **Potassium phosphate**	*Add 20-40 meq/l to IV fluid when K+<5.5. Use KCl/KPi 2:1 if phosphate depletion*

Bicarbonate rarely needed for DKA and AKA. Consider bicarbonate if pH<7.1
Caution: intracellular acidosis, worsening respiratory acidosis, hypocalcemia

2.13   Metabolic Alkalosis

2.13.1   Chloride-dependent Metabolic Alkalosis

	Isotonic saline solution (Cl⁻ replacement)	**Normal Saline 0.9%** (154meq/l)	*1-2l IV*
If low K⁺	**Potassium chloride solution** (K⁺ replacement)	**K⁺Cl⁻ solution** (injectable, 1.5 or 2 meq/ml)	*20-40meq in 1l NS at 10-20meq/h*
sos	**Carbonic anhydrase inhibitor** (inhibition of $H^+CO_3^-$ reabsorption)	**Acetazolamide** (Diamox, Gens)	*250mg PO qd or bid*
sos	**Acid** (pH neutralization)	**Hydrochloric acid** (150meq/l)	*H^+Cl^- (meq buffers 50% bicarb excess) IV via central line over 8-24h*

Na⁺Cl⁻ only effective in chloride dependent forms, not in mineralocorticoid excess

Bicarb excess (meq)= (bicarb-24) x 0.5 x kg

2.13.2   Chloride-independent Metabolic Alkalosis (Primary Aldosteronism)

	Aldosterone antagonist (mineralocorticoid steroid effects ↓)	**Spironolactone** (Aldactone, Gens)	*25-100mg q8h*

3.   Hematology

Tracey Walsh, Pharm.D., BCOP
Department of Pharmacy, Tripler Army Medical Center,
Honolulu, HI
Cesar O. Freytes, MD, FACP
Adult Bone Marrow Transplant Program,
University of Texas Health Science Center at San Antonio &
South Texas Veterans Health Care System, TX

3.1   Hemophilia
3.1.1   Hemophilia A

Mild to moderate form

	Vasopressin analogue (release of factor VIII from endothelial cells ⇒ factor VIII ↑ 2-4 fold)	**Desmopressin** (Concentraid, DDAVP, Stimate, Gens)	*0.3µg/kg IV/SC or nasal spray 150 µg (<50kg), 300µg (>50 kg) q12-24h; no more therapeutic response after 3-5 doses*
or	**Antifibrinolytic** (inhibits systemic and local fibrinolysis at sites of vascular injuries)	**E-aminocaproic acid** (Amicar, Gens)	*h1 5g IV/PO, then 1.0-1.25g/h IV for 8h or until bleeding stops; max 30g/d; DARF: red by 15-25%*
		Tranexamic acid (Cyklokapron)	*10mg/kg IV prior surgery, then 25 mg/kg tid-qid for 2-8d; DARF: adj dose*

Severe form

	Coagulation factor (substitution)	**Recombinant Factor VIII** (Helixate FS, Kogenate FS, Recombinate, ReFacto, Bioclate, Kogenate)	*Factor VIII dose: (target Factor VIII − baseline Factor VIII) x weight in kg/2 IV; target factor level in hemarthrosis 40%, in tooth extraction 60-80%, in minor surgery 60-80%, in major surgery 100%; rep dose q12h*
or	**Coagulation factor** (substitution)	**Plasma-derived concentrates** (Alphanate, Hemofil M, Koate-DVI, Monoclate P)	

3.1.2   Hemophilia B

	Coagulation factor (substitution)	Recombinant Factor IX (BeneFix)	*Factor IX dose: (target factor IX − baseline Factor IX) x weight in kg IV; target Factor IX level similar to Hemophilia A; rep dose q24h*
or	Coagulation factor (substitution)	Plasma-derived concentrates (Mononine, AlphaNine SD, Profilnine DS, Bebulin VH)	

3.1.3   Hemophilia with Inhibitors

	Coagulation factor (substitution)	Porcine factor VIII (Hyate C)	*For Factor VIII inhibitor only: 100-150 U/kg IV if antibody level < 50 Bethesda U; rep q6-8h*
or	Coagulation factor (substitution)	Recombinant Factor VIIa (NovoSeven)	*For Factor VIII or IX inhibitor 90µg/kg IV q2h until hemostasis*
or	Coagulation factor (substitution)	Anti-inhibitor coagulant complex (Autoplex T, Feiba VH Immuno)	*25-100 U/kg IV prn, rep in 12h sos*

Immune tolerance induction should be considered in severe cases.

6. Kroll MH. Hemophilia and other coagulation disorders in: Manual of Coagulation Disorders, Blackwell Science, Williston, 2001, 196-209.
7. Shapiro AD. Coagulation factor concentrates in:Goodnight SH and Hathaway WE, Disorders of Hemostasis and thrombosis, McGraw-Hill, New York, 2001, 505-16.

3.2   Von Willebrand's Disease

Non-transfusional Tx in mild cases and before minor surgery

Vasopressin analogue (release of factor VIII from endothelial cells ⇒ factor VIII ↑ 2-4 fold)	Desmopressin (Concentraid, DDAVP, Stimate, Gens)	*0.3µg/kg IV/SC or nasal spray 150 µg (<50kg), 300µg (>50 kg) q12-24h; no more therapeutic response after 3-5 doses.*

Note: desmopressin effective in type 1, contraindicated in type 2B

or	Antifibrinolytic (inhibits systemic and local fibrinolysis at sites of vascular injuries)	E-aminocaproic acid (Amicar, Gens)	h1 5g IV/PO, then: 1.0-1.25g/h IV for 8h or until bleeding stops; max 30g/d; DARF: red by 15-25%
		Tranexamic acid (Cyklokapron)	10mg/kg IV prior surgery, then 25 mg/kg tid-qid for 2-8d; DARF: adj dose
or	vWF-enriched preparations (substitution)	vWF (Humate-P)	25-100 U/kg IV prn, rep in 12h sos

8.   Kroll MH. Hemophilia and other coagulation disorders in: Manual of Coagulation Disorders, Blackwell Science, Williston, 2001, 196-209.
9.   Shapiro AD. Coagulation factor concentrates in: Goodnight SH and Hathaway WE, Disorders of Hemostasis and thrombosis, McGraw-Hill, New York, 2001, 505-16.
10. Mannucci PM. How I treat patients with von Willebrand disease. Blood 2001;97: 1915-9.

3.3   Anemias

3.3.1   Iron Deficiency

Iron preparation (substitution)	Ferrous Sulfate (Feosol, Feratab, Fer-In-Sol, Fer-Iron, Slow FE, ED-IN-SOL, Fe^{50}, Fergensol, Gens)	300mg PO tid, preferably on an empty stomach for 3–6mo
	Iron dextran (InFed, Dexferrum)	IV dose (mg) = 0,3 x weight (lbs) x (100-(Hgb x 100/14.8)) for total dose infusion

11. Brittenham GM. Disorders of iron metabolism in: Hematology Basic Principles and Practice, 3rd ed., Churchill Livingstone, New York, 2000, 397-427
12. Auerbach M et al. Clinical use of the total dose intravenous infusion of iron dextran. J Lab Clin Med 1988; 111: 566-70

Anemias 63

3.3.2 Megaloblastic Anemia

Vitamin B12 deficiency (pernicious anemia)

| | Vitamin B12 (substitution) | Hydroxocobalamin (Hydro Cobex, Hydro – Crysti-12, LA-12, Gens) | wk1: 1000µg IM qd, wk2: 1000µg IM tiw wk3-6: 1000µg IM qwk, then 1000µg qmo for life |
| or | | Cyanocobalamin (Crystamine, Cristi 1000, Cyanoject, Cyomin, Rubesol-1000, Gens) | wk1: 1000µg IM qd, wk2: 1000µg IM biw wk3-6: 1000µg IM qwk, then 1000µg qmo for life |

13. Antony AC. Megaloblastic anemias in: Hematology Basic Principles and Practice, 3rd ed., Churchill Livingstone, New York, 2000, 397-427.

Folic acid deficiency

| | Folic acid (substitution) | Folic acid (Folvite, Gens) | 1–5mg PO qd |

Therapeutic doses of folate will partly correct the abnormalities of B12 deficiency, but neurologic manifestations will progress. It is essential to also evaluate patients for B12 deficiency.

14. Antony AC. Megaloblastic anemias in: Hematology Basic Principles and Practice, 3rd ed., Churchill Livingstone, New York, 2000, 397-427.

3.3.3 Hemolytic Anemias

Beta-Thalassemia major

| | Antidote (complexes with ferric ions → renal elimination) | Deferoxamine (Desferal) | 1–2g IV or SC qd over 8 –12h (long-term Tx) |

15. Brittenham GM. Disorders of iron metabolism in: Hematology Basic Principles and Practice, 3rd ed., Churchill Livingstone, New York, 2000, 397-427.

3.3.4 Autoimmune Hemolytic Anemia

IgG warm autoantibodies

| | Glucocorticoid (anti-inflammatory, immunosuppressive) | Prednisone (Deltasone, Orasone, Liquid Pred, Sterapred DS, Panasol-S, Meticorten, Prednicen-M, Gens) | 1-2mg/kg PO qd, red slowly when adequate Hb level achieved |

poss.	**Alkylating agent** (immunosuppressive)	**Cyclophosphamide** (Cytoxan, Neosar, Gens)	2mg/kg/d PO (for patients unresponsive to prednisone)
or	**Purine antagonist** (immunosuppressive)	**Azathioprine** (Imuran, Gens)	1.5mg/kg/d PO

IgM cold autoantibodies (cold agglutinins)

	Alkylating agent	**Cyclophosphamide** (Cytoxan, Neosar, Gens)	2mg/kg/d PO
or		**Chlorambucil** (Leukeran)	0.1mg/kg/d PO

16. Schwartz RS et al. Autoimmune hemolytic anemias in: Hematology Basic Principles and Practice, 3rd ed., Churchill Livingstone, New York, 2000, 611-30.

3.3.5 Anemia of Chronic Renal Failure

	Erythrocyte colony stimulating factor (RBC production↑, maturation, activation↑)	**Erythropoietin** (Epogen, Procrit)	50-100 U/kg SC or IV tiw
or		**Darbepoetin alfa** (Aranesp)	0.45µg/kg/wk SC, target dose to maint Hb at 12g/dl

17. Dainiak N. Hematologic complications of renal disease in: Hematology Basic Principles and Practice, 3rd ed., Churchill Livingstone, New York, 2000, 2357-73.

3.3.6 Anemia in Non-myeloid Cancer Patients on Chemotherapy

	Erythrocyte colony stimulating factor (RBC production↑, maturation, activation)	**Erythropoietin** (Epogen, Procrit)	40,000-60,000 U SC qwk
		Darbepoetin (Aranesp)	200µg SC

18. Gabrilove JL, et al. Clinical evaluation of once-weekly dosing of epoetin alfa in chemotherapy patients: improvements in hemoglobin and quality of life are similar to three-times-weekly dosing. J Clin Oncol 2001;19(11):2875-82.
19. Schwartzberg LS et al. A randomized comparison of every-2-week darbepoietin alfa and weekly epoietin alfa for the treatment of chemotherapy-induced anemia in patients with breast, lung or gynecologic cancer. The Oncologist 2004;9:696-707

3.3.7 Aplastic Anemia

	Anti-lymphocyte antibodies (immunosuppressive)	**Lymphocyte immune globulin** (ATGAM)	40mg/kg/d IV for 4d

plus	**Glucocorticoid** (anti-inflammatory, immunosuppressive)	**Prednisone** (Deltasone, Orasone, Liquid Pred, Sterapred DS, Panasol-S, Meticorten, Prednicen-M, Gens))	*60–100mg/d PO for 2wk, taper dose to discontinue on d30*
plus	**Inhibition of interleukin-2 activation of T-lymphocytes** (immunosuppressive)	**Cyclosporine** (Gengraf, Neoral, Sandimmune, SangCya, Gens)	*10–12mg/kg/d PO for 6mo to maintain serum levels of 200–400ng/ml*

20. Rosenfeld SJ et al. Intensive immunosuppression with antithymocyte globulin and cyclosporine as treatment of severe acquired aplastic anemia. Blood 1995;85:3058-65.

3.4   Agranulocytosis

poss.	**Granulocyte colony stimulating factor** (neutrophil production↑, maturation, activation↑)	**Filgrastim** (Neupogen)	*5.75–11.5µg/kg/d SC until ANC ≥ 1500/mm^3 (then maint Tx)*

21. Dale DC, et al. A randomized controlled phase III trial of recombinant human granulocyte colony-stimulating factor (filgrastim) for treatment of severe chronic neutropenia. Blood 1993:81(10):2496-2502.
22. Welte K, Boxer LA. Severe chronic neutropenia: pathophysiology and therapy. Seminars in Hematology 1997:34(4):267-78.

3.5   Idiopathic Thrombocytopenic Purpura
3.5.1   In General

	Glucocorticoid (anti-inflammatory, immunosuppressive)	**Prednisone** (Deltasone, Orasone, Liquid Pred, Sterapred DS, Panasol-S, Meticorten, Prednicen-M, Gens)	*1-1.5mg/kg/d PO qd for 3wk then taper slowly*
or	**Anti-D immune globulin** (saturate spleen capacity to clear antibody coated platelets)	**Anti-D immune globulin** (WinRho SDF)	*Ini 50µg/kg IV, then 40-60µg/kg; only in non-splenectomized, Rh (D) positive patients*

or	**Immune globulin** (Fc receptor saturation of reticuloendothelial system)	**Immune globulin** (Gamimune N, Gammagard S/D, Gammar- P IV, Iveegam, Panglobulin, PolygamS/D, Venoglobulin-S, Sandoglobulin)	*1g/kg IV qd for 2-3d*

3.5.2 For Patients Resistant to Prednisone Administration after Splenectomy

	Androgen (platelet clearance↓)	**Danazol** (Danocrine, Gens)	*10-15mg/kg/d PO; maint dose as low as 50mg/d*
or	**Decreases platelet clearance**	**Dapsone** (Gens)	*75mg/d PO*
or	**Anti-CD20 monoclonal antibody** (immunomodulation)	**Rituximab** (Rituxan)	*375mg/m² IV qwk for 2-4wk*
or	**Purine antagonist** (immunosuppression)	**Azathioprine** (Imuran, Gens)	*1-4mg/kg PO qd*
or	**Alkylating agent** (immunosuppression)	**Cyclophosphamide** (Cytoxan, Neosar, Gens)	*1-2mg/kg/d PO*

23. Cines DB et al. Immune thrombocytopenic purpura. N Engl J Med 2002;346:995-1008.

3.6 Polycythemia Vera

poss	**Antiplatelet drug** (phosphodiesterase/ platelet aggregation-adhesion inhibition)	**Aspirin – ASA** (Ascriptin, Asprimox, Bayer Aspirin, Bufferin, Easprin, Ecotrin, Empirin, Genprin, Halfprin, St. Joseph Pain Reliever, Zorprin, Gens)	*81-325mg PO qd; only for Tx of erythromyalgia*
poss	**Interferon** (immune modulation)	**IFN–alpha-2a/b** (Roferon A, Intron A)	*2-5 M U SC tiw; only to control intractable pruritis, thrombocytosis and extramedullary hematopoiesis*

poss.	**Cytostatic** (phospholipase A2 inhibition)	**Anagrelide** (Agrylin)	*0.5mg PO qid; incr dose by 0.5mg/d qwk prn; usual dose 2-2.5mg/d; only in patients with erythromelalgia*

24. Spivak JL. The optimal management of polycythaemia vera, Br J Hematol 2002;116:243-54.

3.7 Essential Thrombocytosis

poss.	**Cytostatic** (phospholipase A2 inhibition)	**Anagrelide** (Agrylin)	*In younger patients: 0.5mg PO qid; incr dose by 0.5mg/d qwk prn; usual dose 2-2.5mg/d*
poss.	**Interferon** (immunomodulation)	**IFN-alpha-2a/b** (Roferon A, Intron A)	*In younger patients: 2-5 M U SC tiw*
poss.	**Cytostatic** (ribonucleotide diphosphate reductase inhibition)	**Hydroxyurea** (Hydrea, Droxia, Mylocel)	*1 g PO qd; adj according to platelet count*

25. Hoffman R, Primary Thrombocythemia in: Hematology Basic Principles and Practice, 3rd ed., Churchill Livingstone, New York, 2000, 1188-1204.

3.8 Chronic Myeloid Leukemia
3.8.1 Chronic Phase

	Tyrosine kinase inhibitor (white blood cells↓)	**Imatinib mesylate** (Gleevec)	*400-800mg PO qd*
or	**Interferon** (immunostimulation, modulation)	**IFN-alpha-2a/b** (Roferon A, Intron A)	*5 x 10^6 U/m^2 SC qd (long-term Tx)*
+/-	**Cytostatic** (purine antagonist)	**Cytarabine** (Cytosar-U, Cytosine Arabinoside, Ara-C)	*20mg/m^2 IV qd for 10d (q4wk)*
or	**Cytostatic** (ribonucleotide diphosphate reductase inhibition)	**Hydroxyurea** (Hydrea, Droxia, Mylocel)	*40-50 mg/kg PO qd*

poss.	**Xanthine oxidase inhibitor** (uric acid production ↓)	**Allopurinol** (Aloprim, Zyloprim, Gens)	300-600mg PO/IV qd
poss.	**Urine hydration + alkalinization** (solubility of uric acid ↑)	Hydration +/- Sodium bicarbonate	150-200ml/h; start 24-48h prior to chemo-Tx

3.8.2   Accelerated/Blast Phase

	Tyrosine kinase inhibitor	**Imatinib mesylate** (Gleevec)	600mg PO qd
or	**Interferon** (immunostimulation, modulation)	**IFN-alpha-2a/b** (Roferon A, Intron A)	5 x 10⁶ U/m² SC qd (long-term Tx)
+/-	**Cytostatic** (ribonucleotide diphosphate reductase inhibition)	**Hydroxyurea** (Hydrea, Droxia, Mylocel)	40-50mg/kg PO qd
poss.	**Xanthine oxidase inhibitor** (uric acid production ↓)	**Allopurinol** (Aloprim, Zyloprim, Gens)	300-600mg PO/IV qd
poss.	**Urine hydration + alkalinization** (solubility of uric acid ↑)	Hydration +/- Sodium bicarbonate	150-200ml/h; start 24-48h prior to chemo-Tx

26. Guilhot F, et al. Interferon alfa-2b combined with cytarabine versus interferon alone in chronic myelogenous leukemia. N Engl J Med 1997;337:223-9.
27. Silver RT, et al. An evidence-based analysis of the effect of busulfan, hydroxyurea, interferon, and allogeneic bone marrow transplantation in treating the chronic phase of chronic myeloid leukemia: developed for the American Society of Hematology. Blood 1999;94(5):1517-36.
28. Talpaz M, et al. Imatinib induces durable hematologic and cytogenetic responses in patients with accelerated phase chronic myeloid leukemia: results of a phase 2 study. Blood 2002;99(6):1928-37.
29. Kantarjian H et al. High-dose imatinib mesylate therapy in newly diagnosed Philadelphia chromosome-positive chronic phase chronic myeloid leukemia. Blood 2004;103:2873-8
30. O'Brien SG et al. Imatinib compared with interferon and low-dose cytarabine for newly diagnosed chronic-phase chronic myeloid leukemia. N Engl J Med 2003;348:994-1004

3.9　Myelofibrosis with Myeloid Metaplasia

poss.	**Interferon** (immunomodulation)	**IFN-alpha-2a/b** (Roferon A, Intron A)	*2-5 M U SC tiw*
poss.	**Cytostatic** (ribonucleotide diphosph. reductase inhib.)	**Hydroxyurea** (Hydrea, Droxia, Mylocel)	*20-30mg/kg PO biw or tiw*
poss.	**Androgen** (erythropoiesis↑)	**Danazol** (Danocrine, Gens)	*200mg PO bid or tid*
poss.	**Anabolic steroid** (erythropoiesis↑)	**Oxymetholone** (Anadrol-50)	*50mg PO tid*

31.　Tefferi A et al. Myelofibrosis with myeloid metaplasia. N Engl J Med 2000;342:1255-65.

3.10　Myelodysplastic Syndromes

poss.	**Antidote** (complexes with ferric ions and elimination through kidneys)	**Deferoxamine** (Desferal)	*2g IV after each unit of blood + 1-2g SC over 8-24h qd or 1g SC bid*
poss.	**Erythrocyte colony stimulating factor** (RBC production↑, maturation, activation)	**Erythropoietin** (Epogen, Procrit)	*150-300 U/kg SC tiw or 40,000-60,000 U SC qwk*
poss.	**Granulocyte colony stimulating factor** (neutrophil production↑, maturation, activation↑)	**Filgrastim** (Neupogen)	*0.3-5µg/kg/d SC*
poss.	**Azacytidine** **antimetabolite** (pyrimidine antagonist)	**Azacitidine, 5-AZC, 5-azacytidine** (Vidaza)	*75mg/m² SC qd x 7d repeat every 28 days*

32.　Franchini M, Gandini G, de Gironcoli M, et al. Safety and efficacy of subcutaneous bolus injection of deferoxamine in adult patients with iron overload. Blood 2000;95(9):2776-9.
33.　Hellstrom-Lindberg E. Efficacy of erythropoietin in the myelodysplastic syndromes: meta-analysis of 205 patients from 17 studies. Br J Haematol 1995;89:67-71.
34.　Negrin RS, Haeuber DH, Nagler A, et al. Maintenance treatment of patients with myelodysplastic syndromes using recombinant human granulocytic colony-stimulating factor. Blood 1990;76(1):36-43.
35.　Ozer H, Armitage J, Bennett C, et al. 2000 Update of recommendations for the use of hematopoietic colony-stimulating factors: evidence-based, clinical practice guidelines. J Clin Oncol 2000;18(20):3558-85.

3.11 Acute Leukemia
3.11.1 Acute Myelogenous Leukemia (AML)

Induction (7+3)

	Antimetabolite (purine antagonist)	**Cytarabine** (Cytosar-U, Tarabine PFS)	*100mg/m² /d continuous IV Inf d1-7*
plus	**Anthracycline** (DNA intercalation, topoisomerase II inhibition)	**Daunorubicin** (Cerubidine)	*45-60mg/m²/d IV d1-3 (may consider other anthracyclines)*
poss.	**Granulocyte colony stimulating factor** (neutrophil production ↑, maturation, activation ↑)	**Filgrastim** (Neupogen)	*5μg/kg SC qd beginning 24h after chemo-Tx through neutrophil recovery*
or	**Granulocyte and macrophage colony stimulating factor** (neutrophil/macrophage production ↑, maturation, activation)	**Sargramostim** (Leukine)	*250μ/m² SC qd beginning 24h after chemo-Tx through neutrophil recovery*
poss.	**Xanthine oxidase inhibitor** (uric acid production ↓)	**Allopurinol** (Aloprim, Zyloprim, Gens)	*300-600mg PO/IV qd*
poss.	**Urine hydration + alkalinization** (solubility of uric acid ↑)	**Hydration +/– Sodium bicarbonate**	*150-200ml/h; start 24-48h prior to chemo-Tx*

Consolidation (histone deacetylase, HDAC)

	Antimetabolite (purine antagonist)	**Cytarabine** (Cytosar-U, Tarabine PFS)	*1-3g/m² IV q12h on d1, d3, and d5; rep q28d*

36. Arlin Z, Case D, Moore J, et al. Randomized multicenter trial of cytosine arabinoside with mitoxantrone or daunorubicin in previously untreated adult patients with acute nonlymphocytic leukemia (ANLL). Leukemia 1990;4(3):177-183.
37. Mayer RJ, Davis RB, Schiffer CA, et al. Intensive post-remission chemotherapy in adults with acute myeloid leukemia. N Engl J Med 1994;331:896-903.

3.11.2 Acute Lymphocytic Leukemia (T-ALL)

Induction (Linker)

	Anthracycline (DNA intercalation, topoisomerase II inhibition)	**Daunorubicin** (Cerubidine)	*50mg/m² IV d1-3*
plus	**Antimitotic** (Mitotic spindle poison)	**Vincristine** (Oncovin, Vincasar PFS, Gens)	*2mg IV d1, d8, d15, and d22*
plus	**Glucocorticoid** (anti-inflammatory, immunosuppressive, lympholytic)	**Prednisone** (Deltasone, Orasone, Liquid Pred, Sterapred DS, Panasol-S, Meticorten, Prednicen-M, Gens)	*60 mg/m² PO d1-28*
plus	**Enzyme** (asparagine deamination, ⇒ protein synthesis ↓)	**L-asparaginase** (Elspar)	*6000 U/m² IM d17-28 (test dose prior to 1st dose)*
poss.	**Granulocyte colony stimulating factor** (neutrophil production↑, maturation, activation↑)	**Filgrastim** (Neupogen)	*5µg/kg SC qd beginning 24h after chemo-Tx through neutrophil recovery*
or		**Sargramostim** (Leukine)	*250µg/m² SC qd; start 24h after chemo-Tx through neutrophil recovery*
poss.	**Xanthine oxidase inhibitor** (uric acid production↓)	**Allopurinol** (Aloprim, Zyloprim, Gens)	*300-600mg PO/IV qd*
poss.	**Urine hydration + alkalinization** (solubility of uric acid↑)	**Hydration +/- Sodium bicarbonate**	*150-200ml/h; start 24-48h prior to chemo-Tx*

Consolidation (Linker – cycle 1, 3, 5, 7)

	Anthracycline (DNA intercalation, topoisomerase II inhibition)	**Daunorubicin** (Cerubidine)	*50mg/m² IV d1-2*
plus	**Antimitotic** (Mitotic spindle poison)	**Vincristine** (Oncovin, Vincasar PFS, Gens)	*2mg IV d1, d8*

plus	**Glucocorticoid** (anti-inflammatory, immunosuppressive, lympholytic)	**Prednisone** (Deltasone, Orasone, Liquid Pred, Sterapred DS, Panasol-S, Meticorten, Prednicen-M, Gens)	*60mg/m² PO d1-14*
plus	**Enzyme** (asparagine deamination, resulting in decreased protein synthesis)	**L-asparaginase** (Elspar)	*12000U/m² IM d2, 4, 7, 9, 11, 14*

Consolidation (Linker – cycle 2, 4, 6, 8)

	Topoisomerase II inhibition	**Etoposide** (VePesid, Etopophos, Toposar) – takes place of teniposide	*100mg/m² IV d1, 4, 8, 11*
plus	**Antimetabolite** (purine antagonist)	**Cytarabine** (Cytosar-U, Tarabine PFS)	*300mg/m² IV d1, 4, 8, 11*

Consolidation (Linker – cycle 9)

	Antimetabolite (folic acid antagonist)	**Methotrexate** (Gens)	*690mg/m² IV over 42h x 1 dose*
plus	**Reduced folate** (normal cell rescue)	**Leucovorin** (Wellcovorin, Folinic acid)	*15mg/m² IV q6h x12h beginning h 42 (adj based on MTX levels)*

Maintenance (Linker)

	Antimetabolite (folic acid antagonist)	**Methotrexate** (Rheumatrex, Gens)	*20mg/m² PO q wk until 30mo of CR*
plus	**Antimetabolite** (purine antagonist)	**6-Mercaptopurine** (Purinethol)	*75mg/m² PO qd until 30mo of CR*

Note: Consolidation treatments given approximately monthly

38. Linker CA, Levitt LJ, O'Donnell M, et al. Treatment of adult acute lymphoblastic leukemia with intensive cyclical chemotherapy: a follow-up report. Blood 1991;78(11):2814-22.

3.11.3 Acute Lymphocytic Leukemia (B-ALL)

Induction/Consolidation (hyperCVAD – cycle 1, 3, 5, 7)

	Alkylating agent (DNA cross-linking)	**Cyclophosphamide** (Cytoxan, Neosar, Gens)	*300mg/m² IV q12h x 6 doses, d1-3*
plus	**Antimitotic** (Mitotic spindle poison)	**Vincristine** (Oncovin, Vincasar PFS, Gens)	*2mg IV d4, d11*

| plus | **Anthracycline** (DNA intercalation, topoisomerase II inhib.) | **Doxorubicin** (Adriamycin PFS, Adriamycin RDF, Rubex, Gens) | *50mg/m² IV d4* |
| plus | **Glucocorticoid** (anti-inflammatory, immunosuppressive, lympholytic) | **Dexamethasone** (Decadron, Dexameth, Dexone, Hexadrol, Gens) | *40mg/d PO d1-4, d11-14* |

Induction/Consolidation (hyperCVAD – cycle 2, 4, 6, 8)

	Antimetabolite (folic acid antagonist)	**Methotrexate** (Gens)	*200mg/m² IV over 2h, then 800mg/m² IV over 22h x1 dose on d1*
plus	**Reduced folate** (normal cell rescue)	**Leucovorin** (Wellcovorin, Folinic acid)	*15 mg IV/PO q6h x 8 doses. Begin 24h after MTX complete (adj based on MTX levels)*
plus	**Antimetabolite** (purine antagonist)	**Cytarabine** (Cytosar-U, Tarabine PFS)	*3g/m² IV q12h x 4 doses on d2-3*
plus	**Glucocorticoid** (anti-inflammatory, immunosuppressive)	**Methylprednisolone** (Solu-Medrol, A-Methapred)	*50mg IV q12h d1-3*
poss.	**Granulocyte colony stimulating factor** (neutrophil production↑, maturation, activation↑)	**Filgrastim** (Neupogen)	*5µg/kg SC qd; start 24h after chemo-Tx through neutrophil recovery*
or	**Granulocyte and macrophage colony stimulating factor** (neutrophil /macrophage prod.↑, maturation, activ.)	**Sargramostim** (Leukine)	*250µg/m² SC qd; start 24h after chemo-Tx through neutrophil recovery*
poss.	**Xanthine oxidase inhibitor** (uric acid production↓)	**Allopurinol** (Aloprim, Zyloprim, Gens)	*300-600mg PO/IV qd*
poss.	**Urine hydration + alkalinization** (solubility of uric acid↑)	**Hydration +/- Sodium bicarbonate**	*150-200ml/h; start 24-48h prior to chemo-Tx*

Note: Subsequent treatments given upon WBC and platelet recovery per protocol.

39. Garcia-Manero G, Kantarjian HM. The Hyper-CVAD regimen in adult acute lymphocytic leukemia. Hematol Oncol Clin North Am 2000;14(4):1381-96.

Central nervous system IT therapy

poss.	**Antimetabolite** (folic acid antagonist)	**Methotrexate** (Methotrexate LPF)	*12-15mg intrathecal (lower doses for age < 3y old)*
poss.	**Antimetabolite** (purine antagonist)	**Cytarabine** (Cytosar-U, Tarabine PFS)	*50-100mg intrathecal (lower doses for age < 3y old)*
poss.	**Glucocorticoid** (anti-inflammatory, immunosuppressive)	**Hydrocortisone acetate** (preservative-free)	*12-35mg intrathecal (lower doses for age < 3y old)*

Note: Frequency of therapy depends on protocol and if patient has active CNS involvement of leukemia.

40. Hoelzer D. Treatment of acute lymphoblastic leukemia. Semin Hematol 1994;31:1-15.
41. Steinherz PG. CNS leukemia: problem of diagnosis, treatment and outcome. J Clin Oncol 1995;13(2):310-13.

3.11.4   Acute Promyelocytic Leukemia (APL, M3 AML)

Induction

	Retinoid (APL cell maturation, cytodifferentiation, decreases proliferation)	**Tretinoin** (Vesanoid, ATRA, All-*trans*-retinoic acid)	*45mg/m²/d PO (divided bid)*
plus	**Anthracycline** (DNA intercalation, topoisomerase II inhibition)	**Idarubicine** (Idamycin)	*12mg/m²/d IV on d 2, 4, 6, 8 (may consider other anthracyclines)*

Consolidation (cycle 1)

	Retinoid (APL cell maturation, cytodifferentiation, decreases proliferation)	**Tretinoin** (Vesanoid, ATRA, All-*trans*-retinoic acid)	*45mg/m²/d PO (divided BID)*
plus	**Anthracycline** (DNA intercalation, topoisomerase II inhib.)	**Idarubicine** (Idamycin)	*5mg/m²/d IV x 4d (may consider other anthracyclines)*
poss.	**Granulocyte colony stimulating factor** (neutrophil production ↑, maturation, activation ↑)	**Filgrastim** (Neupogen)	*5µg/kg SC qd; start 24h after chemo-Tx through neutrophil recovery*

or	**Granulocyte and macrophage colony stimulating factor** (neutrophil/macrophage production ↑, maturation, activation)	**Sargramostim** (Leukine)	*250µ/m² SC qd; start 24h after chemo-Tx through neutrophil recovery*
poss.	**Xanthine oxidase inhibitor** (uric acid production ↓)	**Allopurinol** (Aloprim, Zyloprim, Gens)	*300-600mg PO/IV qd*
poss.	**Urine hydration + alkalinization** (solubility of uric acid ↑)	**Hydration +/− Sodium bicarbonate**	*150-200ml/h; start 24-48h prior to chemo-Tx*

Consolidation (cycle 2)

	Retinoid (APL cell maturation, cytodifferentiation, decreases proliferation)	**Tretinoin** (Vesanoid, ATRA, All-*trans*-retinoic acid)	*45mg/m²/d PO (divided BID)*
plus	**Anthracenedione** (inhibition of DNA and RNA synthesis by DNA intercalation)	**Mitoxantrone** (Novantrone)	*10mg/m²/d IV x 5d*
+/−	**Antimetabolite** (purine antagonist)	**Cytarabine** (Cytosar-U, Tarabine PFS)	*1-2g/m² IV q12h d1-4*

Consolidation (cycle 3)

	Anthracycline (DNA intercalation, topoisomerase II inhibition)	**Idarubicine** (Idamycin)	*12mg/m²/d IV x 1d*

Maintenance

	Retinoid (APL cell maturation, cytodifferentiation, decreases proliferation)	**Tretinoin** (Vesanoid, ATRA, All-*trans*-retinoic acid)	*45mg/m²/d PO for 15d (q3mo x 2y)*
+/−	**Antimetabolite** (purine antagonist)	**6-Mercaptopurine** (Purinethol)	*90mg/m²/d PO (x2y)*
+/−	**Antimetabolite** (folic acid antagonist)	**Methotrexate** (Rheumatrex, Gens)	*15mg/m²/wk PO(x2y)*

42. Fenaux P, Chastang C, Chevret S, et al. A randomized comparison of all transretinoic acid (ATRA) plus chemotherapy and the role of maintenance therapy in newly diagnosed acute promyelocytic leukemia. Blood 1999;94(4):1192-1200.
43. Sanz MA, Martin G, Rayon C, et al. A modified AIDA protocol with anthracycline-based consolidation results in high antileukemia efficacy and reduced toxicity in newly diagnosed PML/RARa-positive acute promyelocytic leukemia. Blood 1999;94(9):3015-21.
44. Tallman MS, Nabhan C, Feusner JH, et al. Acute promyelocytic leukemia: evolving therapeutic strategies. Blood 2002;99(3):759-67.

3.12 Non-Hodgkin Lymphoma

3.12.1 Low-grade

Single agent

	Alkylating agent (DNA cross-linking)	Chlorambucil (Leukeran)	6-14mg PO qd until symptoms improve, then cont as intermittent Tx: 0.7mg/kg PO over 2-4d; rep q3wk until stabilized

COP (repeat every 21 days)

	Alkylating agent (DNA cross-linking)	Cyclophosphamide (Cytoxan, Neosar, Gens)	800mg IV on d1
plus	Antimitotic (Mitotic spindle poison)	Vincristine (Oncovin, Vincasar PFS, Gens)	1.4mg/m² IV on d1 (max 2mg)
plus	Glucocorticoid (anti-inflammatory, immunosuppressive, lympholytic)	Prednisone (Deltasone, Orasone, Liquid Pred, Sterapred DS, Panasol-S, Meticorten, Prednicen-M, Gens)	60mg/m² PO, d1-5

Rituximab

	Anti-CD20 monoclonal antibody (antineoplastic)	Rituximab (Rituxan)	375mg/m² IV qwk x 4 wk

45. Roeser HP, et al. Advanced non-Hodgkin's lymphomas: response to treatment with combination chemotherapy and factors influencing prognosis. Br J Haematol 1975;30(2):233-47.
46. McLaughlin et al: Rituximab chimeric anti-CD20 monoclonal antibody therapy for relapsed indolent lymphoma: half of patients respond to a four-dose treatment program. J Clin Oncol 1998;16:2825-33.

3.12.2 Chronic Lymphocytic Leukemia, Small Lymphocytic Lymphoma

	Alkylating agent (DNA cross-linking)	**Chlorambucil** (Leukeran)	*0.1mg/kg/d PO until counts improve or symptoms subside*
OR	**Alkylating agent** (DNA cross-linking)	**Chlorambucil** (Leukeran)	*0.3mg/kg/d PO qd x 5d; rep q28 d*
plus	**Glucocorticoid** (anti-inflammatory, immunosuppressive, lympholytic)	**Prednisone** (Deltasone, Orasone, Liquid Pred, Sterapred DS, Panasol-S, Meticorten, Prednicen-M, Gens)	*40mg/m² PO qd x 5d; rep q28 d*
OR	**Antimetabolite** (purine antagonist)	**Fludarabine** (Fludara)	*25 mg/m² IV qd x 5d; rep q28 d*
OR	**Monoclonal antibody** (inhibition of CD52 and subsequent cell lysis)	**Alemtuzumab** (Campath)	*Taper slowly over 3-7d; ini 3mg/d until tolerated, then 10mg/d until tolerated, then 30 mg/d; max single dose 30mg, max cumulative dose 90 mg; maint Tx 30 mg IV tiw on alternate days for up to 12wk*

47. Dighiero G et al: Chlorambucil in indolent chronic lymphocytic leukemia, N Engl J Med 1998; 338:1506-14.
48. Rai KR et al: Fludarabine compared with chlorambucil as primary therapy for chronic lymphocytic leukaemia. N Engl J Med 2000;343:1750-7.
49. Keating MJ et al: Therapeutic role of alemtuzumab (Campath IH) in patients who failed fludarabine: results of a large international study. Blood 2002;99:3554-61.

3.12.3 Intermediate-grade Lymphoma

CHOP-R (repeat every 21 days)

	Alkylating agent (DNA cross-linking)	**Cyclophosphamide** (Cytoxan, Neosar, Gens)	*750mg/m² IV on d1*
plus	**Anthracycline** (DNA intercalation, topoisomerase II inhibition)	**Doxorubicin** (Adriamycin PFS, Adriamycin RDF, Rubex, Gens)	*50mg/m² IV on d1*
plus	**Antimitotic** (Mitotic spindle poison)	**Vincristine** (Oncovin, Vincasar PFS, Gens)	*1.4mg/m² IV (max 2mg) on d1*

plus	**Glucocorticoid** (anti-inflammatory, immunosuppressive, lympholytic)	**Prednisone** (Deltasone, Orasone, Liquid Pred, Sterapred DS, Panasol-S, Meticorten, Prednicen-M, Gens)	*40mg/m² qd x 5d*
plus	**Anti–CD20 monoclonal antibody** (antineoplastic)	**Rituximab** (Rituxan)	*375mg/m² IV on d1*

50. Coiffier B et al: CHOP chemotherapy plus rituximab compared with CHOP alone in elderly patients with diffuse large-B-cell lymphoma. N Engl J Med 2002;346:235-42.

3.12.4   High-grade Lymphoma

Induction/Consolidation (hyperCVAD - cycle 1,3,5,7)

	Alkylating agent (DNA cross-linking)	**Cyclophosphamide** (Cytoxan, Neosar, Gens)	*300mg/m² IV q12h x 6 doses, d1-3*
plus	**Antimitotic** (Mitotic spindle poison)	**Vincristine** (Oncovin, Vincasar PFS, Gens)	*2mg IV d4, d11*
plus	**Anthracycline** (DNA intercalation, topoisomerase II inhibition)	**Doxorubicin** (Adriamycin PFS, Adriamycin RDF, Rubex, Gens)	*50mg/m² IV d4*
plus	**Glucocorticoid** (anti-inflammatory, immunosuppressive, lympholytic)	**Dexamethasone** (Decadron, Dexameth, Dexone, Hexadrol, Gens)	*40mg/d PO d1-4, d11-14*

Induction/Consolidation (hyperCVAD - cycle 2,4,6,8)

	Antimetabolite (folic acid antagonist)	**Methotrexate** (Gens)	*200mg/m² IV over 2h, then 800mg/m² IV over 22h x1 dose on d1*
plus	**Reduced folate** (normal cell rescue)	**Leucovorin** (Wellcovorin, Folinic acid)	*15mg IV/PO q6h x 8 doses. Begin 24h after MTX complete (adj based on MTX levels)*
plus	**Antimetabolite** (purine antagonist)	**Cytarabine** (Cytosar-U, Tarabine PFS)	*3g/m² IV q12h x 4 doses on d2-3*

plus	Glucocorticoid (anti-inflammatory, immunosuppressive, lympholytic)	Methylprednisolone (Solu-Medrol, A-Methapred)	*50mg IV q12h d1-3*
poss.	Granulocyte colony stimulating factor (neutrophil production↑, maturation, activation↑)	Filgrastim (Neupogen)	*5µg/kg SC qd; start 24h after chemo-Tx through neutrophil recovery (dose modification from publication)*
or	Granulocyte and macrophage colony stimulating factor (neutrophil/macrophage production↑, maturation, activation)	Sargramostim (Leukine)	*250µg/m² SC qd; start 24h after chemo-Tx through neutrophil recovery*
poss.	Xanthine oxidase inhibitor (uric acid production↓)	Allopurinol (Aloprim, Zyloprim, Gens)	*300-600mg PO/IV qd*
poss.	Urine hydration + alkalinization (solubility of uric acid↑)	Hydration +/- Sodium bicarbonate	*150-200ml/h; start 24-48h prior to chemo-Tx*

Note: Subsequent treatments given upon WBC and platelet recovery per protocol.

51. Thomas DA, et al. Hyper-CVAD program in Burkitt's-type adult acute lymphoblastic leukaemia. J Clin Oncol 1999;17(8):2461-70.

3.13 Hodgkin Disease
3.13.1 ABVD

Repeat cycle every 28 days

	Anthracycline (DNA intercalation, topoisomerase II inhibition)	Doxorubicin (Adriamycin PFS, Adriamycin RDF, Rubex, Gens)	*25mg/m² IV d1 and d15*
plus	Antitumor antibiotic	Bleomycin (Blenoxane)	*10 U/m² IV d1 and d15 (1 U test dose prior to 1ˢᵗ dose)*

plus	**Antimitotic** (mitotic spindle poison)	**Vinblastine** (Velban)	*6mg/m² IV d1 and d15*
plus	**Pseudo-alkylating agent**	**Dacarbazine** (DTIC-Dome)	*375mg/m² IV d1 and d15*

52. Canellos GP, et al. Chemotherapy of advanced Hodgkin's disease with MOPP, ABVD, or MOPP alternating with ABVD. N Engl J Med 1992;327:1478-84.
53. Duggan D, et al. MOPP/ABV versus ABVD for advanced Hodgkin's disease – a preliminary report of CALGB 8952 (with SWOG, ECOG, NCIC). Proc Amer Soc Clin Oncol 1997;16:12a.

3.14 Multiple Myeloma
3.14.1 General Therapy

Repeat after 14d rest

	Glucocorticoid (anti-inflammatory, immunosuppressive)	**Dexamethasone** (Decadron, Dexameth, Dexone, Hexadrol, Gens)	*20mg/m² PO qd d1-4, 9-12, and 17-20*

Or VAD, repeat cycle every 28 days

	Antimitotic (Mitotic spindle poison)	**Vincristine** (Oncovin, Vincasar PFS, Gens)	*0.4mg/d continuous IV Inf d1-4*
plus	**Anthracycline** (DNA intercalation, topoisomerase II inhibition)	**Doxorubicin** (Adriamycin PFS, Adriamycin RDF, Rubex, Gens)	*9mg/m²/d continuous IV Inf d1-4*
plus	**Glucocorticoid** (anti-inflammatory, immunosuppressive)	**Dexamethasone** (Decadron, Dexameth, Dexone, Hexadrol, Gens)	*40mg PO qd d1-4, 9-12, and 17-20*

Or MP, repeat cycle every 28 days

	Alkylating agent	**Melphalan** (Alkeran)	*8-10mg/m² PO qd d1-4*
plus	**Glucocorticoid** (anti-inflammatory, immunosuppressive)	**Prednisone** (Deltasone, Orasone, Liquid Pred, Sterapred DS, Panasol-S, Meticorten, Prednicen-M, Gens)	*60mg/m² PO qd d1-4*

Or Thalidomide +/- Dexamethasone			
	Immunomodulator	**Thalidomide** (Thalomid)	*200-800mg/d PO*
+/-	**Glucocorticoid** (anti-inflammatory, immunosuppressive)	**Dexamethasone** (Decadron, Dexameth, Dexone, Hexadrol, Gens)	*Variable dosing strategies, e.g. 20mg/m² PO qd d1-5, d15-18 (rep qmo)*
poss.	**Bisphosphonate** (osteoclast inhibition)	**Pamidronate** (Aredia)	*90mg IV qmo (long term)*
or poss.	**Bisphosphonate** (osteoclast inhibition)	**Zolendronate** (Zometa)	*4mg IV qmo (long term)*
poss.	**Erythrocyte colony stimulating factor** (RBC production ↑, maturation, activation)	**Erythropoietin** (Procrit, Epogen)	*150 U/kg SC tiw or 40000 U SC qwk; DARF: lower doses*

54. Alexanian R, Dimopoulos M, Delasalle K, et al. Primary dexamethasone treatment of multiple myeloma. Blood 1992;80(4):887-90.
55. Alexanian R, Barlogie B, Tucker S, et al. VAD-based regimens as primary treatment for multiple myeloma. Am J Hematol 1990;33:86-9.
56. Tricot G, Multiple myeloma and other plasma cell disorders in: Hematology Basic Principles and Practice, 3rd ed., Churchill Livingstone, New York, 2000, 1398-1416.
57. Singhal S, Mehta J, Desikan R, et al. Antitumor activity of thalidomide in refractory multiple myeloma. N Engl J Med 1999;341:1565-71.
58. Weber DM, Rankin K, Gavino M, et al. Thalidomide with dexamethasone for resistant multiple myeloma. Blood 2000;96(11):167a (abstract #719).
59. Berenson JR, Lichtenstein A, Porter L, et al. Efficacy of pamidronate in reducing skeletal events in patients with advanced multiple myeloma. N Engl J Med 1996;334:488-93.

4.   Respiratory System

Charles L. Daley, MD
Professor of Medicine
Division of Mycobacterial and Respiratory Infections,
National Jewish Medical and Research Center,
Denver, CO

4.1   Asthma

4.1.1   Long-Term Therapy and Quick Relief Therapy

Step 1 (mild intermittent)

Beta$_2$-agonist, short acting (bronchodilating)	**Albuterol** (Proventil, Proventil HFA, Ventolin HFA 90µg/puff)	*2 puffs tid-qid prn*
or	**Metaproterenol** (Alupent, 650µg/puff)	*2 puffs tid-qid prn*
or	**Pirbuterol** (Maxair Autoinhaler, 200µg/puff)	*2 puffs tid-qid prn*

Step 2 (mild persistent) - Step 1 plus:

Corticosteroid, inhaled, low doses (anti-inflammatory)	**Beclomethasone** (Qvar 40µg/puff)	*168-480µg/d: 4-12 puffs qd (40µg/puff)*
or	**Budesonide** (Pulmicort Turbohaler, 200µg/dose)	*200-400µg/d: 1-2 inhs qd*
or	**Flunisolide** (Aerobid, 250µg/puff)	*500-1000µg/d: 2-4 puffs qd*
or	**Fluticasone** (Flovent MD, 44, 110, 220µg/puff)	*88-264µg/d: 2-6 puffs qd (44µg/puff) or 2 puffs qd (110µg/puff)*
or	**Triamcinolone acetonide** (Azmacort, 100µg/puff)	*400-1000µg/d: 4-10 puffs qd*
OR	**Mast cell stabilizer** (mediator release ↓)	**Cromolyn sodium** (Intal, 1mg/puff)	*2-4 puffs tid -qid*
or		**Nedocromil** (Tilade, 1.75mg/puff)	*2-4 puffs bid-qid*

OR	**Leukotriene modifiers** (bronchodilating)	**Zafirlukast** (Accolate, 20mg)	*20mg PO bid*
or		**Zileuton** (Zyflo, 600mg)	*600mg PO qid*
		Montelukast (Singulair, 10mg)	*10mg PO qd in evening*

Step 3 (moderate persistent) – Step 1 plus			
Either	**Corticosteroid, inhaled, medium dose** (anti-inflammatory)	**Beclomethasone** (Qvar 40µg/puff)	*504-800µg/d: 12-20 puffs qd (40µg/puff)*
or		**Budesonide** (Pulmicort Turbohaler, 200µg/dose)	*400-600µg/d: 2-3 inhs qd*
or		**Flunisolide** (Aerobid, 250µg/puff)	*1000-2000µg: 4-8 puffs qd*
or		**Fluticasone** (Flovent MD, 110, 220µg/puff)	*264-660µg/d: 2-6 puffs qd (110µg(puff) or 2-3 inhs qd (220µg/puff)*
or		**Triamcinolone acetonide** (Azmacort, 100µg/puff)	*1000-2000µg/d: 10-20 puffs qd*
OR	**Corticosteroid, inhaled, low-medium dose** (anti-inflammatory)	See above, →82	
plus	**Beta₂-agonist, long-acting inhaled** (bronchodilating)	**Salmeterol** (Serevent Diskus, 50µg/blister)	*Diskus: 1 inh q12h*
or		**Formoterol** (Foradil Aerolizer, 12µg/Cap)	*1 inh q12h*
poss	**Methylxanthines** (bronchodilating, central respiratory stimulation)	**Theophylline-sustained release** (multiple preparations)	*Ini dose 10mg/kg/d up to 300mg div over 24h; max 800mg/d; adj dose to serum level (5-15µg/ml)*
or	**Beta₂-agonist, long-acting tablets**	**Albuterol - sustained release** (Volmax)	*4-8mg PO q12h*
or		**Terbutaline** (Brethine, Gens)	*2.5-5.0mg PO tid*

Consider for allergic asthma not controlled by inhaled corticosteroids			
	Monoclonal antibody	Omalizumab (Xolair)	150-375µg q2-4wk, dose based on pre-treatment, IgE level and body weight

Step 4 (severe persistent)			
	Corticosteroid, inhaled, high dose (anti-inflammatory)	Beclomethasone (Qvar 40µg/puff)	>800 µg/d: >20 puffs qd (40µg/puff)
or		Budesonide (Pulmicort Turbohaler, 200µg/dose)	>600µg/d: >3 inh qd
or		Flunisolide (Aerobid, 250µg/puff)	>2000µg/d: >8 puffs qd
or		Fluticasone (Flovent MD, 110, 220µg/puff)	>660µg/d: >6 puffs qd (110µg/puff) or >3 puffs qd (220µg/puff)
or		Triamcinolone acetonide (Azmacort, 100µg/puff)	>2000µg/d: >20 puffs qd
and	Beta₂-agonist, long-acting inhaled (bronchodilating)	Salmeterol (Serevent Diskus, 50µg/blister)	1 inh q12h
		Salmeterol + Fluticasone (Advair, 100/ 50, 250/50, 500/50 µg/ dose)	1 inh q12h
or		Formoterol (Foradil Aerolizer, 12µg/Cap)	1 inh q12h
poss	Methylxanthines (bronchodilating, central respiratory stimulation)	Theophylline-sustained release (multiple preparations)	Ini dose 10mg/kg/d up to 300mg in div doses over 24h: max dose 800mg/d; adj dose to serum level (5-15µg/ml)
or	Beta₂-agonist, long-acting tablets	Albuterol - sustained release (Volmax)	4-8mg PO q12h
		Terbutaline (Brethine, Gens)	2.5-5.0mg PO tid

and	Corticosteroid, oral (anti-inflammatory)	Methylprednisolone (Gens)	7.5-60mg qd or qid prn OR short-course "burst": 40-60mg qd or div bid for 3-10d
		Prednisolone (Gens)	
		Prednisone (Gens)	

Consider for allergic asthma not controlled by inhaled corticosteroids

	Monoclonal antibody	Omalizumab (Xolair)	150-375µg q2-4wk, dose based on pre-treatment, IgE level and body weight

4.1.2 Prophylaxis of Exercise or Irritant-Induced Asthma

	Beta₂-agonist, short acting (bronchodilating)	Albuterol (Proventil, Proventil HFA, Ventolin HFA, 90µg/puff)	2 puffs prior to exercise or allergen exposure
or		Metaproterenol (Alupent, 650µg/puff)	2 puffs prior to exercise or allergen exposure
or		Pirbuterol (Maxair Autoinhaler, 200µg/puff)	2 puffs prior to exercise or allergen exposure
OR	Long-acting inhaled beta₂-agonist	Salmeterol (Serevent Diskus, 50µg/blister)	2 puffs or 1 inh at least 30min prior to excercise
or		Formoterol (Foradil Aerolizer, 12µg/Cap)	1 inh at least 15min prior to excercise
OR	Mast cell stabilizer (mediator liberation inhibition)	Cromolyn sodium (Intal, 1mg/puff)	2 puffs qid or one puff prior to exercise or allergen exposure

4.1.3 Asthma Exacerbations in Emergency Medical Care or Hospital

	Beta₂-agonist, short acting (bronchodilating)	Albuterol (Proventil, Ventolin, Gens; Nebulizer Sol - 5mg/ml, MDI - 90µg/puff)	2.5-5mg q20min x 3, then 2.5-10mg q1-4h prn or 10-15mg/h cont; 4-8 puffs q20min up to 4h, then q1-4h prn (use spacer device)
or		Pirbuterol (Maxair, Maxair Autoinhaler, 200µg/puff)	
or		Levalbuterol (Xopenex)	0.63-1.25mg nebulized q6-8h

poss	**Methylxanthines** (bronchodilating, central respiratory stimulation)	**Aminophylline** (Gens)	*5mg/kg as short-inf over 30 min, then 1mg/kg/h, after 12h 0.8mg/kg/h (serum level = 5-15)*
and	**Corticosteroid** (anti-inflammatory) betarecept. ↑)	**Prednisone** (Gens) **Methylprednisolone** (Gens) **Prednisolone** (Gens)	*120-180mg/d in 3-4 div doses for 48h, then 60-80mg/d until PEF 70% of predicted/personal best*
poss	**Beta₂-agonist, systemic** (bronchodilating)	**Terbutaline** (Brethine, 1mg/ml)	*0.25mg SC q20min for 3 doses*
or	**Alpha-beta-adrenergic agonist** (bronchodilating)	**Epinephrine** (1:1000, 1mg/ml)	*0.3-0.5mg SC q20min for 3 doses*
poss	**Anticholinergic** (bronchodilating)	**Ipratropium bromide** (Atrovent Nebulizer Sol - 250µg/ml, Atrovent MDI - 18µg/puff)	*0.5mg q30min for 3 doses, then q2-4h prn 4-8 puffs prn*
and	**Gas** (blood oxygenation)	**Oxygen**	*Prn to maintain O_2 saturation of ≥ 90%*

60. National Institutes of Health. National Heart, Lung, and Blood Institute. Guidelines for the Diagnosis and Management of Asthma. 1997:1-86.

4.2 Chronic Obstructive Pulmonary Disease (COPD)
4.2.1 In General

Smoking cessation is critical!

Gas (blood oxygenation)	**Oxygen**	*If pO_2 < 55mmHg at rest or < 60mmHg with exercise, sleep, chronic cor pulmonale or secondary polycythemia; Caution when pCO_2↑*

4.2.2   Long-Term Therapy

Stage 1 (mild COPD – FEV$_1$ > 80% predicted)

	Beta$_2$-agonist, short acting (bronchodilating)	**Albuterol** (Proventil, Proventil HFA, Ventolin HFA, 90μg/puff)	*2 puffs tid-qid prn*
or		**Metaproterenol** (Alupent, 650μg/puff)	*2 puffs tid-qid prn*
or		**Pirbuterol** (Maxair Autoinhaler, 200μg/puff)	*2 puffs tid-qid prn*
OR	**Anticholinergic** (bronchodilating)	**Ipratropium bromide** (Atrovent MDI, 18μg/puff)	*2-4 puffs tid-qid*
OR	**Beta$_2$-agonist + Parasympatholytic** (bronchodilating)	**Albuterol + Ipratropium bromide** (Combivent, 103μg+18μg/puff)	*2 puffs qid*

Stage 2 (moderate COPD – 30% < FEV$_1$ < 80% predicted) – Stage 1 plus

	Beta$_2$-agonist, long-acting inhaled (bronchodilating)	**Salmeterol** (Serevent Diskus, 50μg/blister)	*2 puffs q12h* / *1 inh q12h*
or		**Formoterol** (Foradil Aerolizer, 12μg/Cap)	*1 inh q12h*
or	**Methylxanthines** (bronchodilating, central respiratory stimulation)	**Theophylline-sustained release** (multiple preparations)	*Ini dose 10mg/kg/d up to 300mg, max 800mg/d; adj dose to serum level (5-15μg/ml)*
poss	**Corticosteroid, inhaled**	If significant symptoms and spirometric response or if repeated excerbations; low to moderate doses, see Asthma →82	
and	**Rehabilitation**	Refer for pulmonary rehabilitation if available	

Stage 3 (severe COPD – FEV$_1$ < 30% predicted) – Stage 2 plus

	Gas (blood oxygenation)	Oxygen	*If pO$_2$ < 55mmHg at rest or < 60mmHg with exercise, sleep, chronic cor pulmonale or secondary polycythemia; Caution when pCO$_2$↑*
and	Rehabilitation	Refer for pulmonary rehabilitation if available	
and	Surgery	Consider for surgical treatments	

4.2.3   Acute Exacerbations of Chronic Bronchitis

Simple, uncomplicated AECB

Any age, 4 exacerbations per year, no co-morbid illness, FEV$_1$ >50%

	Macrolide	Azithromycin (Zithromax)	*d1: 500mg PO, d2-5: 250mg/d*
		Clarithromycin (Biaxin, Biaxin XL)	*250-500mg PO bid*
or	Cephalosporin	Cefpodoxime (Vantin)	*200mg PO q12h*
		Cefuroxime-Axetil (Ceftin, Veftin)	*250-500mg PO bid*
		Cefprozil (Cefzil)	*500mg q12h for 10d*
or	Tetracycline	Doxycycline (Vibramycin, Gens)	*d1: 200mg PO, then 100mg PO qd*

Complicated AECB

Patient >64y, > 4 exacerbations per year, serious co-morbid illness, chronic oral steroids, FEV$_1$ <50%

	Fluorquinolones	Moxifloxacin (Avelox, Avelox I.V.)	*400mg PO/IV q24h for 5d*

Complicated AECB at risk for P. aeruginosa

Patients with chronic bronchial sepsis, need for chronic corticosteroid therapy and frequent (>4/y) courses of antibiotics, FEV$_1$ <35%

	Fluorquinolones	Ciprofloxacin (Cipro, Cipro I.V.)	*750mg PO q12h for 7-14d, 400mg IV q8h for 7-14d*

61. Niederman MS, et al. Consultant 2002; 42, 39-43

4.3   Pneumonia
4.3.1   General Measures

poss	**Gas** (blood oxygenation)	Oxygen	*Prn to maintain O_2 saturation of $\geq 90\%$*
poss	**Aniline derivative** (anlagesic, antipyretic)	Acetaminophen (Tylenol, Gens)	*500-1000mg PO/PR q6-8h*

The recommended dosages are meant for adults with normal renal and hepatic function. The duration of therapy is 7-14 days unless specified otherwise.

4.3.2   Community-acquired Pneumonia (CAP)

Otherwise healthy outpatients

first-line	**Macrolide**	Azithromycin (Zithromax)	*500mg PO qd on d1, then 250mg qd on d2-5*

Alternative first-line antibiotic therapy

	Ketolide	Telithromycin (Ketek)	*800mg PO qd*
or	**Fluoroquinolone**	Moxifloxacin (Avelox)	*400mg PO qd*
		Levofloxacin (Levaquin)	*500mg PO qd*
		Gatifloxacin (Tequin)	*400mg PO qd*
or	**Macrolide**	Clarithromycin (Biaxin, Biaxin XL)	*500mg PO bid or 1g XL PO qd*
or	**Tetracycline**	Doxycycline (Vibramycin, Gens)	*100mg PO bid*

Outpatients with comorbidity

First-line antibiotic therapy

	Fluoroquinolone	Moxifloxacin (Avelox)	*400mg PO qd*
or	**Ketolide**	Telithromycin (Ketek)	*800mg PO qd*

Alternative first-line antibiotic therapy

	Fluoroquinolone	Levofloxacin (Levaquin)	*500mg PO qd*
or	**Macrolide – advanced generation**	Azithromycin (Zithromax)	*500mg PO qd on d1, then 250mg qd on d2-5*
		Clarithromycin (Biaxin, Biaxin XL)	*500mg PO bid or 1g XL PO qd*
or	**Fluoroquinolone**	Gatifloxacin (Tequin)	*400mg PO qd*

In-Hospital (not in ICU) underlying risk factors or comorbid conditions

First-line antibiotic therapy

	Cephalosporin	**Ceftriaxone** (Rocephin)	*1-2.0g IV qd*
plus	Macrolide	**Azithromycin** (Zithromax)	*500mg IV qd on d1, then 250mg qd on d2-5*

Alternative first-line antibiotic therapy

	Fluoroquinolone	**Moxifloxacin** (Avelox)	*400mg IV qd*
		Levofloxacin (Levaquin)	*500mg IV qd*
		Gatifloxacin (Tequin)	*400mg IV qd*

CAP acquired in the nursing home environment

First-line antibiotic therapy

	Cephalosporin	**Ceftriaxone** (Rocephin)	*1-2.0g IV qd*
plus	Macrolide	**Azithromycin** (Zithromax)	*500mg IV qd on d1, then 250mg qd on d2-5*

Alternative first-line antibiotic therapy

	Fluoroquinolone	**Moxifloxacin** (Avelox)	*400mg IV qd*
		Levofloxacin (Levaquin)	*500mg IV qd*
		Gatifloxacin (Tequin)	*400mg IV qd*

CAP in the elderly individual with chronic alcoholism

First-line antibiotic therapy

	Cephalosporin	**Ceftriaxone** (Rocephin)	*1-2.0g IV qd*
plus	Macrolide	**Azithromycin** (Zithromax)	*500mg IV qd on d1, then 250mg qd on d2-5*

Alternative first-line antibiotic therapy

	Cephalosporin	**Ceftriaxone** (Rocephin)	*1-2.0g IV qd*
plus	Macrolide	**Azithromycin** (Zithromax)	*500mg IV qd on d1, then 250mg qd on d2-5*
plus	Lincosamide	**Clindamycin** (Cleocin)	*200-600mg IV tid-qid*
OR	Fluoroquinolone	**Levofloxacin** (Levaquin)	*500mg IV qd*

Severe bacteremic CAP with documented S. pneumoniae species showing high-level resistance

First-line antibiotic therapy

	Cephalosporin	**Ceftriaxone** (Rocephin)	*1-2.0g IV qd*
plus	Fluoroquinolone	**Moxifloxacin** (Avelox)	*400mg IV qd*

Alternative first-line antibiotic therapy

	Cephalosporin	**Ceftriaxone** (Rocephin)	*1-2.0g IV qd*
plus	Fluoroquinolone	**Levofloxacin** (Levaquin)	*500mg IV qd*

Severe CAP complicated by structural disease of the lung

First-line antibiotic therapy

	Cephalosporin	**Ceftazidime** (Ceptaz, Fortaz, Tazicef, Tazidime, Gens)	*2g IV q8h*
plus	Aminoglycoside	**Tobramycin** (Nebcin, Gens)	*7mg/kg IV qd*
		Gentamicin (Garamycin, Gens)	*7mg/kg IV qd*
		Amikacin (Amikin)	*20mg/kg IV qd*
plus	Macrolide	**Azithromycin** (Zithromax)	*500mg IV qd on d1, then 250mg qd on d2-5*
OR	Carbapenem	**Imipenem** (Primaxin)	*500mg IV q6h*
plus	Aminoglycoside	**Tobramycin** (Nebcin, Gens)	*7mg/kg IV qd*
		Gentamicin (Garamycin, Gens)	*7mg/kg IV qd*
		Amikacin (Amikin)	*20mg/kg IV qd*
plus	Fluoroquinolone	**Moxifloxacin** (Avelox)	*400mg IV qd*

Alternative first-line antibiotic therapy

	Cephalosporin	**Ceftazidime** (Ceptaz, Fortaz, Tazicef, Tazidime, Gens)	*2g IV q8h*
plus	Aminoglycoside	**Tobramycin** (Nebcin, Gens)	*7mg/kg IV qd*
		Gentamicin (Garamycin, Gens)	*7mg/kg IV qd*
		Amikacin (Amikin)	*20mg/kg IV qd*
plus	Fluoroquinolone	**Levofloxacin** (Levaquin)	*500mg IV qd*
OR	Penicillin	**Piperacillin** (Pipracil)	
plus	Macrolide	**Azithromycin** (Zithromax)	*500mg IV qd on d1, then 250mg qd on d2-5*
plus	Aminoglycoside	**Tobramycin** (Nebcin, Gens)	*7mg/kg IV qd*
		Gentamicin (Garamycin, Gens)	*7mg/kg IV qd*
		Amikacin (Amikin)	*20mg/kg IV qd*

CAP in patient with suspected aspiration

First-line antibiotic therapy

	Cephalosporin	**Ceftriaxone** (Rocephin)	*1-2.0g IV qd*
plus	Macrolide	**Azithromycin** (Zithromax)	*500mg PO/IV qd on d1, then 250mg qd on d2-5*
plus	Lincosamide	**Clindamycin** (Cleocin)	*200-600mg IV tid-qid*

Alternative first-line antibiotic therapy

	Fluoroquinolone	**Moxifloxacin** (Avelox)	*400mg IV qd*
plus	Lincosamide	**Clindamycin** (Cleocin)	*200-600mg IV tid-qid*
OR	Carbapenem	**Ertapenem** (Invanz)	*1g IV qd*
plus	Macrolide	**Azithromycin** (Zithromax)	*500mg PO/IV qd on d1, then 250mg qd on d2-5*
OR	Fluoroquinolone	**Gatifloxacin** (Tequin)	*400mg IV qd for 7-14d*
plus	Lincosamide	**Clindamycin** (Cleocin)	*200-600mg IV tid-qid*

Suspected MRSA CAP (i.e. severe CAP in a compromised host)

First-line antibiotic therapy

	Fluoroquinolone	Moxifloxacin (Avelox)	400mg IV qd
plus	Oxazolidinone	Linezolid (Zyvox)	600mg IV bid for 7-28d
OR	Fluoroquinolone	Moxifloxacin (Avelox)	400mg IV qd
plus	Glycopeptide	Vancomycin (Vancocin, Vancoled, Gens)	1g IV bid as short infusion for 7-28d

Alternative first-line antibiotic therapy

	Fluoroquinolone	Levofloxacin (Levaquin)	500mg IV qd
plus	Glycopeptide	Vancomycin (Vancocin, Vancoled, Gens)	1g IV bid as short infusion for 7-28d
OR	Cephalosporin	Ceftriaxone (Rocephin)	1-2.0g IV qd
plus	Macrolide	Azithromycin (Zithromax)	500mg IV qd on d1, then 250mg qd on d2-5
plus	Oxazolidinone	Linezolid (Zyvox)	600mg IV bid for 7-28d

CAP with severe pneumonia requiring ICU hospitalization

First-line antibiotic therapy

	Cephalosporin	Ceftriaxone (Rocephin)	1-2.0g IV qd
plus	Fluoroquinolone	Levofloxacin (Levaquin)	500mg IV qd
OR	Cephalosporin	Ceftriaxone (Rocephin)	1-2.0g IV qd
plus	Fluoroquinolone	Moxifloxacin (Avelox)	400mg IV qd

Alternative first-line antibiotic therapy

	Cephalosporin	Ceftriaxone (Rocephin)	1-2.0g IV qd
plus	Macrolide	Azithromycin (Zithromax)	500mg IV qd on d1, then 250mg qd on d2-5

CAP with severe pneumonia requiring ICU hospitalization (Pseudomonas is highly suspected)

First-line antibiotic therapy

	Cephalosporin	**Ceftazidime** (Ceptaz, Fortaz, Tazicef, Tazidime, Gens)	*2g IV q8h*
plus	Aminoglycoside	**Tobramycin** (Nebcin, Gens)	*7mg/kg IV qd*
		Gentamicin (Garamycin, Gens)	*7mg/kg IV qd*
		Amikacin (Amikin)	*20mg/kg IV qd*
plus	Macrolide	**Azithromycin** (Zithromax)	*500mg IV qd on d1, then 250mg qd on d2-5*
OR	Carbapenem	**Imipenem** (Primaxin)	*500mg IV q6h*
plus	Aminoglycoside	**Tobramycin** (Nebcin, Gens)	*7mg/kg IV qd*
		Gentamicin (Garamycin, Gens)	*7mg/kg IV qd*
		Amikacin (Amikin)	*20mg/kg IV qd*
plus	Fluoroquinolone	**Levofloxacin** (Levaquin)	*500mg IV qd*

Alternative first-line antibiotic therapy

	Cephalosporin	**Ceftazidime** (Ceptaz, Fortaz, Tazicef, Tazidime, Gens)	*2g IV q8h*
plus	Aminoglycoside	**Tobramycin** (Nebcin, Gens)	*7mg/kg IV qd*
		Gentamicin (Garamycin, Gens)	*7mg/kg IV qd*
		Amikacin (Amikin)	*20mg/kg IV qd*
plus	Fluoroquinolone	**Levofloxacin** (Levaquin)	*500mg IV qd*
OR	Penicillin	**Piperacillin** (Pipracil)	*3-4g IV q4-6h*

plus	Aminoglycoside	Tobramycin (Nebcin, Gens)	7mg/kg IV qd
		Gentamicin (Garamycin, Gens)	7mg/kg IV qd
		Amikacin (Amikin)	20mg/kg IV qd
plus	Macrolide	Azithromycin (Zithromax)	500mg IV qd on d1, then 250mg qd on d2-5

62. Year 2005 Antibiotic Selection for Community-Aquired Pneumonia Guidelines

4.3.3 Hospital-acquired Pneumonia (HAP)

HAP without risk factors for multidrug-resistant pathogens, early onset and any disease severity
Possible organisms: Streptococcus pneumoniae, Haemophilus influenzae, methicillin-sensitive Staphylococcus aureus, antibiotic-sensitive enteric gram-negatives, Enterobacter species, Escherichia coli, Klebsiella pneumoniae, Proteus spp., Serratia marcescens,

or	Cephalosporin – nonpseudomonal 3rd gen.	Cefotaxime (Claforan)	1-2g IV q4-8h
		Ceftriaxone (Rocephin)	1-2g IV q12h
or	Penicillin + beta-lactamase inhibitor	Ampicillin + Sulbactam (Unasyn)	1+0.5g - 2+1g IV q6h
	Nonpseudomonal fluoroquinolone	Levofloxacin (Levaquin)	750mg IV qd
		Moxifloxacin (Avelox)	400mg IV qd
		Ciprofloxacin (Cipro)	400mg IV q8h

HAP with risk factors for multidrug-resistant pathogens or late-onset and any disease severity
Possible organisms: as above plus methicillin-resistant Staphylococcus aureus (MRSA), Legionella pneumophilia, and multidrug-resistant pathogens: Pseudomonas aeruginosa, Klebsiella pneumoniae, and Acinetobacter species

	Cephalosporin – antipseudomonal	Cefepime (Maxipime)	1-2.0g IV q12h
		Ceftazidime (Ceptaz, Fortaz, Tazicef, Tazidime, Gens)	2g IV q8h
or	Carbapenem – antipseudomonal	Imipenem (Primaxin)	500mg IV q6h or 1g IV q8h
		Meropenem (Merrem)	1g IV q8h

or	Penicillin + beta-lactamase inhibitor	Piperacillin + Tazobactam (Zosyn)	3+0.375g IV q6h
Plus	Nonpseudomonal fluoroquinolone	Levofloxacin (Levaquin)	750mg IV qd
		Ciprofloxacin (Cipro)	400mg IV q8h
or	Aminoglycoside	Amikacin (Amikin)	20mg/kg IV qd
		Tobramycin (Nebcin, Gens)	7mg/kg IV qd
		Gentamicin (Garamycin, Gens)	7mg/kg IV qd
plus	Glycopeptide	Vancomycin (Vancocin, Vancoled, Gens)	15mg/kg IV q12h until methicillin-resist. Staph. aureus is ruled out; Caution: DARF, also check peak and trough serum levels to adj dose
or	Oxazolidinone	Linezolid (Zyvox)	600mg IV/PO q12h
poss Legionella spp			
	Macrolide	Azithromycin (Zithromax)	500mg IV qd
or	Nonpseudomonal fluoroquinolone	Levofloxacin (Levaquin)	750mg IV qd
		Ciprofloxacin (Cipro)	400mg IV/PO q8h

63. American Thoracic Society and Infectious Disease Society of America. Guidelines for the Management of Adults with Hospital-aiqured, Ventilator-associated, and Healthcare-associated pneumonia. Am J Respir Crit Care Med 2005;171:388-416

4.4   Pleural Disease
4.4.1   Pleurisy

	Aniline derivative (analgesic, antipyretic)	Acetaminophen (Tylenol, Gens)	500-1000mg PO/PR qid
or	NSAID (analgesic, antipyretic)	Ibuprofen (Advil, Motrin, Gens)	400-800mg PO tid-qid
poss	Opioid (antitussive, analgesic)	Codeine (Gens)	30-50mg PO bid, max. 150mg/d prn

4.4.2   Pleural Infections

Empiric Treatment: In general, treat as for pneumonia and alter Tx if a specific pathogen is isolated. Include antibiotics with anaerobic coverage in the Tx regimen unless a specific pathogen is identified. Complicated parapneumonic effusions and empyemas require chest tube drainage and prolonged antibiotic Tx (e.g., 1+ mo).

Consider			
	Lincosamide	**Clindamycin** (Cleocin)	*900mg IV q8h*

4.4.3   Specific Pathogens

Streptococcus pneumoniae			
1st choice	Benzylpenicillin	**Penicillin G** (Gens)	*1-2 M U IV q4-6h*
If penicillin allergic			
	Macrolide	**Azithromycin** (Zithromax)	*500mg IV qd*
or	Glycopeptide	**Vancomycin** (Vancocin, Vancoled, Gens)	*15mg/kg IV q12h*
or	Oxazolidinone	**Linezolid** (Zyvox)	*600mg IV/PO q12h*
If penicillin resistant			
	Fluoroquinolone	**Levofloxacin** (Levaquin)	*500-750mg IV qd*
		Moxifloxacin (Avelox)	*400mg IV qd*
		Gatifloxacin (Tequin)	*400mg IV qd*
or	Cephalosporin	**Ceftriaxone** (Rocephin)	*1-2g IV q12h*

Streptococcus spp.			
	Benzylpenicillin	**Penicillin G** (Gens)	*1-2 M U IV q4-6h*

Staphylococcus aureus			
1st choice	Penicillin – 2nd gen.	**Nafcillin** (Nallpen, Unipen, Gens)	*1-2g IV q4-6h*
If methicillin resistant			
	Glycopeptide	**Vancomycin** (Vancocin, Vancoled, Gens)	*15mg/kg IV q12h*
or	Oxazolidinone	**Linezolid** (Zyvox)	*600mg IV/PO q12h*

Pseudomonas aeruginosa			
	Cephalosporin – 3rd gen.	Ceftazidime (Ceptaz, Fortaz, Tazicef, Tazidime, Gens)	1-2g IV q8-12h
or	Carbapenem	Imipenem (Primaxin)	500-1000mg IV q6-8h
		Meropenem (Merrem)	1g IV q8h
plus	Aminoglycoside	Tobramycin (Nebcin)	2-3mg/kg IV loading dose, then 1.0-1.7mg/kg IV q8h
or	Fluoroquinolone	Ciprofloxacin (Cipro)	200-400mg IV bid
Haemophilus influenzae			
	Aminopenicillin (if β-lactamase negat.)	Ampicillin (Gens)	250-500mg IV q6h
or	Cephalosporin – 3rd gen.	Cefotaxime (Claforan)	1.0-2.0g IV q4-8h
		Ceftriaxone (Rocephin)	1.0-2.0g IV qd
		Ceftizoxime (Cefizox)	1.0g IV q8-12h to 4.0g IV q8h
Klebsiella			
	Cephalosporin – 3rd gen.	Cefotaxime (Claforan)	1.0-2.0g IV q4-8h
		Ceftriaxone (Rocephin)	1.0-2.0g IV qd
		Ceftizoxime (Cefizox)	1.0g IV q8-12h to 4.0g IV q8h

4.5 Pulmonary Thromboembolism (PE)
4.5.1 General measures

Gas (blood oxygenation)	Oxygen		Prn to maintain O_2 saturation of $\geq$ 90%

4.5.2 Anticoagulation

Heparin, low-molecular-weight (LMWH)	Enoxaparin (Lovenox)	1mg/kg SC q12h or 1.5mg/kg SC qd; single dose max. 180mg
	Tinzaparin (Innohep)	175 anti-Xa IU/kg SC qd
	Dalteparin (Fragmin)	200 anti-Xa IU/kg SC qd

or	Heparin – unfractionated	Heparin (Gens)	5000 U bolus IV, then maint inf 18 U/kg/h IV; rebolus 80 U/kg IV prn; adj dose based on PTT (2-3) or plasma heparin level (0.2-0.4 U/ml)
and	Oral anticoagulant (carboxylation of coagulation factors in liver ↓)	Warfarin (Coumadin, Gens)	Ini 5mg PO, adj dose based on INR (2.0); stop LMWH or UFH, when INR in therapeutic range (INR 2) for 4d

Continue for 3mo with INR 2.5 (2-3) in first PE with reversible risk or time-limited factors; for 6 mo in first PE without risk factors; or 12mon/permanent after recurrence or continuous risk factor

4.5.3   Thrombolysis in PE

The use of thrombolytics in treating PE must be individualized. Thrombolysis is generally indicated in hypotension or other signs of systemic hypoperfusion. In right ventricular dysfunction, consider thrombolysis if there are no contraindications.

	Tissue Plasminogen activator (thrombolytic)	rt-PA (Alteplase)	100mg continuous IV inf over 2h; then heparin IV to maintain a PTT of 1.5-2.5
or	Plasminogen activator (thrombolytic)	Streptokinase (Streptase)	250,000 U loading dose over 30 min, then 100,000 U/h over 24h; then heparin IV to maintain a PTT of 1.5-2.5
		Urokinase (Abbokinase)	4400U/kg loading over 10min, then 4400U/kg/h for 12h

IVC Filter: Consider with: 1) proximal vein thrombosis or PE or with high risk for these conditions, when anticoagulant Tx has failed or is contraindicated or has resulted in a complic.; 2) recurrent thromboembolism that occurs despite adequate anticoagulation, with chronic recurrent embolism and pulmonary hypertens., and with concurrent surgical pulmonary embolectomy or pulm. thromboendarterectomy.

	IVC Filter	IVC filter should be placed by experienced practit.

64. The American College of Chest Physicians. Sixth ACCP consensus conference on antithrombotic therapy. Chest 2001;119;16-20.

4.6   Primary Pulmonary Hypertension

4.6.1   In General

Gas (blood oxygenation)	**Oxygen**	*If pO_2 < 55mmHg at rest or < 60mmHg with exercise, sleep, chronic cor pulmonale or secondary polycythemia; Caution when $pCO_2\uparrow$*

4.6.2   PPH Patients with Significant Pulmonary Vasoreactivity

Patients with primary pulmonary hypertension should be assessed for evidence of vasoreactivity by undergoing right heart catheterization with acute vasoreactivity testing (inhaled nitrious oxide, epoprostenol, or adenosine). Responders (e.g., = 10% decrease in mean pulmonary arterial pressure (MPAP) with either no change or an increase in cardiac output and/or a decrease in pulmonary vascular resistance (PVR) of approximately 20%) should have a hemodynamically monitored trial of calcium channel blockers.

Calcium–channel blocker (inotropic ↓, afterload ↓)	**Nifedipine** (Procardia, Procardia XL, Gens)	*Ini 20mg, incr dose qh up to a 20% decr in MPAP and PVR; then admin 50% of effective dose q6-8h*
or	**Diltiazem** (Cardiazem CD, Cardizem SR, Gens)	*Ini 60mg, incr dose qh up to a 20% decr in MPAP and PVR, then admin 50% of effective dose q6-8h*

4.6.3   PPH Patients without Pulmonary Vasoreactivity

For patients who do not respond to acute vasoreactivity testing, consider other vasodilator drugs. The drugs should be titrated to the desired effect.

Endothelin receptor antagonist (vasodilation)	**Bosentan** (Tracleer)	*62.5mg bid PO for 4wk, then incr to maint dose 125mg bid; monitor liver function tests, Hb, HCG*
or	**Direct vasodilator** (peripheral resistance ↓)	**Epoprostenol** (Flolan)	*Ini 2 ng/kg/min cont inf, then titrate in increments of 2 ng/kg/min q15 min*

Or poss	**Direct vasodilator** (peripheral resistance ↓)	**Treprostinil** (Remodulin)	*Ini 1.25 ng/kg/min via SC inf pump; adj dose to 0.625 ng/kg/min if inability to tolerate ini dose or in mild/moderate hepatic insuff. or renal impairment; incr inf rate in increments of 0.625ng/kg/min qwk*
or	**Prostaglandin**	**Iloprost** (Ventavis)	*Ini 2.5μg/dose inh, if tolerated incr to 5μg/dose adm 6–9 times daily*
and	**Oral anticoagulant** (carboxylation of coagulation factors ↓)	**Warfarin** (Coumadin, Gens)	*Ini 5mg PO, adj to maintain INR of 2.0*

65. Pass SE, Dusing ML. Current and Emerging Therapy for Primary Pulmonary Hypertension. Ann Pharmacother 2002; 36:1430–42

4.6.4 Right Heart Failure

	Aldosterone antagonist (renal H$_2$O and NaCl loss, K$^+$ secretion ↓)	**Spironolactone** (Aldactone, Gens)	*25–100mg PO qd or bid*
and/or	**Loop diuretic**	**Furosemide** (Lasix, Gens)	*10–240mg PO qd-qid*
and/or	**Cardiac glycoside**	**Digoxin** (LanoxiCap, Lanoxin, Gens)	*0.125–0.375mg PO qd; monitor levels*

4.7 Cystic Fibrosis (CF)
4.7.1 In General

The primary goals of Tx are to **treat infections**, decrease the burden of infections, aid in the clearance of secretions, and improve bronchopulmonary hygiene. **Nutrition** is critical for both the pulmonary and nonpulmonary manifestations of CF.

| | **Gas** (blood oxygenation) | **Oxygen** | *If pO$_2$ < 55mmHg at rest or < 60mmHg with exercise, sleep, chronic cor pulmonale or secondary polycythemia; Caution when pCO$_2$↑* |

Mucolytic (sputum viscosity ↓)	**Dornase alpha**	*2.5mg q12-24h via nebulizer*
Beta$_2$-agonist, short acting (bronchodilating)	**Albuterol** (Proventil, Proventil HFA, Ventolin, 90µg/puff; Ventolin Rotacaps, 200µg/puff)	*2 puffs tid-qid prn*
or	**Metaproterenol** (Alupent, 650µg/puff)	*2 puffs tid-qid prn*
or	**Pirbuterol** (Maxair, Maxair Autoinhaler, 200µg/puff)	*2 puffs tid-qid prn*

4.7.2 Infections

Suppressive Regimen

Aminoglycoside	**Tobramycin** (Nebcin, Gens)	*300mg bid via nebulizer x 28d*

4.7.3 Acute Infection

For acute infections, a prolonged course of oral antibiotics is recommended. If the patient does not respond or has a severe exacerbation, consider IV antibiotics. The antibiotic regimen should cover for Pseudomonas aeruginosa. If a specific pathogen is identified, that pathogen should be treated based on drug-susceptibility results.

Haemophilus influenzae

Aminopenicillin	**Ampicillin** (Gens)	*2-3g IV q4-6h*
or	Folate antagonist + p-Aminobenzoic acid antagonist (Cotrimoxazole)	**Sulfamethoxazole + Trimethoprim** (Bactrim, Cotrim, Septra, Sulfamethoprim, Sulfatrim, Gens)	*160+800mg PO bid or 5mg/kg IV q8h*

Staphylococcus aureus

Penicillin – 2nd gen.	**Nafcillin** (Nallpen, Unipen, Gens)	*2mg IV q4h*
Cephalosporin – 1st gen.	**Cefazolin** (Ancef, Kefzol, Gens)	*1-2g IV q4-6h*
or	Glycopeptide (if methcillin resistant)	**Vancomycin** (Vancocin, Vancoled, Gens)	*1g q12h*
or	Oxazolidinone	**Linezolid** (Zyvox)	*600mg IV/PO q12h*

Pseudomonas aeruginosa			
	Cephalosporin – 3rd/4th gen. (antipseudomonal)	Ceftazidime (Ceptaz, Fortaz, Tazicef, Tazidime, Gens)	*2g IV q8h*
or		Cefepime (Maxipime)	*2g IV q12h*
or	Penicillin – antipseudomonal	Piperacillin (Pipracil)	*100mg/kg IV q6h*
or		Ticarcillin (Ticar)	*100mg/kg IV q6h*
Plus	Quinolone – antipseudomonal	Ciprofloxacin (Cipro)	*400mg IV q8-12h*
or	Aminoglycoside	Tobramycin (Nebcin)	*3mg/kg IVq8h*

4.8   Sarcoidosis
4.8.1   Relief of Musculoskeletal Symptoms

poss	NSAID – acetic acid derivative (analgesic, antipyretic)	Indomethacin (Indocin, Indocin SR, Gens)	*25-50mg PO bid-tid*

4.8.2   In Symptomatic Systemic Disease

In cardiac, neurologic, progressive pulmonary disease and eye disease not responding to topical therapy, and in hypercalcemia

	Corticosteroid (anti-inflammatory)	Prednisone (Prednisone Intensol, Gens)	*Ini 20-40mg PO qod for 1-3mon: red to 5-10mg qod for 12mon, then reassess*
or/plus	Immunosuppressant (cytokine synthesis ↓)	Methotrexate (Rheumatrex, Trexall, Gens)	*10-25mg/wk PO*
or		Azathioprine (Imuran, Gens)	*50-200mg PO qd*
or	Immunosuppressant (alkylating agent)	Cyclophosphamide (Cytoxan)	*50-100mg PO qd or 500-2000mg q2wks IV (more toxic than above drugs)*
poss	Antirheumatic (stabilizat. lyso. mebrane)	Hydroxychloroquine (Plaquenil, Gens)	*200-400mg PO qd*

66.   American Thoracic Society. Statement on Sarcoidosis. Am J Respir Crit Care 1999;160:736-755.

5. Rheumatology

Gary Gilkeson, MD
Division of Rheumatology and Immunology, Department of Medicine
Medical University of South Carolina, Charleston, SC

5.1 Raynaud Syndrome

	Calcium antagonist (vasodilation)	Nifedipine (Adalat, Adalat cc, Procardia, Procardia XL, Gens)	5mg PO tid, up to max. 180mg/d; Caution: cimetidine/grape fruit juice increase levels, toxicity of vincristine↑, digoxin level ↑
		Any calcium channel blocker	
poss	Isosorbide dinitrate (vasodilation)	Isosorbide dinitrate cream	Admin cream 1% for acute episodes
poss	Antiplatelet drugs (phosphodiesterase/ platelet aggregation-adhesion inhibition)	Aspirin – ASA (Ascriptin, Asprimox, Bayer Aspirin, Bufferin, Easprin, Ecotrin, Empirin, Genprin, Halfprin, St. Joseph Pain Reliever, Zorprin, Gens)	85mg PO qd
		Dipyridamole (Persantine, Gens)	75mg qid

5.2 Fibromyalgia

poss	Tricyclic Antidepressant (distancing from pain, sleep inducing)	Amitriptyline (Clavil, Elavil, Endep, Gens)	25mg PO qd qpm, incr dose prn until sleep achieved; Caution: with digitalis increased danger of arrhythmias
		Other tricyclics	
plus	physical Tx + psychosomatic care + endurance sports!		

5.3 Osteoarthritis
5.3.1 In Activated Arthrosis

poss	**Analgesic – aniline derivative** (inhibits cyclooxygenase ⇒ prostaglandins ↓)	**Acetaminophen** (Tylenol, Gens)	*1000mg PO qid*
poss	**NSAID** (inhibits cyclooxygenase ⇒ prostaglandins ↓⇒ anti-inflammatory, analgesic)	**Diclofenac** (Voltaren, Voltaren-XR, Gens)	*50mg qd-tid (max. 150mg/d)*
		Ibuprofen (Advil, Children's advil, Motrin, Gens)	*800-1600mg/d PO div tid-qid; well tolerated*
		Indomethacin (Indocin SR, Indocin, Gens)	*25mg PO bid-tid, max 200mg/d;* **Note:** *strongest analgesic EF, highest rate of AE*

NSAID ⇒ methotrexate levels ↑ ⇒ liver toxicity↑; interaction with warfarin!

poss	**Local anesthetic** (muscle relaxation in tenseness)	**Bupivacaine 0.25%** (Marcaine HCT, Sensorcaine, Gens)	*2-5ml Inj IM*
poss	**Glucocorticoid** (anti-inflammatory, immunosuppressive)	**Triamcinolone acetonide** (Aristocort, Kenalog) **+ Lidocaine** (Gens)	*Intraarticular Inj: large joint: 10-20mg, middle size joint: 5-10mg, small joint: 2-5mg; max. 4 Inj/y, at least 3-4wk apart*
poss	**Viscous compounds** (structure modifying)	**Hyaluronic acid** (Hyalgan, Synvisc)	*Intraarticular Inj qwk for 3-4wk*
		Glucosamine sulfate (Gens)	*500mg PO tid*

5.4 Rheumatoid Arthritis
5.4.1 Symptomatic Therapy (Acute Episode)

In General

	NSAID (inhibits cyclooxygenase ⇒ prostaglandins ↓ ⇒ anti-inflammatory, analgesic, antipyretic)	**Naproxen** (Anaprox, Naprelan, Naprosyn, Gens)	*500mg PO bid*
		Indomethacin (Indocin SR, Indocin, Gens)	*25-50mg PO bid-tid, 75mg (SR) PO qd-bid, 50-100mg PR qd-bid prn*
		Diclofenac (Voltaren, Voltaren-XR, Gens)	*50mg PO qd-tid (max 150mg)*
		Ibuprofen (Advil, Children's advil, Motrin, Gens)	*1-2 SR Tab PO bid-qid, max. 1600mg/d;* **Note:** *well tolerated*

NSAID ⇒ methotrexate levels ↑ ⇒ liver toxicity↑; interaction with warfarin!

In ventricular/duodenal ulcers

	NSAID – Cyclooxygenase-2-Inhibitor (inhibits cyclooxygenase-2 ⇒ prostaglandins ↓ ⇒ anti-inflammatory, analgesic)	**Celecoxib** (Celebrex)	*100-200mg PO bid, max. 400mg/d*
poss	**Glucocorticoid** (anti-inflammatory, immunosuppressive)	**Prednisolone** (Onapred, Pediapred, Prelone, Gens)	*40mg PO qd; ini dose depending on symptoms*
or	**Opioid** (analgesia)	**Tramadol** (Ultram)	*Up to 50-100mg PO qid* **Caution:** *IA with other psychotropic drugs; with MAOIs severe CNS-AEs*

Intraarticular injections

poss	**Glucocorticoid** (anti-inflammatory, immunosuppressive)	**Triamcinolone acetonide** (Aristocort, Kenalog) **+ Lidocaine** (Gens)	*Intraarticular Inj: large joint: 10-20mg, middle size joint: 5-10mg, small joint: 2-5mg (max. 2 Inj/y, 3-4wk apart)*

5.4.2	Basal Therapy in Mild Courses		
	Antirheumatic (stabilization of lysosome membrane, influence on BG-metabolism)	Hydroxychloroquine (Plaquenil, Gens)	*Long-term Tx: 200-400mg PO qd (at least 3mo, if successful maint.Tx)*

5.4.3	Basal Therapy in Moderately Severe Courses		
	Antirheumatic - acetic acid derivative (prostaglandin synthesis ↓)	Sulfasalazine (Azulfidine, Azulfidine en-tabs, Gens)	*Wk 1: 500mg PO qd, wk 2: 500mg PO bid, wk 3: 500mg PO tid, wk 4: 500mg PO qid; at least 3mo, if successful, maint.Tx; IA: EF of warfarin, antidiabetics↑, iron absorption↓*
	Antibiotic (tetracycline)	Minocycline (Dynacin, Minocin, Vectrin, Gens)	*100mg IV/PO qd*

5.4.4	Basal Therapy in Severe Courses		
	Immunosuppressant (cytokine synthesis ↓)	Methotrexate (Folex, Rheumatrex, Gens)	*7.5-20mg/wk PO, incr up to 25mg/wk prn as SC Inj*
In intolerance plus			
	Vitamin	Folic acid (Folicet, Gens)	*1mg PO qd*
In CI against methotrexate and failure with other basal therapeutics			
1st choice	Disease-modifiying antirheumatic (inhibition of T-cell pyrimidine biosynthesis ⇒ immunomodulation)	Leflunomide (Arava)	*d1-3: 100mg, from d4 10-20mg qd (at least 4-6wk until results, then maint Tx); no simultan. live vaccination*
2nd choice	(monoclonal Ab against TNFα)	Infliximab (Remicade)	*3mg/kg IV over 2h, poss rep at 2wk, 6wk, then q8wk*
		Adalimumab (Humira)	*40mg SQ q2wk*
or	(soluble TNFα-Receptor)	Etanercept (Enbrel)	*25mg SC biw or 50mg qw*
or	(IL1 Receptor antagonist)	Anakinra (Kineret)	*100mg SC qd*

5.5   Ankylosing Spondylitis
5.5.1   Symptomatic Therapy (Acute Episode)

NSAID (inhibits cyclooxygenase ⇒ prostaglandins ↓⇒ anti-inflammatory, analgesic, antipyretic)	**Indomethacin** (Indocin SR, Indocin, Gens)	*25-50mg PO bid-tid, 75mg (SR) PO qd-bid, 50-100mg PR qd-bid*
	Other NSAIDs	

5.5.2   Peripheral Joint Involvement

poss	**Antirheumatic – acetic acid derivative** (prostaglandin synthesis ↓)	**Sulfasalazine** (Azulfidine, Azulfidine en-tabs, Gens)	*Wk 1: 500mg PO qd, wk 2: 500mg PO bid, wk 3: 500mg PO tid, wk 4: 500mg PO qid*
poss	**Glucocorticoid** (anti-inflammatory, immunosuppressive)	**Prednisone** (Deltasone, Meticorten, Gens)	*40mg PO qd (ini dose depending on symptoms)*
poss	**Immunosuppressant** (cytokine synthesis ↓)	**Methotrexate** (Folex, Rheumatrex, Gens)	*7.5-20mg/wk PO*

In intolerance plus

Vitamin	**Folic acid** (Gens)	*1mg qd*

5.5.3   Involvement of the Axial Skeleton

Clinical studies

Disease-modifiying antirheumatic (monoclonal antibody against TNFα)	**Infliximab** (Remicade)	*3-5mg/kg IV over 2h, rep at 2wk, 6wk and then q8wk*
(soluble TNFα-Receptor)	**Etanercept** (Enbrel)	*25mg SC biw or 50mg qw*

5.6   Reactive Arthritis, Reiter's Syndrome
5.6.1   Symptomatic Therapy (Acute Episode)

NSAID (inhibits cyclooxygenase ⇒ prostaglandins ↓⇒ anti-inflammatory, analgesic, antipyretic)	**Indomethacin** (Indocin SR, Indocin, Indo-lemmon, Indomethagan, Gens)	*25-50mg PO bid-tid, 75mg (SR) PO qd-bid, 50-100mg PR qd-bid*
	Other NSAIDs	

poss	Glucocorticoid (anti-inflammatory, immunosuppressive)	Prednisone (Deltasone, Meticorten, Gens)	40mg PO qd (ini dose depending on symptoms)

5.6.2	Chronic Course		
poss	Antirheumatic – acetic acid derivative (prostaglandin synthesis ↓)	Sulfasalazine (Azulfidine, Azulfidine en-tabs, Gens)	Wk 1: 500mg PO qd, wk 2: 500mg bid, wk 3: 500mg tid, wk 4: 500mg qid (at least 3mo)
poss	Immunosuppressant (cytokine synthesis ↓)	Methotrexate (Folex, Rheumatrex, Gens)	7.5-20mg/wk PO

In intolerance plus			
	Vitamin	Folic acid (Gens)	1mg PO qd

5.6.3	Enteropathic Form		
Chlamydia, Mykoplasma			
	Tetracycline (antibiosis)	Doxycycline (Doryx, Vibramycin, Gens)	100mg PO qd; IA: milk + antacid resorbtion↓, safety of contracept.↓, EF of digoxin ↑
Yersinia			
	Fluoroquinolone (antibiosis)	Ciprofloxacin (Cipro)	250-750mg PO bid
	IA with NSAIDs: spasmophilia ↑, half-life of diazepam ↑		

5.7 Psoriatic Arthritis
5.7.1 Symptomatic

	NSAID (inhibits cyclooxygenase ⇒ prostaglandins ↓⇒ anti-inflammatory, analgesic, antipyretic)	Indomethacin (Indocin SR, Indocin, Gens)	25-50mg PO bid-tid, 75mg (SR) PO qd-bid, 50-100mg PR qd-bid

5.7.2	Basal Therapy		
poss	**Antirheumatic – acetic acid derivative** (prostaglandin synthesis ↓)	**Sulfasalazine** (Azulfidine, Azulfidine en-tabs, Gens)	*Wk 1: 500mg PO qd, wk 2: 500mg bid, wk 3: 500mg tid, wk 4: 500mg qid (at least 3mo)*
or poss	**Immunosuppressant** (cytokine synthesis ↓)	**Methotrexate** (Folex, Rheumatrex, Gens)	*7.5-20mg/wk PO*
	Anti-TNF therapy (soluble TNFα-Receptor)	**Etanercept** (Enbrel)	*25mg SC biw or 50mg qwk*
	Anti-CD20 monoclonal antibody (immunomodulation)	**Rituximab** (Rituxan)	*3-5mg/kg IV over 2h, rep at 2wk, 6wk and then q8wk*
In intolerance plus			
	Vitamin	**Folic acid** (Gens)	*1mg PO qd*

5.8 Systemic Lupus Erythematosus
5.8.1   In Skin Involvement

poss	**NSAID** (inhibits cyclooxygenase ⇒ prostaglandins ↓ ⇒ anti-inflammatory, analgesic)	**Diclofenac** (Voltaren, Voltaren-XR, Gens)	*50mg PO/PR qd-tid, 100mg (SR) PO qd or 75mg IM qd*
		Any NSAID	
poss	**Antirheumatic** (stabilization of lysosome membrane)	**Hydroxychloroquine** (Plaquenil, Gens)	*200mg PO bid*
poss	**Glucocorticoid** (anti-inflammatory, immunosuppressive)	**Prednisone** (Deltasone, Meticorten, Gens)	*1mg/kg PO qd (ini dose depending on symptoms)*

5.8.2   Slight Visceral Involvement (Pleuritis, Pericarditis)

poss	**NSAID** (inhibits cyclooxygenase ⇒ prostaglandins ↓ ⇒ anti-inflammatory, analgesic)	**Diclofenac** (Voltaren, Voltaren-XR, Gens)	*50mg PO bid-tid or 100mg PO qd*

poss	**Glucocorticoid** (anti-inflammatory, immunosuppressive)	**Prednisolone** (Onapred, Pediapred, Prelone, Gens)	*1mg/kg PO qd (ini dose depending on symptoms, red slowly)*
poss	**Antirheumatic** (stabilization of lysosome membrane)	**Hydroxychloroquine** (Plaquenil, Gens)	*Long-term Tx: 200mg PO bid*

5.8.3   Severe Visceral Involvement (Lupus Nephritis, Myocarditis)

Tx of choice	**Alkylating agent** (immunosuppression)	**Cyclophosphamide** (Cytoxan, Neosar)	*0.5-1g/m² q4wk IV, or 2-4mg/kg PO qd*
plus	**Acrolein neutralisation** (reacts with urotoxic metabolites of cyclophosphamide ⇒ cystitis PRO)	**Mesna** (Uromitexan, Mesnex)	*200-400mg IV before, 4h + 8h after cyclophosphamide Inf (prn, in most patients not needed)*
poss	**Glucocorticoid** (anti-inflammatory, immunosuppressive)	**Prednisone** (Deltasone, Meticorten, Gens)	*1mg/kg, red slowly*
poss	**Immunosuppressant** (cytokine synthesis ↓)	**Cyclosporine** (Neoral, Sandimmune, Gens)	*1-3mg/kg/d PO (not in combination with cyclophosphamide)*

5.9   Progressive Systemic Sclerosis

5.9.1   In Skin Involvement

poss	**Immunosuppressant** (cytokine synthesis ↓)	**Methotrexate** (Folex, Rheumatrex, Gens)	*7.5-20mg/wk PO/IM*
poss		**Cyclosporine** (Neoral, Sandimmune, Gens)	*3mg/kg/d PO div bid*

No proven effective Tx! No influence on organic changes.

5.9.2   In Pulmonary Involvement

	Alkylating agent (immunosuppression)	**Cyclophosphamide** (Cytoxan, Neosar)	*2-4mg/kg qd or 500-1000mg/m² IV q4wk*

5.9.3   In Pulmonary Hypertension

Direct vasodilator (prostaglandin-I2-analogue)	Epoprostenol (Flolan)	2ng/kg/min constant IV Inf with initial ICU monitoring
Endothelin-1 receptor antagonist	Bosentan (Tracleer)	62.5mg PO bid for 4wk, then 125mg bid

Do right coronary catheter to test effectiveness before administration

5.10   Temporal Arteritis

Glucocorticoid (anti-inflammatory, immunosuppressive)	Prednisone (Deltasone, Meticorten, Gens)	Ini 60mg PO qd until results, then taper over 2-3mo until < 10mg/d, then red by 1mg/d q4-8wk; in loss of vision Pulse Tx: 1g IV for 3d (maint. for 6-12 mo)

5.11   Polymyalgia Rheumatica

Glucocorticoid (anti-inflammatory, immunosuppressive)	Prednisone (Deltasone, Meticorten, Gens)	Ini 10-20mg qd, then taper slowly over 8-12mo

5.12   Panarteritis Nodosa

5.12.1   Slight

poss	Glucocorticoid (anti-inflammatory, immunosuppressive)	Prednisone (Deltasone, Meticorten, Gens)	Ini 40mg PO qd, red by 10mg q5d to 20mg qd, then red by 5mg q3-4wk

5.12.2   Severe (Systemic Involvement)

Glucocorticoid (anti-inflammatory, immunosuppressive)	Prednisolone (Onapred, Pediapred, Prelone, Gens)	1mg/kg PO qd (ini dose depending on symptoms, red slowly)
Alkylating agent (immunosuppression)	Cyclophosphamide (Cytoxan, Neosar)	0.5g/m^{2}q 3-4wk IV or 2-4mg/kg qd PO

| plus | **Acrolein neutralisation** (reacts with urotoxic metabolites of cyclophosphamide ⇒ cystitis PRO) | **Mesna** (Uromitexan, Mesnex) | *200-400mg IV before, 4h + 8h after cyclophosphamide Inf (prn)* |

5.13 Wegener's Granulomatosis
5.13.1 Localized Initial Stage

| poss rarely ind | **Antibiotic** (folate antagonist + p-aminobenzoic acid antagonist) | **Sulfamethoxazole + Trimethoprim** (Bactrim, Septra, Sulfamethoprim, Sulfatrim, Gens) | *160+800mg PO bid; IA: EF of anticoagulants, antidiabetics, phenytoin, MTX, thiazides↑; risk of thrombopenia↑* |

5.13.2 Generalized Stage

	Glucocorticoid (anti-inflammatory, immunosuppressive)	**Prednisolone** (Onapred, Pediapred, Prelone, Gens)	*1-2mg/kg PO qd q1-2wk red by 10mg to 20mg qd, then red by 5mg q2-3wk; poss pulse Tx: 500-1000mg for 3d IV*
	Alkylating agent (immunosuppression)	**Cyclophosphamide** (Cytoxan, Neosar)	*0.5-1g/m² /3-4wk IV or 2-4mg/kg PO qd*
plus	**Acrolein neutralisation** (reacts with urotoxic metabolites of cyclophosphamide ⇒ cystitis PRO)	**Mesna** (Uromitexan, Mesnex)	*200-400mg IV before, 4h + 8h after cyclophosphamide Inf (prn, in most patients not needed)*

5.14 Sjögren's Syndrome

	Film builder (artificial tears)	**Hypromellose 5%** (Ocucoat)	*Apply prn*
	Epithelializing agent (corneal protection/care)	**Dexpanthenol** (Bepanthen, Panthenol)	*Apply bid-qid*
	Salivary stimulant	**Cevimeline** (Evoxac)	*30mg tid*

6. Metabolic, Endocrine

Ehud Ur, MB, FRCP
Head, Division of Endocrinology & Metabolism
Dalhousie University, Halifax, Nova Scotia, Canada

6.1 Diabetes Mellitus

6.1.1 Type 1 (formerly IDDM)

Conventional insulin therapy (strict insulin administrations)

e.g.	**Intermediate-acting insulin or biphasic insulins** (glucose resorption in muscle and fat cells↑ ⇒ anabolism↑ (glycogen-, lipid- and protein synthesis), catabolism↓ (glycogenolysis, lipolysis, proteolysis)	**Insulin NPH** (Humulin N, Novolin N) **Insulin NPH + Insulin Regular** (Humulin 70/30, Novolin 70/30)	*2/3 of needs qam, 1/3 qpm(e.g. comb. 2/3 intermediate + 1/3 regular insulin) (outdated approach!)*

Intensive insulin therapy (basal/bolus concept) (specialist may be required!)

e.g.	**Long-acting insulin + regular insulin** (substitution according to circadian rhythm of insulin needs)	**Insulin lente** (Novolin L) **+ Insulin Regular** (Novolin L)	*R= regular insulin, L= long-acting insulin; R: 50% of daily needs, 10-20% of total daily insulin requirement at each meal; L: 50% of the total dose: of this 50% at night, of the other 50%, 30% am and 70% at noon; am: R>L, noon: R<L, pm R, qhs (10pm) L*

Basal needs managed with long-acting insulin (L), with regular insulin at meals (R) according to circadian rhythm of insulin needs. High insulin requirement am and a little less pm, low insulin around noon and from midnight until 4am.

Short-acting insulin analogue (monom. insulin anal.)	**Insulin lispro** (Humalog) **Insulin aspart** (Novolog)	*Effect maximum 1h after inj, inj immediately after eating*

Long-acting insulin analogue (precipitation of insulin Glargine in neutral pH of SC tissue ⇒ release into circulation ↓)	**Insulin Glargine** (Lantus)	*Inj around 10pm, duration of action about 24h, almost constant absorption rate*

67. Bolli B. How to ameliorate the problem of hypoglycemia in intensive as well as non intensive treatment of type 1 diabetes; Diabetes care, 22 Suppl 2 B43–B52, 1999
68. American Diabetes Association: Clinical practice recommendations. Diabetes Care 1998; 21(Supplement 1): s1–s70

Diabetic Ketoacidosis (ICU, specialist required!)

	Isotonic saline solution (volume + electrolyte substitution)	**Saline 0.9%** (if Na > 150mmol/l ⇒ 0.45%)	*1l in 1h, then 500ml/h over the next 6h, then 250ml/h over 4h*
plus	**Insulin** (substitution)	**InsulinRegular**	*0.1U/kg/h in IV; at BS of 250mg/dl add gluc. 5%*
sos	**K⁺Cl⁻ solution** (substitution)	**K⁺Cl⁻ 7.45%** (1ml = 1mmol)	*K⁺ < 3mmol/l: 40mmol/h; K⁺ < 4mmol/l: 30mmol/h; K⁺ < 5mmol/l: 20mmol/h*
sos	**Buffer** (acidosis therapy, pH neutralisation)	**Sodium bicarbonate 8.4%** (100ml = 100mmol HCO³⁻)	*BE x 0.3 x kg = mmol, only give 1/3 of calculated need (starting at pH < 6.9)*
sos	**Phosphate** (substitution)	**Potassium phosphate**	*2mmol/h in 500ml saline 0.9% over 6h (prn)*
sos	**Low-dose heparin** (low-molecular; thrombosis PRO)	**Dalteparin** (Fragmin)	*2850 IU SC qd (prn)*

69. Fleckmann AM, Diabetic ketoacidosis, Endocrin Metab Clin North Am, 1993, 22, 181–207
70. Kitabchi AE, Wall BM: Diabetic ketoacidosis. Med Clin North Am 1995 Jan; 79(1): 9–37

Hypoglycemic coma

	Glucose (substitution)	**Glucose 40%, then Glucose 5%**	*20-50ml 40% IV, then 5% (until BS 200mg/dl)*
sos	**Antihypoglycemic** (hepat. glycogenolysis ↑, gluconeogenesis ↑ ⇒BS ↑)	**Glucagon** (GlucaGen, Gens)	*0.5-1mg SC, IM, IV*

71. Service FJ, Hypoglycemic disorders, N Eng J Med, 1995, 332, 1144-52

6.1.2 Type 2 (formerly NIDDM)

1. Biguanide and/or Glucosidase inhibitor (if diet is not sufficient)

1sr choice	**Biguanide** (glucose uptake into cell ↑, gluconeogenesis in liver ↓, glucose transport into muscle/fat tissue ↑)	**Metformin** (Glucophage, Glucophage XR)	*500-1500mg PO qam, max. 2500mg/d (tid); Caution: extensive CI, lactic acidosis, creatinine > 130μmol/l*
or / sos plus	**Glucosidase inhibitor** (intestinal glucose release ↓)	**Acarbose** (Precose)	*50-200mg PO tid, incr slowly; Caution: poor compliance due to AE*

Generally Metformin is first choice over Acarbose especially in obese patients.

2. Other Oral Antidiabetics

	Sulfonylurea (blockade of ATP dependent K^+ channels, insulin release from pancreas beta-cells ↑)	**Glyburide** (DiaBeta, Glynase, Micronase, Gens)	*Ini 1.25-10mg PO qam, max. 10mg bid; Caution: not > 65y: severe protracted hypoglycemias; Tx break in unstable AP, before PTCA, very acute MI – temporary insulin Tx)*
or	**Sulfonylurea** (frequency of hypoglycemia ↓)	**Glimepiride** (Amaryl)	*1-4mg qd qam*
or	**Meglitinide** (insulin secretagogue, acts like sulfonylureas, short EHL ⇒ admin ac)	**Repaglinide** (Prandin)	*Up to 8mg PO tid within 30min ac; max 16mg/d*
or	**Thiazolidinedione** ("insulin sensitizer" binds to (PPA)-receptor in insulin target tissue ⇒ insulin effectiveness ↑ ⇒ cellular glucose uptake ↑, hepatic glucose output ↓)	**Rosiglitazone** (Avandia)	*4-8mg PO qd or 2-4mg PO bid*
		Pioglitazone (Actos)	*15-45mg PO qd caution: hepatotoxicity, fluid retention, weight gain (especially when combined with insulin)*

3. Useful: combination of Meglitinide (insulin secretagogue) and Thiazolidinedione (insulin sensitizer)

4. Combination therapy: Insulin + Metformin (biguanide) or sulfonylurea

Intermediate–acting insulin	Insulin NPH (Humulin N, Novolin N)	*HPH (basal) insulin qhs, sos 2nd insulin inj qam*

5. Insulin monotherapy (if 28 IU in comb. with sulfonylureas is not sufficient)

Biphasic insulins (glucose resorption in muscle and fat cells↑ ⇒ anabolism↑ (glycogen-, lipid- and protein synthesis), catabolism↓ (glycogenolysis, lipolysis, proteolysis))	Insulin NPH + Insulin Regular (Humulin 70/30, Novolin 70/30)	*0.14–0.24 IU/kg qam, 0.07–0.12 IU/kg qpm IU according to BS profile, disadvantage: strict system; Intensified insulin Tx: ac admin of regular insulin. Starting total dose = fasting BS x 0.2, div in 3 regular insulin doses ac in relationship 3:1:2 per BU more IU qam 2 IU; In increased fasting BS additional NPH Insulin qpm or metformin admin*

72. Williams G., Management of non-insulin depent diabetes mellitus, Lancet, 1994, 343, 95-100
73. UK Prospective Diabetes Study Group, Effect of intensive blood-glucose control with metformin on complications in overweight patients with type 2 diabetes, UKPDS 34, Lancet, 1998, 352, 854-65
74. UK Prospective Diabetes Study Group, Intensive blood-glucose control with sulphonylureas or insulin compared with conventional treatment and risk of complications in patients with type 2 diabetes, UKPDS 33, Lancet, 1998, 352, 837-53

6.2   Hyperlipidemias
6.2.1   Hypercholesterolemia (Hereditary/Polygenic)

HMG-CoA-reductase inhibitor (intracell. cholesterol synthesis ↓, LDL ↓, HDL ↑)	Lovastatin (Altocor, Mevacor)	*20-40mg PO qd qpm*
	Atorvastatin (Lipitor)	*10-80mg PO qd*
	Fluvastatin (Lescol)	*20-40mg PO qd*
	Pravastatin (Pravachol)	*10-40 mg PO qd*
	Simvastatin (Zocor)	*20-80mg PO qd*

poss.	Bile acid sequestrant (intestinal bile acid binding ↑ ⇒ bile acid production from cholesterol ↑ ⇒ serum cholesterol ↓ ⇒ hepat. LDL uptake ↑)	Cholestyramine (Locholest, Locholest Light, Prevalite, Questran, Questran Light, Gens)	4-16g PO qd, incr slowly; Caution: sufficient distance to ingestion of other drugs (e.g. warfarin, digitalis, thiazides)
sos	Fat soluble vitamins (parenteral substitution)	Vitamins A, D, E, K	1ml/2wk IM (prn)

75. Illingworth DR: Management of hypercholesterolemia. Med Clin North Am 2000 Jan; 84(1): 23-42

6.2.2   Hereditary Lipoprotein Lipase Deficiency

sos	Fat soluble vitamins (parenteral substitution)	Vitamins A, D, E,K	1ml/2wk IM (prn)

6.2.3   Hereditary Dysbetalipoproteinemia

	Fibric acid (lipoprotein lipase activity ↑ ⇒ LDL ↓, HDL ↑, triglycerides ↓)	Fenofibrate (Tricor)	67-200 mg PO qd ac
		Gemfibrozil (Lopid, Gens)	300-600mg PO bid
sos	Nicotinic acid derivative (triglyceride lipase activity ↓, lipoprotein lipase activity ↑ ⇒ triglycerides ↓, cholesterol ↓)	Inositol nicotinate (Hexopal, No-Flush Niacin)	600-800mg PO bid-tid
sos	HMG-CoA-reductase inhibitor (intracell. cholesterol synthesis ↓, LDL↓, HDL↑)	Lovastatin (Mevacor, Altocor)	20-40mg PO qd qpm
		Atorvastatin (Lipitor)	10-80mg PO qd
		Fluvastatin (Lescol)	20-40mg PO qd
		Pravastatin (Pravachol)	10-40 mg PO qd
		Simvastatin (Zocor)	20-80mg PO qd

Caution if combining HMG-CoA-reductase inhibitors with fibrates due to increased risk of rhabdomyolysis!

6.2.4   Hereditary Hypertriglyceridemia

Fibric acid (lipoprotein lipase activity ↑ ⇒ LDL ↓, HDL ↑, triglycerides ↓)	**Fenofibrate** (Tricor)	*67-200 mg PO qd ac*
	Gemfibrozil (Lopid, Gens)	*300-600mg PO bid*
possibly in combination with	**Nicotinic acid derivative** (triglyceride lipase activity ↓, lipoprotein lipase activity ↑ ⇒ triglycerides ↓, cholesterol ↓)	**Inositol nicotinate** (Hexopal, No-Flush Niacin)	*600-800mg PO bid-tid*

6.2.5   Hereditary Combined Hyperlipidemia

	HMG-CoA-reductase inhibitor (intracelluläre cholesterol synthesis ↓, LDL ↓, HDL ↑)	**Lovastatin** (Mevacor, Altocor)	*20-80mg PO qd qpm*
sos	**Fibric acid** (lipoprotein lipase activity ↑ ⇒ LDL ↓, HDL ↑, triglycerides ↓)	**Fenofibrate** (Tricor)	*67-200 mg PO qd ac*
		Gemfibrozil (Lopid, Gens)	*300-600mg PO bid*
sos	**Nicotinic acid derivative** (triglyceride lipase activity ↓, lipoprotein lipase activity ↑ ⇒ triglycerides ↓, cholesterol ↓)	**Inositol nicotinate** (Hexopal, No-Flush Niacin)	*600-800mg PO bid-tid*

76. Betteridge DJ, Management of hyperlipidaemia: guidelines of the British Hyperlipidaemia Association, Postgrad Med J, 1993, 69, 359-69
77. Oster G, Cholesterol-Reduction Intervention study. A randomized trial to assess effectivness and costs in clinical practice, Arch Intern Med, 1996, 156, 731-9

6.3   Gout
6.3.1   Long-Term Therapy

Xanthine oxidase inhibitor (Xanthine oxidase inhibition ⇒ uric acid production ↓)	**Allopurinol** (Alloprin, Lopurin, Zyloprim, Gens)	*100-300mg PO qd (UA in serum < 6.5mg/dl)*
Uricosuric (tubular uric acid reabsorption ↓)	**Probenecid** (Probalan, Probampacin, Gens)	*50-100mg PO qd*
sos **Urine alkalinization** (uric acid solubility ↑)	**K^+Na^+-hydrogen citrate**	*2.5g PO qid, target urine pH 6.5 - 7.5*

6.3.2   Acute Gout Attack

NSAID – acetic acid derivative (cyclooxygenase inhibitor ⇒ anti-inflammatory, analgesic, antipyretic)	**Indomethacin** (Indocin, Indocin SR, Indo-lemmon, Indomethagan, Gens)	*25-50mg PO bid-tid, 75mg/d (SR) PO qd-bid, 50-100mg/d PR qd-bid*
Other antigout drug (phagocytosis of urate crystals by leukocytes ↓ ⇒release of inflammatory mediators; antimitotic)	**Colchicine** (Gens)	*1mg PO, max. 8mg/d in first 4h, qh 1mg PO, then q2h 0.5 -1mg PO*

78. Emmerson BT, The management of gout, N Eng J Med, 1996, 334, 445-51
79. Pittman JR, Bross MH, Diagnosis and management of gout. Am Fam Physician. 1999 Apr 1;59(7):1799-806
80. Shrestha M, Randomized double blind comparison of the analgesic efficacy of IM ketordac and oral indomethacin in the treatment of acute gouty arthritis, Ann Emerg Med, 1995, 26, 682-86
81. Wallace ST, Cholchicine gem in Arthritis, Rheum, 1974, 3, 369-81

6.4 Porphyrias
6.4.1 Porphyria Cutanea Tarda (Chronic Hepatic)

	Aminoquinoline derivative (builds chloroquine porphyrin complexes ⇒ renal elimination)	**Chloroquine** (Aralen, Gens)	*2 x 125mg/wk (8-12mo)*

6.4.2 Acute Intermittent Porphyria (Acute Hepatic; Specialist Required!)

	Delta aminolevulic acid reactivity ↓ (δ-aminolevulic acid ↓, porphobilinogen ↓)	**Glucose 20%**	*2l/d IV*
plus	**Heme analogue** (heme synthesis ↓)	**Hemin** (Panhematin)	*4mg/kg/d as short inf. over 15min for 4d*
plus	**Loop diuretic** (forced diuresis)	**Furosemide** (Lasix, Gens)	*40-80mg IV qd*
sos	**Neuroleptic** (sedation)	**Chlorpromazine** (Sonazide, Sparine, Thorazine, Gens)	*25-50mg PO tid, 25-50mg IM, IV tid after dilution with saline*
sos	**Betablocker** (cardiac output ↓ (neg. chrono-/inotropic), central sympathetic activity ↓)	**Propranolol** (Inderal, Inderal LA, Gens)	*40-80mg PO bid-tid, 1mg slowly IV qd, max. 10mg IV (prn)*
sos	**Parasympatholytic** (spasmolysis)	**Scopolamine** (Hypodermic, Transderm Scop, Transderm-V, Gens)	*3-5 x 10-20mg/d PO, up to 5 x 20mg slowly IV (prn)*
sos	**Opioid** (analgesia)	**Meperidine** (Demerol, Gens)	*25-100mg PO, PR up to qid, or 25-100mg slowly IV up to qid, max. 500mg/d (prn)*

82. Elder G, The acute porphyrias, Lancet, 1997, 349, 1613-161
83. Sassa S, Diagnosis and therapy of acute intermittent porphyria, Blood Rev, 1996, 10, 53-8

6.5 Osteoporosis
6.5.1 In General

	Calcium preparation (substitution)	**Calcium** (Alka-Mints, Calci-Chew, Calci-Mix, Caltrate, Chooz, Liqui-Cal, Nephro-Calci, Os-Cal, Titralac, Tums, Gens)	*500-1000mg PO qd*
sos	**Hormone** (mostly analgesia, osteoclast inhibition)	**Calcitonin** (Calcimar, Miacalcin)	*100IU SC, IM or 200IU intranasal (1-2y)*
sos	**Vitamin D** (calcium resorption ↑)	**Vit D3**	*500-2000IU PO qd*
sos	**Bisphosphonate** (osteoclast inhibition)	**Alendronate** (Fosamax)	*10mg PO qd (30min before breakfast; optimal duration not known)*
		Etidronate (Didronel)	*400mg qd over 14d, then 1g calcium qd over 11wk (repeat cycle q3mo)*

6.5.2 Postmenopausal Patients

	Estrogen (hormone replacement)	**Estrogen, conjugated** (Premarin)	*0.3-1.25mg*
		Estradiol valerate (Delestrogen, Gens)	*1-2mg*
		Estradiol (Estrace)	*2-4mg*
		Estradiol (Estring - ext.rel, vag)	*1mg*
	Estrogens in patients with personal or family history of breast CA.		
plus sos	**Progesterone**	**Medroxyprogesterone acetate** (Depo-provera, Amen, Provera, Gens)	*5mg d1-d10 of calendar month or 2.5mg continuously*
		Progesterone Prometrium	*200-300mg*
	Addition of Progesterone in patients with intact uterus.		

poss.	Selective estrogen receptor modulator (bone density ↑, total + LDL cholesterol ↓)	Raloxifene (Evista)	*Osteoporosis PRO/Tx: 60mg PO qd; breast CA PRO: 60–120mg PO qd*
sos	Fluoride preparation (osteoblast stimulation)	Sodium fluoride (Flura-Drops, Fluorodex, Fluoritab, Flura, Pediaflor, Luride, Luride-Sf)	*75mg qpm (plus qam 1g calcium plus 1000IU Vit D; for 3-4y, yearly x-ray controls)*
sos	Cyclooxygenase inhibitors (anti-inflammatory, antipyretic, analgesic)	Diclofenac (Voltaren, Voltaren-XR, Gens)	*50mg PO, PR qd-tid, 100mg (SR) PO qd, 75mg IM qd (prn)*
sos	Opioid (analgesic, sedating, respiratory depressive, antitussive, constipating)	Tramadol (Ultram)	*50-100mg PO, IV, IM, SC, up to qid; 100-200mg SR PO qd-bid (prn)*
sos	Conjugated estrogen-progestogen combination (calciumresorption ↑, osteoblast activity ↑)	Conjugated estrogen + Medroxyprogesterone	*0.6mg estrogen qd + 2.5mg medroxy-progesterone qd for max. 4y*

84. AAC Clinical Practise Guidelines for the Prevention and Treatment of Postmenopausal Osteoporosis 1966 AACE
85. Avioli L, Salmon Calcitonine Nasal Spray (Review), Endocrine, 1996, 2, 115-127
86. Bamighade T, Tramadol hydrochloride. An overview of current use, Hospital Medicine, 5/98, Vol 59, No 5, 373-76
87. Black BM, Randomised trial of effect of alendronate on risk of fracture in women with exsisting vertebral fractures, Lancet, 1996, 348, 1535-41
88. Gennari C, Use of calcitonin in treatment of bone pain associated with osteoporosis, Calcif Tissue Int, 1991, 49, Supp 2, 9-13
89. Hanson T, The effect of fluoride and calcium on spinal bone mineral content. a controlled prospective study (3 years), Calcif Tissue Int, 1987, 40(6), 315-7
90. Recker RR, Correcting calcium nutritional deficiency prevents spine fractures in elderly women, J Bone Miner res, 1996, 11, 1961-6
91. Sahota O. et al, A comparison of continous Atendronate, cyclical Atendronate and cyclical Etidronate with calcitriol in the treatment of postmenopausal vertebral osteoporosis: A randomized Controlled Trial, Osteoporos Int 2000 11: 959-966
92. The Writing Group for the PEPI trial, Effects of hormone therapy on bone mineral density: results from the Postmenopausal Estrogen/Progestin Interventions Trial (PEPI), JAMA, 1996, 276, 1389-96

6.6   Osteomalacia

6.6.1   In General

	Calcium preparation (substitution)	**Calcium** (Alka-Mints, Calci-Chew, Calci-Mix, Caltrate, Chooz, Liqui-Cal, Mallamint, Nephro-Calci, Os-Cal, Titralac, Tums, Gens)	*1000-1500mg PO qd*
sos	**Vitamin D** (calcium resorption ↑)	**Cholecalciferol**	*Ini 0.25µg PO qid, then 2-3 x 0.25µg/wk (prn, calcitriol in renal osteomalacia)*

6.6.2   Anticonvulsive Drug Induced Rickets

	Vitamin D (calcium resorption ↑)	**Cholecalciferol**	*2000-5000IU qd over 5wk, then 1000IU qd*

6.6.3   Malabsorbtion Syndrome

	Fat soluble vitamins (parenteral substitution)	**Vitamins A, D, E, K**	*Once a wk IM*

6.6.4   Chronic Renal Failure

	1,2 (OH)$_2$D$_3$ (prophylaxis)	**Calcitriol** (Calcijex, Rocaltrol)	*0.25µg qd*
plus	**Phosphate binder**	**Calcium carbonate** (Mylanta, Titralac, Tums)	*1-2g qd*

6.6.5   Manifest Osteomalacia

	1,25 (OH)$_2$D$_3$	**Calcitriol** (Calcijex, Rocaltrol)	*0.25-1µg qd*
plus	**Phosphate binder**	**Calcium carbonate** (Mylanta, Titralac, Tums)	*1-2g qd*

93. Hutchison F, Osteomalacia and Rickets, Seminars in Nephrology, 1992, Vol 12 (2), 127-45

6.7   Paget's Disease of Bone (Osteitis Deformans)

	NSAID – acetic acid derivative (cyclooxygenase inhibitor ⇒ anti-inflammatory, analgesic, antipyretic)	**Indomethacin** (Indocin, Indocin SR, Indolemmon, Indomethagan, Gens)	*25-50mg PO bid-tid, 75mg/d (SR) PO qd-bid, 50-100mg PR qd-tid*
SOS	**Hormone** (analgesic, osteoclast inhibition)	**Calcitonin** (Calcimar, Miacalcin)	*100IU SC, IM (6wk)*
SOS	**Biphosphonate** (osteoclast inhibition)	**Alendronate** (Fosamax)	*40mg PO qd (3-6mo)*

94. Meunier PJ, Therapeutic Strategy in Paget's disease of bone, Bone, 1995, 17 (5 Suppl), 489S-91S
95. Siris E, Comparative study of alendronate versus etidronate for the treatment of Paget's disease of bone, J Clin Endocrinol Metabol, 1996, 81, 961-7
96. Tiegs RD: Paget's disease of bone: indications for treatment and goals of therapy. Clin Ther 1997 Nov-Dec; 19(6): 1309-29

6.8   Wilson's Disease

Complex builder (copper elimination ↑)	**Penicillamine** (Cuprimine, Depen)	*1-2wk: 150mg PO qd, incr qwk by 150mg up to 450-900mg PO qd; add pyridoxine supplement 25mg qd*
Complex builder (intestinal copper resorptioning ↓)	**Zinc**	*75-300mg qd; not in acute hepatic or neurologic symptoms*

97. Gitlin N, Wilson's disease: the scourge of copper, J Hepatol, 1998, 28, 734-9

6.9   Hemochromatosis

SOS	**Complex builder** (iron elimination ↑)	**Deferoxamine** (Desferal)	*25-50mg, 1g/kg as SC inf over 24h;* **Caution:** *q(1/2)y eye/ear exams*

98. Kirking MH, Treatment of chronic iron overload, Clin Pharm, 1991, 10, 775-83

6.10 Nontoxic Goiter
6.10.1 In General

	Potassium iodide (substitution)	Potassium iodide (iodine)	*200µg PO qd (at first for 6-12mo)*
or	Thyroid hormone (hormone substitution ⇒ TSH↓)	Levothyroxine (Levo-T, Levoxyl, Unithroid)	*25-100µg PO qd, incr dose up to 200µg PO sos; adj to low normal range 0.3-0.8 mV/l*

Ind: manifest/subclinical hypothyroidism, patients > 40y, patients with evidence of thyroid antibodies, insufficient effects of iodine Tx after 1y

or	Potassium iodide + thyroid hormone (substit. of synthesis comp.+hormone ⇒TSH↓)	Iodine + Levothyroxine (100µg I⁻ + 100µg T4)	*Iodine: 100-200µg PO qd (at first for 6-12mo) + Levothyroxine: 50-75µg PO qd*

6.10.2 Relapse-/Prophylaxis

Potassium iodide (substitution of synthesis component)	Potassium iodide (iodine)	*100-200µg PO qd*

6.10.3 Objectives of Therapy with Iodine

- Children, teens: complete regression of goiter
- Adults < 40y: Volume reduction of 30%, sonographic control after 0.5, 1y

99. Perrild H, Hansen JM, Hegedus L: Triiodothyronine and thyroxine treatment of diffuse non-toxic goiter evaluated by ultrasonic scanning. Acta Endocrinol (Copenh) 1982 Jul; 100: 382-7
100. Ross DS: Thyroid hormone suppressive therapy of sporadic nontoxic goiter. Thyroid 1992 Fall; 2(3): 263-9

6.11 Hyperthyroidism
6.11.1 Grave's Disease, Thyrostatic

Antithyroid (peroxidase inhibition ⇒ hormone synthesis ↓)	Methimazole (Tapazole, Gens)	*Ini 10-20mg PO qd, maint dose 10mg/d PO qd; euthyroid usually after 2-8wk, try to discontinue after 12-18mo;* **Caution:** *check blood count due to AE (agranulocytosis 0.1-1%)*

| or sos | **Antithyroid** (conversion T4 → T3 ↓, peroxidase inhibition ⇒ hormone synthesis ↓) | **Propylthiouracil** (Gens) | *ini 150-400mg div into bid, maint dose 50-150mg qd* |

101. Leech NJ, Controversies in the management of Graves' disease, Clinical Endocrinology, 1998, 49, 273-80
102. Reinwein D, A prospective randomized trial of antithyroid drug dose in Grave's disease therapy, J Clin Endocrinol Metabol, 1993, 76, 1516-21
103. Weetman AP: Graves' disease. N Engl J Med 2000 Oct 26; 343(17): 1236-48

6.11.2 Functional Autonomy, Thyrostatic

	Antithyroid (peroxidase inhibition ⇒ hormone synthesis ↓)	**Methimazole** (Tapazole, Gens)	*Ini 20mg PO qd-bid, maint dose 5-20mg PO qd*
or sos	**Radio-iodine** beta (90%)/gamma (10%) emission ⇒ destruction of hormone active cells	**I 131 radio-iodine**	*In isolation according to thyroid volume*

6.11.3 Symptomatic (Tachycardia, Hypertension)

| | **Betablocker** (conversion T4 → T3 ↓, cardiac output ↓ (neg. chronotropic/inotropic), central symp. activity ↓) | **Propranolol** (Inderal, Inderal LA, Gens) | *10-40mg PO bid-tid (prn)* |

6.11.4 Inoperability/Relapse after Operation

| | **Radio-iodine** beta (90%)/gamma (10%) emission ⇒ destruction of hormone active cells | **I 131 radio-iodine** | *In isolation according to thyroid volume* |

6.11.5 Thyrotoxicosis (Specialist Required!)

1. Thyrostatic

	Antithyroid (peroxidase inhibition ⇒ hormone synthesis ↓)	**Methimazole** (Tapazole)	*40-80mg slowly IV q6-8h*
or sos	**Antithyroid** (conversion T4 → T3 ↓, peroxidase inhibition ⇒ hormone synthesis ↓)	**Propylthiouracil** (Gens)	*Ini 150-400mg div into bid, maint dose 50-150mg qd*

2. Symptomatic

Calorie substitution (nutrient substitution)	**Glucose 20–50%**	*Approx. 4000-6000KJ/d (prn)*
Isotonic saline solution, cristalloid plasma expander (volume + electrolyte substitution)	**Saline 0.9%, Ringer's solution**	*Approx. 4-6l/d IV according to CVP (prn)*
Betablocker (conversion T4 → T3 ↓, cardiac output ↓ (neg. chronotropic, neg. inotropic), central sympathic activity ↓)	**Propranolol** (Inderal, Inderal LA, Gens)	*40mg IV over 6h (prn)*
Benzodiazepine (sedation)	**Diazepam** (Diastat, Diazepam Intensol, Valium, Gens)	*10mg IV (prn)*
Glucocorticoid (manage associated adrenal cortex failure, conversion T4 → T3 ↓)	**Hydrocortisone** (A-Hydrocort, Cortef, Solu-Cortef, Gens)	*100mg as bolus, then 250mg/24h IV; emerg. thyroid resection in hyperdynamic shock with multiorgan failure*

6.11.6 Prophylaxis of Iodine Induced Hyperthyroidism in Suppressed Basal TSH

Antithyroid (peroxidase inhibition ⇒ hormone synthesis ↓)	**Perchlorate** (Irenat)	*500mg (= 25gtt) 2-4h before CM admin and 2-4h after CM admin, then 3 x 300mg (=15gtt) over 7- 14d; begin before CM admin over 7-14d*
plus **Antithyroid** (peroxidase inhibition ⇒ hormone synthesis ↓)	**Methimazole** (Tapazole)	*20mg over 7-14d, start before CM admin*

104. Gittoes NJ, Franklyn JA: Hyperthyroidism. Current treatment guidelines. Drugs 1998 Apr; 55(4): 543-53

6.12 Hypothyroidism
6.12.1 Chronic Hypothyroidism

Thyroid hormone (hormone substitution ⇒ TSH ↓)	**Levothyroxine** (Levo-T, Levoxyl, Unithroid)	*Ini 50µg PO qd, incr by 25µg q1-3wk up to maint dose: 100-150µg qd; in older patients with CHD ini 25µg, incr q4wk cautiously by 12.5µg*

6.12.2 Myxedema Coma (Specialist Required!)

Glucocorticoid (because of possible adrenal cortex failure)	**Hydrocortisone** (A-Hydrocort, Cortef, Solu-Cortef, Gens)	*100-200mg/24h IV*
Thyroid hormone (hormone substitution ⇒ TSH ↓)	**Levothyroxine** (Levo-T, Levoxyl, Unithroid)	*d1: 500µg IV, d2-7: 100µg IV qd, from d8: 100µg PO qd*
Calorie substitution (symptomatic Tx, ICU)	**Glucose 20-40%**	

Electrolyte balance: fluid restriction due to dilution hyponatremia (depending on CVP)

Circulation support: catecholamine admin, possibly relief of a pericardial effusion, slow warming (1°C/h)

105. Nicoloff JT, Myxedema coma, Endocrin Metabol Clin North Am, 1993, 2, 279-90

6.13 Thyroiditis
6.13.1 Hashimoto's Thyroiditis (Chronic Lymphocytic Thyroiditis)

sos	**Thyroid hormone** (hormone substitution ⇒ TSH ↓)	**Levothyroxine** (Levo-T, Levoxyl, Unithroid)	*Ini 50-100µg PO qd, maint dose 1.5-2µg/kg qd; **Caution:** in older patients with CHD incr dose cautiously*

106. Dayan CM, Daniels GH: Chronic autoimmune thyroiditis. N Engl J Med 1996 Jul 11; 335(2): 99-107

6.13.2 Riedel's Thyroiditis (Invasive Fibrous Thyroiditis)

Glucocorticoid (anti-inflammatory, immunosuppressive)	**Prednisolone** (Econopred, Econopred Plus, Pred Forte, Pred Mild)	*80mg PO qd, red gradually to 5mg qd*

107. Vaidya B, Corticosteroid therapy in Riedel's thyroiditis, Postgrad Med J, 1997, 73, 817-9

6.13.3 Subacute Thyroiditis (De Quervain's Thyroiditis)

Mild

NSAID – acetic acid derivative (cyclooxygenase inhibitor ⇒ anti-inflammatory, analgesic, antipyretic)	**Indomethacin** (Indocin, Indocin SR, Indo-lemmon, Indomethagan, Gens)	*25-50mg PO bid-tid, 75mg (SR) PO qd-bid, 50-100mg PR qd-bid*

Severe

sos	**Glucocorticoid** (anti-inflammatory, immunosuppressive)	**Prednisolone** (Econopred, Econopred Plus, Pred Forte, Pred Mild)	*Ini 40mg PO qd for 4-6 wk, then reduce q3d by 8mg until 16mg/d, then qwk by 4mg; sos pulse Tx 500-1000mg on d3 IV*

108. Hamburger JI: The various presentations of thyroiditis. Diagnostic considerations. Ann Intern Med 1986 Feb; 104(2): 219-24

6.14 Cushing Syndrome

6.14.1 ACTH–Producing Pituitary Tumor

1st choice	**Transsphenoidal surgery**, if failure, bilateral adrenalectomy – preoperative normalisation of hypercortisolism		
	Inhibition of 11-/ and 18-beta-hydroxylase (blocking of cortisone synthesis)	**Ketoconazole** (Nizoral, Gens)	*200-1200mg qd*

6.14.2 Ectopic ACTH Production and ACTH Independent Cushing Syndrome

sos	**Inhibition of 3beta-dehydrogenase** (cytotoxic, cortisol synthesis ↓)	**Mitotane** (Lysodren)	*0.5-4g qd (glucocorticoid substitution sos; in LDL cholesterol ↑, HMG-CoA reductase inhibitor)*

sos	Inhibition of 11-/ and 18-beta-hydroxylase (blocking of cortisone synthesis)	Ketoconazole (Nizoral, Gens)	200-1200mg qd
sos	Inhibition of 11-/ and 18-beta-hydroxylase (blocking of cortisone synthesis)	Metyrapone (Metopirone)	1.5g PO qd div tid-qid (AE limit use)
sos	Aromatase inhibitor (cortisol synthesis ↓)	Aminoglutethimide (Cytadren)	Adrenal cortex adenoma: 250mg PO bid-tid, in ect. ACTH prod. qid-7x/d

109. Trainer PJ, Cushing´s syndrome. Therapy directed at the adrenal gland, Endocrin Metab Clin North Am, 1994, 23, 571-84
110. Yanovski JA, Cutler GB Jr: Glucocorticoid action and the clinical features of Cushing's syndrome. Endocrinol Metab Clin North Am 1994; 23(3): 487-509

6.15 Aldosteronism

| sos | Thiazide diuretic (elimination of Na^+, Cl^-, H_2O and K^+ ↑) | Hydrochlorothiazide (Esidrix, Hydrodiuril, Microside, Oretic, Gens) | 12.5-50mg PO qd |
| plus | Aldosterone antagonist (mineralocorticoid steroid effects ↓) | Spironolactone (Aldactone, Gens) | D1-5: 50-100mg bid-qid, then 50-100mg PO qd-bid |

6.16 Adrenal Insufficiency
6.16.1 Long-Term Therapy

Primary (Addison disease)

| | Glucocorticoid (substitution) | Hydrocortisone (A-Hydrocort, Cortef, Solu-Cortef, Gens) | 10-12mg/m² PO bid-qid, adj replacement dose based on cortisol day curve, e.g. 15-5-5mg, 10-10-5mg or 15-10-0mg |
| plus | Mineralocorticoid (substitution) | Fludrocortisone (Florinef) | 50-200µg qd qam |

6.16.2   Addison Crisis (Specialist Required!)

	Glucocorticoid (substitution)	Hydrocortisone (A-Hydrocort, Cortef, Solu-Cortef, Gens)	100mg IV q6h, when stabilized 50mg IV q6h; maint dose from d4/d5
	Isotonic saline solution + glucose (volume + glucose + electrolyte substitution)	Saline 0.9% + Glucose 40%	Ini 500ml saline 0.9% + 40ml glucose 40%, then glucose 5%
sos	Low dose heparin (low molecular heparin, embolism PRO)	Dalteparin (Fragmin)	2850 IU SC qd

111. Werbel S, Acute adrenal insufficiency, Endocrin Metab Clin North Am, 1993, 22, 303-28

6.17   Pheochromocytoma

6.17.1   Long-Term Therapy, Preoperative Preparation

	Alpha-blocker, non competitive (vasodilation ↑, afterload ↓, preload ↓)	Phenoxybenzamine (Dibenzyline)	10mg PO bid, max. 30mg tid (sos until OP; hematocrit ↓, normotension)
plus	Betablocker (cardiac output ↓ (neg. chrono-/inotropic), renin secretion ↓, central sympathetic activity ↓)	Propranolol (Inderal, Inderal LA, Gens)	40-80mg PO bid-tid, 80-320mg (SR) PO qd; tachycardia Tx only after sufficiently long alpha-blockade (otherwise paradox BP ↑)
or sos	Alphablocker, reversible (reversible blockage of alpha1-receptor)	Prazosin (Minipress, Minipress XL, Gens)	1mg tid-qid up to 20mg

6.17.2   Hypertensive Crisis

	Alphablocker, imidazole derivative (vasodilation ↑, afterload ↓, preload ↓)	Phentolamine (Regitine, Rogitine, Gens)	5-10mg IV, then 0.25-1mg/min inf, max. dose 120mg/h; duration of BP↓ 20min

| sos plus | **Betablocker** (cardiac output ↓ (neg. chrono-/inotropic), renin secretion ↓, central sympathetic activity ↓) | **Propranolol** (Inderal, Inderal LA, Gens) | *1 x 1mg slowly IV, repeat sos* |

112. Bravo E, Pheochromocytoma, Endocrin Metab Clin North Am, 1993, 22, 329-41

6.18 Hyperparathyroidism
6.18.1 Primary Hyperparathyroidism (Adenoma, Hypertrophy)

Mild

| sos | **Isotonic saline solution** (rehydratation) | **Saline 0.9%** | *D1: 4-6l, then 3-4l/d* |
| sos | **Loop diuretic** (calcium excretion) | **Furosemide** (Lasix, Gens) | *50-100mg IV* |

Hypercalcemic crisis

	Isotonic saline solution (rehydratation)	**Saline 0.9%**	*1-2l IV*
sos	**Loop diuretic** (calcium excretion)	**Furosemide** (Lasix, Gens)	*40-120mg IV*
sos	**Potassium chloride solution** (substitution)	**K⁺Cl⁻ 7.45%** ($1ml = 1mmol$)	*20-40ml in 1l istotonic sol in 10-20mmol/h, max. 100-200mmol/d (prn)*
sos	**Biphosphonate** (osteoclast inhibition in tumor hypercalcemia)	**Pamidronate** (Aredia)	*60mg as single dose if Ca < 3.38mmol/l, 90mg if Ca > 3.38mmol/l, inf over 4-24h*
		Ibandronate (experimental)	*1mg/ml, 4mg in 500ml saline 0.9% over 2h*
sos	**Glucocorticoid** (resorption ↓, mobilisation ↓)	**Prednisone** (Deltasone, Meticorten, Prednisone Intensol, Gens)	*100-200mg qd*
sos	**Hormone** (osteoclast inhibition, only slightly effective)	**Calcitonin** (Calcimar, Miacalcin)	*Ini 3-4IU/kg slowly IV, then 4IU/kg SC qd*

| sos | Cytostatic (osteoclast inhibition) | Mithramycin (Mithracin) | 25ng/kg IV, final resort |

113. Bilezikian JP: Clinical review 51: Management of hypercalcemia. J Clin Endocrinol Metab 1993 Dec; 77(6): 1445-9
114. Bushinsky DA, Calcium, Lancet, 1998, 352, 306-11
115. Edelson GW, Kleerekoper M: Hypercalcemic crisis. Med Clin North Am 1995 Jan; 79(1): 79-92

6.18.2   Secondary Hyperparathyroidism (Circulating Calcium ↓ ⇒ PTH ↑)

In general

| | Calcium preparation (substitution) | Calcium (Alka-Mints, Calci-Chew, Calci-Mix, Caltrate, Chooz, Liqui-Cal, Mallamint, Nephro-Calci, Os-Cal, Titralac, Tums, Gens) | 700-2000mg PO qd (prn) |

In malarbsorbtion

| | Vitamin D$_3$ | Vit D3 | 1000IU qd |

In renal genesis

| | Vit. D (1,25/ OH$_2$) D$_3$ | Calcitriol (Calcijex, Rocaltrol) | 0.25-1µg PO qd |

116. Allerheiligen DA, Schoeber J, Houston RE, et al: Hyperparathyroidism. Am Fam Physician 1998 Apr 15; 57(8): 1795-802, 1807-8

6.19   Hypoparathyroidism
6.19.1   Long-Term Therapy

	Calcium preparation (substitution)	Calcium carbonate (Alka-Mints, Calci-Chew, Calci-Mix, Caltrate, Chooz, Liqui-Cal, Mallamint, Nephro-Calci, Os-Cal, Titralac, Tums, Gens)	1-2g PO qd (prn)
plus	Vitamin D analogue (metabolism influence)	Dihydrotachysterol (DHT)	0.3-1.0mg PO qd (prn)
or	Vitamin D3	Vit D3	500-2500µg qd (depending on Ca level)

6.19.2	Hypocalcemic Crisis		
	Calcium preparation (substitution)	Calcium gluconate 10% (10ml = 2.3mmol)	ini 2.3-4.5mmol slowly IV over 5-15min, then in glucose 5% inf (hospital)

117. Schilling T, Current therapy of hypoparathyroidism, a survey of German endocrinology centers, Exp Clin Endocrinal Diabetes, 1997, 105, 237-41

6.20 Hypopituitarism
6.20.1 Long-Term Therapy (Specialist Required!)

In general

	Glucocorticoid (substitution)	Hydrocortisone (A-Hydrocort, Cortef, Solu-Cortef, Gens)	10-12mg/m² qd, e.g. 10-5-10mg at 7am, 11.30am, 17.30pm (chronic)
plus	Thyroid hormone (substitution)	Levothyroxine (Levo-T, Levoxyl, Unithroid)	Ini 50-100µg PO qd, maint dose: 1.5-2µg/kg qd (after Tx start with steroids)
plus	Growth hormone (substitution)	Somatotropin (Genotropin, Humatrope, Norditropin, Nutropin, Protropin, Saizen)	0.04-0.08mg/kg SC qd, incr slowly (if without benefit discontinue slowly after 6mo)

In women additionally

plus	Estrogen + progestogen (substitution)	Estradiol + Norethindrone	
	Premenopausal: comb. contraceptive with 20 - 35µg ethinyl-estradiol, **postmenopausal:** estradiol valerate 2mg cyclic or cont. with progestogen preparation; if **restitution of fertility** spec. Tx required: pulsatile GnRH inf SC		

In men additionally

plus	Androgen (substitution)	Testosterone depot preparation (Delatestryl, Depo-Testosterone, Testoderm)	1 x 250mg IM q2-4wk or 5mg patch qd (if restitution of fertility spec. Tx required: pulsatile GnRH inf SC)

118. Lamberts SWJ, Pituitary insufficiency, Lancet, 1998, 352, 127-34

6.20.2 Pituitary Coma

Adrenal crisis (Specialist Required!)

	Isotonic saline solution + glucose (volume + glucose + electrolyte substitution)	**Saline 0.9% + Glucose 40%**	*Ini 500ml saline 0.9%+ 40ml glucose 40%, then glucose 5%*
plus	**Glucocorticoid** (substitution)	**Hydrocortisone** (A-Hydrocort, Cortef, Solu-Cortef, Gens)	*Ini 100mg IV, then inf 10mg/h or 100mg IM/IV q6h, then 50mg PO qid, decrease slowly*
sos	**Vasopressor** (dose-depending dopamine-/β- and α-agonism ⇒ cardiac output↓, vasoconstriction renal vasodilation)	**Dopamine** (Intropin, Gens)	*Renal dose: 0.5-5µg/kg/min IV, perf. (250mg) = 5mg/ml ⇒ 1-3.5ml/h, BP dose: 6-10µg/kg/min IV, perf. (250mg) ⇒ 4.5-9ml/h, max. 18ml/h*
sos	**(Beta)sympathomimetic** (inotropic)	**Dobutamine** (Dobutrex, Gens)	*2.5-12µg/kg/min IV*
sos	**Low-molecular heparin** (coagulation factor ↓, embolism PRO)	**Dalteparin** (Fraxiparin) **Enoxaparin** (Lovenox)	*2850 IU SC qd*

Myxedema coma (see Hypothyroidism, →129)

6.21 Hyperpituitarism, Pituitary Tumors
6.21.1 Hyperprolactinemia (Specialist Required!)

Prolactin inhibitor (pituitary dopamine receptor stimulation ⇒ prolactin ↓)	**Bromocriptine** (Parlodel)	*1.25mg PO qhs (in the middle of bedtime snack), incr slowly sos, max 30mg/d in div doses*
	Cabergoline (Dostinex)	*0.25mg PO biw, incr slowly sos, max 1mg biw*

119. Cunnah D, Management of prolactinomas, Clin Endocrinol, 1991, 34, 231-35
120. Serri O: Progress in the management of hyperprolactinemia. N Engl J Med 1994 Oct 6; 331(14): 942-4

6.21.2 Acromegaly (Specialist Required!)

	Prolactin inhibitor (pituitary dopamine receptor stimulation ⇒ prolactin ↓, STH ↓)	**Bromocriptine** (Parlodel)	*1.25mg PO qd, incr slowly sos, max 30mg/d div bid; individual dose!*
or	**Somatostatin analogue** (STH ↓)	**Octreotide** (Sandostatin, Sandostatin LAR Depot)	*Ini 0.05mg SC, then up to 0.5mg SC tid (according to GH level), then depot 20-30mg IM q4wk x 3mo, then q4wk according to GH level*

121. Shimon I, Management of pituitary tumors, Ann Intern Med, 1998, 129, 472-83

6.22 Diabetes Insipidus

6.22.1 Central Diabetes Insipidus

	Hormone (ADH substitution)	**Desmopressin** (Concentraid, DDAVP, Stimate, Gens)	*0.1-0.4mg intranasal tid, SC (chronic)*

6.22.2 Peripheral Diabetes Insipidus

	Thiazide diuretic (GFR ↓, antidiuretic effect)	**Hydrochlorothiazide** (Esidrix, Hydrodiuril, Microside, Oretic, Gens)	*12.5-50mg PO qd*

122. Robertson GL, Diabetes insipidus, Endocrin Metab Clin North Am, 1995, 24, 49-71

6.23 Insulinoma

6.23.1 In General (Specialist Required!)

sos	**Hormone** (antihypoglycemic, gluconeogenesis ↑, glycogenolysis ↑)	**Glucagon** (GlucaGen, Gens)	*According to BS*
sos	**K⁺ channel modulation** (insulin secretion ↓, hepatic glucose output ↑)	**Diazoxide** (Proglycem)	*5mg/kg/d PO in 2-3 single doses*

| sos | Somatostatin analogue (insulin secretion ↓) | Octreotide (Sandostatin, Sandostatin LAR Depot) | *Ini 1-2 x 0.05mg SC, then 0.5mg SC to tid under close supervision, then depot 20-30mg IM q4wk* |

6.23.2 Cytostatic

	Cytostatic, pyrimidine antagonist (thymidine nucleotide synthesis ↓)	5-Fluorouracil (Adrucil)	*400mg/m² IV on d1-d5 (repeat cycle from d43)*
plus	Cytostatic, alkylating (nitrosourea analog, inhibits DNA synthesis)	Streptozocin (Zanosar)	*500mg/m² IV on d1-d5 (repeat cycle from d43)*
plus	Cytostatic antibiotic (DNA damage)	Doxorubicin (Adriamycin)	*50mg/m² IV on d1 + d21 (repeat cycle from d43)*

123. Perry RR, Diagnosis and management of functioning islet-cell tumors, J Endocrin Metab, 1995, 80, 2273

6.24 VIPoma

| | Somatostatin analogue (VIP secretion ↓) | Octreotide (Sandostatin, Sandostatin LAR Depot) | *Ini 1-2 x 0.05mg SC, then 0.5mg SC up to tid under close supervision, then depot 20-30mg IM q4wk* |

124. Arnold R, Management of gastroenteropathic endocrine tumors: The place of Somatostatin Analogues, Digestion, 1994, Suppl 3, 107-13

6.25 Gastrinoma (Zollinger–Ellison Syndrome)

| sos | Proton pump inhibitors (acid secretion ↓) | Omeprazole (Prilosec, Gens) | *20-40mg PO qd, up to max.160mg* |
| sos | Somatostatin analogue (gastrin secretion ↓) | Octreotide (Sandostatin, Sandostatin LAR Depot) | *Ini 1-2 x 0.05mg SC, then 0.5mg SC up to tid under close supervision, then depot 20-30mg IM q4wk* |

125. Meko JB, Management of patients with Zollinger Ellison syndrome, Ann Rev Med, 1995, 46, 395

6.26 Carcinoid Tumor

	Somatostatin analogue (gastrin sekretion ↓)	**Octreotide** (Sandostatin, Sandostatin LAR Depot)	*Ini 1-2 x 0.05mg SC, then 0.5mg SC up to tid under close supervision, then depot 20-30mg IM q4wk*
	Serotonin antagonist (serotonine effects ↓)	**Methysergide** (Sansert)	*4mg (SR) PO bid*
SOS	**Interferon** (immune stimulation/-modulation)	**IFN-alpha-2a/b** (Intron A, Roferon)	*3-5 M IU/wk prn*
SOS	**Antidiarrheal** (stimulation of peripheral opiod receptors)	**Loperamide** (Imodium, Gens)	*Ini 4mg PO, after each episode 2mg, max: 12mg/d (prn)*

126. Kema IP, Willemse PH, De Vries EG: Carcinoid tumors. N Engl J Med 1999 Aug 5; 341(6): 453-4

6.27 Gynecomastia

SOS	**Antiestrogen** (blockade of peripheral estrogen receptors ⇒ estrogen effects ↓)	**Tamoxifen** (Nolvadex)	*20-40mg PO qd (short-term)*

127. Braunstein GD, Gynecomastia, N Engl J Med, 1993, 328, 490-5

7.   Gastroenterology

Stefan Endres, MD
Chief, Division of Clinical Pharmacology
University of Munich, Munich, Germany

7.1   Esophagitis

7.1.1   Gastroesophageal Reflux Disease (GERD)

Grade I/II (endoscopy: erythema – non-confluent erosions)

	Antacid (acid binding)	**Al Hydroxide plus Mg Hydroxide** (Maalox)	*10ml PO qid-6x/d prn*
or	**Proton pump inhibitor** (acid secretion ↓)	**Omeprazole** (Prilosec, Gens)	*20mg PO qd for 4wk, if ineffective for another 4wk; in relapse 40mg qd*
		Lansoprazole (PrevAcid)	*30mg PO qd for 4-8wk*

Grade III/IV (endoscopy: confluent erosions – ulcer, stricture)

	Proton pump inhibitor (acid secretion ↓)	**Omeprazole** (Prilosec, Gens)	*20-40mg PO qd for 12wk*
		Lansoprazole (PrevAcid)	*30mg PO qd for 12wk*

128. Galmiche JP, Letessier E, Scarpignato C. Treatment of gastro-oesophageal reflux disease in adults. BMJ 1998; 316: 1720-1723
129. Moss SF, et al. Consensus Statement for Management of Gastroesophageal Reflux Disease: Result of Workshop Meeting at Yale University School of Medicine, Department of Surgery, November 16 and 17, 1997. J Clin Gastroenterol 1998, 27, 6-12
130. DeVault KR, Castell DO. Updated guidelines for the diagnosis and treatment of gastroesophageal reflux disease. Am J Gastroenterol 2005;100:190-200

Maintenance of Remission

	Proton pump inhibitor (acid secretion ↓)	**Omeprazole** (Prilosec, Gens)	*20mg PO qd, max 40mg qd; try to red after 6mo, sometimes life-long Tx*
		Lansoprazole (PrevAcid)	*30mgPO qd; try to red after 6mo, sometimes life-long Tx*

131. Venables TL, Scand J Gastroenterol, 1997, 32(7), 627-32

7.1.2 Infectious Esophagitis

Candida

	Antifungal (azole derivative)	Fluconazole (Diflucan)	d1: 200mg PO qd, then: 100mg PO qd for 14d

132. Pappas PG, Rex JH, Sobel JD, et al. Practice guidelines for the treatment of candidiasis. Infectious Diseases Society of America. Clin Infect Dis 2004;38:161-89

Herpes simplex

	Antiviral (DNA-polymerase inhib.)	Famciclovir (Famvir)	250mg PO tid for 14d

Caution: Famciclovir is approved only for acute herpes zoster, genital herpes, recurrent herpes simplex in immunocompetent patients and for recurrent orolabial herpes or genital herpes in HIV-infected patients

Cytomegaly virus

	Antiviral (DNA-polymerase inhib.)	Ganciclovir (Cytovene)	5mg/kg IV bid for 14d

7.2 Achalasia

poss	Ca++ channel blocker (muscle relaxation)	Nifedipine (Adalat, Procardia, Gens)	20mg SL ac prn
poss	Nitrate (muscle relaxation)	Isosorbide dinitrate (Isordil, Sorbitrate, Gens)	10mg SL ac prn
poss	Muscle relaxant (acetylcholine release ↓)	Botulinum toxin (Botox)	Endoscopic Inj into lower esophageal sphincter prn, see Prod Info
poss	**Surgical intervention**: Graded pneumatic dilation or surgical myotomy		

133. Vaezi MF, Richter JE. Diagnosis and management of achalasia. Am J Gastroenterol 1999;94:3406-3412

7.3 Gastritis
7.3.1 Acute Erosive Gastritis

	Antacid (acid binding)	Al Hydroxide plus Mg Hydroxide (Maalox)	10ml PO qid-6x/d for a few days
poss	H₂ Antagonist (acid secretion ↓)	Ranitidine (Zantac, Gens)	300mg PO qpm for a few days

7.3.2	Stress Lesion Prophylaxis		
	Antiulcer drug (formation of a film ⇒ mucosa protection)	**Sucralfate** (Carafate, Gens)	*1g PO qid*

7.3.3	Type A in Pernicious Anemia		
poss	**Vitamin B12** (substitution)	**Cyanocobalamin** (Rubramin PC, Vibisone, Gens)	*1000µg/wk IM for 1-3wk, then 1000µg/mo IM (life-long)*

7.4   Peptic Ulcer Disease (PUD)
7.4.1   PUD without Detection of Helicobacter pylori

Uncomplicated

	H₂ Antagonist (acid secretion ↓)	**Ranitidine** (Zantac)	*300mg PO qpm for 3-6wk*
or	**Proton pump inhibitor** (acid secretion ↓)	**Omeprazole** (Prilosec)	*20mg PO qd for 3wk*
		Lansoprazole (PrevAcid)	*30mg PO qd for 3wk*

Complicated (hemorrhage, obstruction, perforation)

	Proton pump inhibitor (acid secretion ↓)	**Omeprazole** (Prilosec, Gens)	*80mg as short IV inf over 30min, then 200mg IV qd for 3d, then 20mg PO qd for 3wk*
or		**Lansoprazole** (PrevAcid)	*30mg PO qd*

Maintenance of Remission

	H₂ Antagonist (acid secretion ↓)	**Ranitidine** (Zantac)	*150mg PO qpm*

134. Schaffalitzky de Muckadell OB, Scand J Gastroenterol, 1997, 32(4), 320-7

7.4.2   PUD with Detection of Helicobacter pylori

„Italian" triple therapy

	Proton pump inhibitor (acid secretion ↓)	**Omeprazole** (Prilosec, Gens)	*20mg PO bid (1h ac) for 7 to 14d*
or		**Lansoprazole** (PrevAcid)	*30mg PO bid (1h ac) for 7 to 14d*

| plus | Macrolide (antibiotic) | Clarithromycin (Biaxin) | *250mg PO bid for 7 to 14d* |
| plus | Nitroimidazole (antibiotic) | Metronidazole (Protostat, Gens) | *500mg PO bid for 14d* |

„French" triple therapy as second therapy in failure

	Proton pump inhibitor (acid secretion ↓)	Omeprazole (Prilosec, Gens)	*20mg PO bid (1h ac) for 10 or 14d*
or		Lansoprazole (PrevAcid)	*30mg PO bid (1h ac) for 10 or 14d*
plus	Macrolide (HP eradication)	Clarithromycin (Biaxin)	*500mg PO bid for 10-14d*
plus	Aminopenicillin (HP eradication)	Amoxicillin (Amoxil, Larotid, Trimox, Wymox)	*1g PO bid for 10 or 14d*

The combination of lansoprazole 30mg, amoxicillin 1g and clarithromycin 500mg is available in a daily dose convenience packaging: Prevpac (TAP Phramaceuticals Inc.); http://www.prevacid.com

Eradication therapy in patients that cannot be treated orally

	Proton pump inhibitor (acid secretion ↓)	Omeprazole (Prilosec)	*200mg IV cont inf qd (switch to PO Tx asap)*
plus	Nitroimidazole (antibiotic)	Metronidazole (Flagyl, Metro, Gens)	*500mg IV tid (switch to PO Tx asap)*
plus	Aminopenicillin (HP eradication)	Amoxicillin (Amoxil, Larotid, Trimox, Wymox, Gens)	*1g IV tid (switch to PO Tx asap)*

135. Soll AH: Consensus conference. Medical treatment of peptic ulcer disease. Practice guidelines. Practice Parameters Committee of the American College of Gastroenterology. JAMA 1996 Feb 28; 275(8): 622-9
136. Salcedo JA, Al-Kawas F: Treatment of Helicobacter pylori infection. Arch Intern Med 1998 Apr 27; 158(8): 842-51
137. Howden CW, Hunt RH. Guidelines for the management of Helicobacter pylori infection. Am J Gastroenterol 1998;93:2330-8

7.5 Diverticular Disease

| | Fluoroquinolone | Ciprofloxacin (Cipro) | *500mg PO bid for 7-10d* |
| plus | Nitroimidazole | Metronidazole (Flagyl, Gens) | *500mg PO tid for 7-10d* |

138. Sanford, Guide to Antimicrobial Therapy, 35th edition, 2005

7.6 Crohn's Disease
7.6.1 Acute Exacerbation

	Glucocorticoid (anti-inflammatory, immunosuppressive)	Prednisolone (Onapred, Pediapred, Prelone, Gens)	60mg PO qd over 6wk, red to 10mg PO qd (wk to mo)
or	Salicylate (anti-inflammatory)	Mesalamine (Asacol/Tab, Pentasa/Cap)	800mg Tab PO tid (Asacol) or 1g Cap PO tid (Pentasa) for 1yr

7.6.2 Acute Exacerbation with Fistulas

plus	Nitroimidazole (antibiotic)	Metronidazole (Flagyl, Metromidol, Gens)	500mg PO tid for <10d

7.6.3 Maintenance of Remission

Salicylate (anti-inflammatory)	Mesalamine (Asacol/Tab, Pentasa/Cap)	800mg Tab PO tid (Asacol) or 1g Cap PO tid (Pentasa) for 1yr

7.6.4 Chronic Active Disease, Refractory Disease

Purine antagonist (immunosuppressive)	Azathioprine (Imuran, Gens)	2.5mg/kg PO qd (effect after 2-4wk)

7.6.5 Refractory Disease with Fistulas

Immunomodulator (anti-TNFα antibody)	Infliximab (Remicade)	5mg/kg IV inf over 2h, rep at 2wk and 6wk prn

139. Hanauer SB and Sandborn W. Management of Crohn's Disease in Adults. Am J Gastroenterol March 2001;96:635-643
140. Schreiber S, et al. Use of anti-tumour necrosis factor agents in inflammatory bowel disease. European guidelines for 2001-2003. Int J Colorectal Dis. 200116:1-11

7.7 Ulcerative Colitis
7.7.1 Acute Exacerbation

Salicylate (anti-inflammatory)	Mesalamine (Asacol/Tab, Canasa/PR, Pentasa/Cap, Rowasa/PR)	Pancolitis: 800mg Tab PO tid or 1g Cap (4 x 250mg) PO tid; in distal involvement: 1g PR qd

In Tx failure plus	Glucocorticoid (anti-inflammatory, immunosuppressive)	Prednisolone (Onapred, Pediapred, Prelone, Gens)	*40mg PO qd over 6wk, red to 10mg PO qd (red further over wk to mo)*

7.7.2 Maintenance of Remission

	Salicylate (anti-inflammatory)	Mesalamine (Pentasa/ Cap)	*500mg Cap PO tid for 2yr*

7.7.3 Refractory Disease

	Purine antagonist (immunosuppressive)	Azathioprine (Imuran, Gens)	*2.0-2.5mg/kg PO qd (effect after 2-4wk)*

141. Sands BE: Therapy of inflammatory bowel disease. Gastroenterology 2000 Feb; 118(2 Suppl 1): S68-82
142. Kornbluth A, Sachar DB: Ulcerative colitis practice guidelines in adults. (Update) American College of Gastroenterology, Practice Parameters Committee. Am J Gastroenterol 2004; 99:1371-85

7.8 Pancreatitis
7.8.1 Acute Pancreatitis

Basic therapy

	Glucose electrolyte solution (volume substitution)	Glucose 5% + Ringer's solution (1:1)	*> 3l/d, according to CVP*
or	Opioid (analgesia without spasmogenic effects on Oddi's sphincter)	Buprenorphine (Buprenex, Gens)	*0.15mg IV q6h prn*
		Meperidine (Demerol, Gens)	*15-35mg/h IV; 50-150mg IM q3-4h*
poss	Calcium preparation (replacement)	Calcium gluconate 10% (4.5meq/ml)	*10-20ml slowy IV prn*
poss	H$_2$ Antagonist (stomach acid secretion ↓ ⇒ pancreas secretion ↓)	Ranitidine (Zantac, Gens)	*50mg IV tid*

In biliary/necrotizing pancreatitis

	Cephalosporin	Ceftriaxone (Rocephin)	*1-2g IV qd (or div bid)*
or	Acylaminopenicillin	Ampicillin (Omnipen, Principen, Totacillin, Gens)	*500-1000mg IV q6h*
or	Acylaminopenicillin + lactamase inhibitor	Ampicillin + Sulbactam (Unasyn)	*2+1g IV q6h*

Banks P. Practice guidelines in acute pancreatitis. Am J Gastroenterology. 1997;92(3):377-386

7.8.2	Chronic Pancreatitis		
	Exocrine pancreatic enzymes (enzyme substitution)	Pancreatin (Creon, Donnazyme, Ultrase)	*1-2 Tab/Cap PO with each meal (100.000IU/d), poss life-long*
poss	Fat soluble vitamins (substitution)	Vitamins A, D, E, K	*1ml q2wk IM prn*
poss	Analgesic (aniline) (inhibits cyclooxygenase)	Acetaminophen (Tylenol, Gens)	*1000mg PO qid*
poss	Opioid (analgesic)	Tramadol (Ultram)	*50-100mg PO qid*

143. Sanford, Guide to Antimicrobial Therapy, 35th edition, 2005

7.9   Hepatitis
7.9.1   Acute Viral Hepatitis A

poss	Bile acid sequestrant (binding of bile acid ⇒ inhibition of pruritus)	Cholestyramine (Locholest, Prevalite, Questran, Gens)	*4-16g PO qd prn*
poss	H₁-antihistamine (inhibition of pruritus)	Loratadine (Claritin)	*10mg PO qd prn*

7.9.2   Chronic Viral Hepatitis B

	Alpha-interferon (immunostimulating and directly antiviral)	IFN Alpha-2A (Roferon A)	*6 M IU tiw SC for 24wk*
or		IFN Alpha-2B (Intron A)	*5 M IU tiw SC for 24wk*
or	Antiviral (nucleoside analogue)	Lamivudine (Epivir-HBV)	*100mg PO qd for 4yr or up to 6mo after anti-HBe seroconversion*

Or when resistance to lamivudine

	Antiviral (nucleotide reverse transcriptase inhibitor)	Adefovir dipivoxil (Hepsera)	*10mg PO qd for 4yr or upto 6mo after anti-HBe seroconversion*
	Peginterferon (immunostimulating, antiviral; complexed to increase half-life)	PEG-IFN Alpha-2A (Pegasys)	*180µg SC qwk for 48wk*

7.9.3 Chronic Viral Hepatitis C

	Peginterferon (immunostimulating, antiviral; complexed to increase half-life)	PEG-IFN Alpha-2A (Pegasys)	*180µg SC qwk*
		PEG-IFN Alpha-2B (Peg-Intron)	*1.5µg/kg SC qwk*

Admin for 24wk for high responders; admin for 48wk for low responders, if genotype 1 or > 2 risk factors (male, > 40yr, signs of liver reorganisation, > 3.5 M copies/ml)

plus	Antiviral (nucleoside analogue, immunostimulating and directly antiviral)	Ribavirin (Rebetol)	*For low responders: 1000mg PO qd (1200mg in BW >75kg; 800mg in BW <60kg); for high responders: 800mg PO qd, fixed dose; Dur of Tx see Interferon*

144. NIH-Consensus 2002
145. Hadziyannis SJ, et al. Peginterferon-(alpha)2a and Ribavirin combination therapy in chronic hepatitis C. Ann Intern Med 2004;140(5):346-55

7.9.4 Autoimmune Hepatitis

	Glucocorticoid (anti-inflammatory, immunosuppressive)	Prednisolone (Onapred, Pediapred, Prelone, Gens)	*40-60mg PO qd over 6wk, red to 10mg PO qd, maint Tx for up to 2yr*
poss	Immunosuppressant (purine antagonist)	Azathioprine (Imuran, Gens)	*2mg/kg PO qd (effects after 2-4mo)*

146. Manns MP, McHutchison JG, Gordon SC, et al. Peginterferon alfa-2b plus ribavirin compared with interferon alfa-2b plus ribavirin for initial treatment of chronic hepatitis C: a randomised trial. Lancet 2001 Sep 22;358(9286):958-965

7.10 Cirrhosis

7.10.1 General Measures

Ascites therapy

	Aldosterone antagonist (volume relief)	**Spironolactone** (Aldactone, Gens)	*d1-5: 50-100mg PO bid-qid, then: 50-100mg PO qd-bid (max BW ↓ 500g/d)*
poss	**Loop diuretic** (volume relief)	**Furosemide** (Lasix, Gens)	*20-40mg PO qd-bid (max BW ↓ 500g/d)*

Vitamin substitution

poss	**Fat soluble Vitamins** (substitution)	**Vitamins A, D, E, K**	*1ml IM q2wk (in proven deficiency)*
poss	**B-Vitamins** (substitution)	**Vitamins B1 + B6 + B12 + Folic acid** (Gens)	*See Prod Info (in proven deficiency)*

Alcoholism, see Psychiatry →229, →232

7.10.2 Primary Biliary Cirrhosis

	Cholic acid derivative (cholesterol secretion ↓, cholesterol resorption ↓)	**Ursodiol** (=ursodeoxycholic acid) (Actigall, Urso)	*15mg/kg PO qd (life-long) in pilot studies: higher doses (20-30mg/kg PO qd)*
poss	**Bile acid sequestrant** (binding of bile acid ⇒ inhibition of pruritus)	**Cholestyramine** (Locholest, Prevalite, Questran, Gens)	*4g PO qd-bid prn, alternating with ursodiol and fat soluble vitamins*
or poss	**H₁-Antihistamine** (inhibition of pruritus)	**Loratadine** (Claritin)	*10mg PO qd prn*

147. Heathcote EJ. Management of primary biliary cirrhosis. The American Association for the Study of Liver Diseases Practice Guidelines. Hepatology 2000;31:1005-13
148. Levy C, Lindor KD. Current management of primary biliary cirrhosis and primary sclerosing cholangitis. J Hepatol 2003;38:24-37

7.10.3 Primary Sclerosing Cholangitis

	Cholic acid derivative (cholesterol secretion ↓, cholesterol resorption ↓)	**Ursodiol** (=ursodeoxycholic acid) (Actigall, Urso)	*15mg/kg PO qd (life-long)*

7.10.4 Portal Hypertension

Primary prophylaxis of bleeding from esophageal varices

poss	**Betablocker** (CO↓, portal vein press.↓)	**Propranolol** (Inderal, Gens)	*Ini 20mg PO tid (goal: HR decrease of 25%)*

Bleeding from esophageal varices

poss	**Somatostatin analogue** (splanchnic vasoconstrict. ⇒ portal vein pressure↓)	**Octreotide** (Sandostatin)	*25µg/h IV*
poss	**Fluoroquinolone** (antibiotic)	**Ciprofloxacin** (Cipro)	*Prophylactic: 500mg PO bid for 7d*

Medical Care
- Initial resuscitation with replacement of blood volume loss
- Endoscopic injection sclerotherapy, balloon-tube tamponade
- Surgical intervention: portal systemic shunts, selective shunts, splenectomy, liver transplantation

149. Garcia-Tsao G. Current management of the complications of cirrhosis and portal hypertension: variceal hemorrhage, ascites, and spontaneous bacterial peritonitis. Gastroenterology 2001;120: 726-48
150. Bosch J, Abraldes JG, Groszmann R. Current management of portal hypertension. J Hepatol 2003;38:54-68

7.10.5 Hepatic Encephalopathy, Hepatic Coma

poss	**Osmotic laxative** (laxative, NH_3 elimination)	**Lactulose** (Cephulac, Cholac, Chronulac, Constilac, Constulose, Enulose, Evalose, Heptalac, Laxilose)	*20-30ml PO tid*
or poss	**Aminoglycoside** (intestinal sterilization)	**Neomycin** (Mycifradin, Neo-rx, Gens)	*2g PO qd-bid*

151. Blei AT, Córdoba J. Hepatic encephalopathy. Am J Gastroenterol, 2001;96:1968-76.

7.11 Cholelithiasis

7.11.1 Oral Bile Acid Dissolution Therapy

Stone: < 10mm, **not** calcareous, **not** > 2 concrements, contractible gall bladder

Cholic acid derivative (cholesterol secretion↓, cholesterol resorption↓)	**Ursodiol** (=ursodeoxycholic acid) (Actigall, Urso)	*10mg/kg PO qd with food (div qid) for up to 3mo after litholysis*

7.11.2 Maintenance of Remission

Cholic acid derivative (cholesterol secretion↓, cholesterol resorption↓)	**Ursodiol** (=ursodeoxycholic acid) (Actigall, Urso)	*300mg PO qd (long-term Tx)*

7.12 Biliary Colic

	Analgesic, NSAID (activity of cyclooxygenase↓)	**Ketorolac** (Acular PF, Toradol, Gens)	*Ini 30-60mg IM, then 15-30mg IM q6h; or 15-30mg IV prn; not to exceed 120mg/d*
plus/or	**Analgesic, opioid** (analgesia without spasmogenic effects on Oddi's sphincter)	**Meperidine** (Demerol, Gens)	*50-150mg PO/IV/IM/SC q3-4h prn*
Plus	**Antiemetic** (dopamine receptor antagonist)	**Metoclopramide** (Reglan, Gens)	*10mg IV q6h prn*
or	**Antiemetic** (inhibits dopamine receptors)	**Prochlorperazine** (Compazine, Compro, Gens)	*5-10mg IM/PO q6h prn; not to exceed 40mg/d*

7.13 Cholecystitis, Cholangitis (bacterial)

Acylaminopenicillin + lactamase inhibitor	**Piperacillin + Tazobactam** (Zosyn)	*3g + 0.375g IV tid*
Antiemetic, antidopaminergic (stimuli to brainstem reticular system↓)	**Promethazine** (Phenergan, Gens)	*12.5-25mg PO/IV/IM/PR q4-6h prn*

7.14 Bowel Preparation for Colonoscopy

	Electrolyte lavage solution (washout of ingested fluids)	**Polyethylene glycol with electrolytes** (Colyte, Golytely)	*one day prior to examination: 240ml PO every 10min till clean, usu 3-4l*
or	**Hyperosmotic laxative** (stimulates fluid secretion and intestinal motility)	**Sodium phosphate** (Fleet enema, Fleet Phospho-Soda)	*one day prior to examination: 45ml PO x 2*
plus sos	**Stimulant laxative** (stimulates colonic peristaltic, antiresorptive, water binding)	**Bisacodyl** (Correctol, Dulcolax, Gens)	*10mg PO*

8.   Nephrology, Urology

Y. Howard Lien, MD
Professor, Section of Nephrology, College of Medicine,
University of Arizona, Tucson, AZ

8.1   Renal Failure
8.1.1   Acute Renal Failure

Volume overload

poss	**Loop diuretic**	**Furosemide** (Lasix)	*50-500mg IV bolus or 40-100mg/h IV infusion*
plus	**Thiazide diuretic**	**Chlorothiazide** (Diazide)	*250-500mg IV with Lasix*

Hyperkalemia

poss	**Cation exchanger** (remove K⁺ from GI)	**Polystyrene sulfonate** (Kayexalate, Kionex, SPS, Gens)	*20g in 100ml 20% sorbitol every 4-6h* **Caution:** *contraindicated in patients with bowel obstruction*
or	**Redistribution** (intracellular shift of K^+)	**Glucose 50% + Regular insulin**	*50ml + 10U IV over 20min*
or	**Redistribution** (intracellular shift of K^+)	**Sodium bicarbonate 8.4%** (1meq/ml)	*50ml IV over 5min*
or	**Membrane antagonism** (inhib. of depolarization)	**Calcium gluconate 10%** (4.5meq/ml)	*10ml IV over 2-3min* **Caution:** *digitalis tox.↑*

Metabolic acidosis

poss	**Buffer** (ph neutralization)	**Sodium bicarbonate 8.4%** (1meq/ml)	*Ini Tx (meq) = (12-bicarb) x 0.7 x kg IV over 4-8h* **Caution:** *may reduce ionized calcium*

8.1.2   Chronic Renal Failure

Anemia

	Erythrocyte colony stimulating factor (RBC production ↑, maturation, activation)	**Erythropoietin** (Epogen, Procrit)	*50-100U/kg SC qwk; iron suppl if iron def. follow hematocrit*
or		**Darbepoetin** (Aranesp)	*0.45µg/kg/wk SC*

Secondary Hyperparathyroidism

poss	Vitamin D (parathyroid hormone ↓)	Calcitriol (Rocaltrol)	0.25-1µg PO tiw. Caution: hypercalcemia
		Doxercalciferol (Hectorol)	2.5-10µg PO tiw

Hyperphosphatemia

poss	Phosphate binder (reduce phosphorus)	Calcium carbonate (Mylanta, Titralac, Tums)	500-1000mg PO tid with meals
		Calcium acetat (Phoslo)	667-2000mg PO tid with meals

Other possible therapies: antihypertensives (esp. ACE inhibitors, caution: hyperkalemia), protein restriction, antilipidemics

8.2 Glomerulonephritis

8.2.1 Goodpasture's Syndrome

	Glucocorticoid (anti-inflammatory, immunosupprressive)	Methylprednisolone (Medrol, Depo-Medrol, Solu-Medrol, Gens)	1g IV qd for 3d, then switch to Prednisone
		Prednisone (Deltasone, Meticorten, Prednisone Intensol, Gens)	1mg/kg PO qd until remission, then taper slowly
plus	Alkylating agent (immunosuppressive)	Cyclophosphamide (Cytoxan, Neosar)	2mg/kg PO qd x 6-12mo Caution: leukopenia
plus	Plasmaphoresis (removes anti-GBM Abs)	Plasmaphoresis	qd till anti-GBM not detected (usu 1-2wk)

8.2.2 Pauci-immune GN (Wegener's Granulomatosis, Microscopic Polyangiitis)

	Glucocorticoid (anti-inflammatory, immunosupprressive)	Methylprednisolone (Medrol, Depo-Medrol, Solu-Medrol, Gens)	1g IV qd for 3d, then switch to Prednisone
		Prednisone (Deltasone, Meticorten, Prednisone Intensol, Gens)	1mg/kg PO qd until remission, then taper slowly

plus	Alkylating agent (immunosuppressive)	Cyclophosphamide (Cytoxan, Neosar)	2mg/kg PO qd x 6-12mo **Caution**: leukopenia
	Plasmaphoresis (removes ANCA)	Plasmaphoresis	qd until pulmonary hemorrhage or ARF improved (usu 1-2wks)

Indications of plasmaphoresis: pulmonary hemorrhage or severe acute renal failure

8.2.3   Idiopathic Cryoglobinemia

	Glucocorticoid (anti-inflammatory, immunosuppressive)	Methylprednisolone (Medrol, Depo-Medrol, Solu-Medrol, Gens)	1g IV qd for 3d, then switch to Prednisone
		Prednisone (Deltasone, Meticorten, Prednisone Intensol, Gens)	1mg/kg PO qd until remission, then taper slowly
plus	Alkylating agent (immunosuppressive)	Cyclophosphamide (Cytoxan, Neosar)	2mg/kg PO qd x 6-12mo **Caution**: leukopenia
plus	Plasma exchange	Plasma exchange replace with FFP	qd until ARF improved (usu 1-2wks)

8.2.4   Lupus Nephritis

	Glucocorticoid (anti-inflammatory, immunosuppressive)	Methylprednisolone (Medrol, Depo-Medrol, Solu-Medrol, Gens)	1g IV qd for 3d, then switch to Prednisone
		Prednisone (Deltasone, Meticorten, Prednisone Intensol, Gens)	1mg/kg PO qd until remission, then taper slowly
plus	Alkylating agent (immunosuppressive)	Cyclophosphamide (Cytoxan, Neosar)	Bolus TX with 0.5-$0.75g/m^2$ IV q1mo x 6, then q3mo x 6, 2yr course **Caution**: leukopenia
or	Purine synthesis inhibitor (immunosuppressive)	Azathioprine (Imuran, Gens)	50-100mg PO qd **Caution**: leukopenia
or		Mycophenolate Mofetil (CellCept)	1g PO bid x 6mo, then 500 mg bid x 6mo; **Caution**: diarrhea, leukopenia

Lupus nephritis WHO classification: Class I: no Tx; Class II: only glucocorticoids; Class III see plan

8.2.5	Acute Post-Streptococcal GN (in active Strep. Infection)		
	Penicillin	**Penicillin V** (Beepen VK, Betapen VK, Ledercillin VK, Pen-vee K, Uticillin VK, V-cillin VK, Veetids)	*500mg PO bid x 10d*
or	Macrolide	**Erythromycin** (E-Base, E-Mycin, Eryc, Ery-Tab, Ilosone, Gens)	*500mg PO qid x 10d, in penicillin allergy*

8.2.6	Minimal Change GN		
Initial treatment			
	Glucocorticoid (anti-inflammatory, immunosupprressive)	**Prednisone** (Deltasone, Meticorten, Prednisone Intensol, Gens)	*1mg/kg PO qd until 1wk after remission, then 1mg/kg PO qod x 1mo, then taper over mo*
Glucocorticoid-resistant or glucocorticoid-dependent			
	Immunosuppressant (Calcineurin inhibitor)	**Cyclosporine** (Neoral, Sandimmune, Gens)	*5mg/kg PO qd x 6mo, taper 25% q3mo.* **Caution**: *nephrotoxic, follow blood level*
or	Alkylating agent (immunosuppressive)	**Cyclophosphamide** (Cytoxan, Neosar)	*2mg/kg PO qd x 8wk*

8.2.7	Membranous GN		
	Glucocorticoid (anti-inflammatory, immunosuppressive)	**Prednisone** (Deltasone, Meticorten, Prednisone Intensol, Gens)	*1mg/kg PO qd x 6mo, then taper over several mo*
plus sos	Alkylating agent (immunosuppressive)	**Cyclophosphamide** (Cytoxan, Neosar)	*1.5mg/kg PO qd x 6m*
or	Immunosuppressant (calcineurin inhibitor, cytokine synthesis ↓)	**Cyclosporine** (Neoral, Sandimmune, Gens)	*5mg/kg PO qd x 6mo, taper 25% q3m;* **Caution**: *nephrotoxic, →blood level*
or	Purine synthesis inhibitor (immunosuppressive)	**Mycophenolate Mofetil** (CellCept)	*500-1000mg PO bid x 12-24 mo* **Caution**: *diarrhea, leukopenia*

8.2.8	Focal Segmental Sclerosing GN		
Initial treatment			
	Glucocorticoid (anti-inflammatory, immunosuppressive)	**Prednisone** (Deltasone, Meticorten, Prednisone Intensol, Gens)	*1mg/kg PO qd x 6 mo, then taper over several months*
Glucocorticoid-resistant			
	Immunosuppressant (calcineurin inhibitor, cytokine synthesis ↓)	**Cyclosporine** (Neoral, Sandimmune, Gens)	*5mg/kg PO qd x 6mo, taper 25% q3m;* **Caution:** *nephrotoxic, →blood level*
or	**Alkylating agent** (immunosuppressive)	**Cyclophosphamide** (Cytoxan, Neosar)	*2mg/kg qd for 8wk* **Caution:** *leukopenia*

8.2.9	IgA Nephropathy		
	Glucocorticoid (anti-inflammatory, immunosuppressive)	**Prednisone** (Deltasone, Meticorten, Prednisone Intensol, Gens)	*1mg/kg PO qd x 6-9mo then taper over several months*
or	**Fish oil** (Omega-3 fatty acid)	**Fish oil** (Omacor, Coromega)	*1.8g EPA and 1.2g DHA PO qd x 24mo*

8.2.10	Idiopathic Membranoproliferative GN (MPGN)		
	Glucocorticoid (anti-inflammatory, immunosuppressive)	**Prednisone** (Deltasone, Meticorten, Prednisone Intensol, Gens)	*1mg/kg PO qd x 6-9mo then taper over several months*
	Alkylating agent (immunosuppressive)	**Cyclophosphamide** (Cytoxan, Neosar)	*2mg/kg qd for 6-12mo* **Caution:** *leukopenia*

8.2.11	Hepatitis C-related MPGN/ Cryoglobulinemia		
	Interferon	**Interferon alpha**	*3MIU IV tiw x 12mo* **Caution:** *neuropsychiatric events, bone marrow toxicity*
		Peginterferon alpha–2b (Peg-Intron)	*1.5µg/kg SC qwk x 12mo*

plus	**Antiviral agent**	Ribavirin	*400mg PO bid x 12 mo* *Contraindication: renal failure;* **Caution**: *hemolytic anemia*

Sustained virological responders have partial or complete remission of MPGN

8.2.12 General Treatment for Nephrotic Syndrome

Intractable edema

	Loop diuretic	**Furosemide** (Lasix, Gens)	*20-40mg PO bid*
plus sos	**Thiazide diuretic**	**Metolazone** (Zaroxolyn)	*2.5-5mg PO given same time as PO furosemide* **Caution**: *hypokalemia*

Hyperlipidemia

	HMG-CoA rductase inhibitor (lipid reduction)	**Simvastatin** (Zocor)	*10-40mg PO qd*
		Atorvastatin (Lipitor)	*10-40mg PO qd*

Caution: rhabdomyelysis, abnormal liver functions

	Cholesterol absorption inhibitor	**Etetimibe** (Zetia)	*10mg PO qd*

Proteinuria

	ACE inhibitor (renoprotective, antihypertensive)	**Benazepril** (Lotensin)	*2.5-20mg PO qd* **Caution**: *coughing;* *Follow renal function*
		Lisinopril (Prinivil, Zestril)	
		Quinapril (Accupril)	
		Ramipril (Altace)	
	Angiotensin II receptor blocker (renoprotective, antihypertensive)	**Candesartan** (Atacand)	*16-32mg PO qd*
		Irbesartan (Avapro)	*75-200mg PO qd*
		Losartan (Cozaar)	*25-100mg PO qd*
		Valsartan (Diovan)	*80-320 mg PO qd*

Blood pressure and blood sugar control important! Follow renal function!

8.3   Acute Tubulointerstitial Nephritis

Glucocorticoid (anti-inflammatory, immunosuppressive)	**Prednisone** (Deltasone, Meticorten, Prednisone Intensol, Gens)	*60mg PO qd x 10d, then taper rapidly*

Stop culprit agent first, glucocorticoid only given for severe acute renal failure or poor response to drug withdrawal

8.4   Hemolytic Uremic Syndrome

	Plasma exchange	**Plasma exchange with FFP**	*4-7x/wk until thrombocytopenia resolved (usu. 1-2wk)*
or/ plus	**Glucocorticoid** (anti-inflammatory, immunosuppressive)	**Prednisone** (Deltasone, Meticorten, Prednisone Intensol, Gens)	*1mg/kg PO qd until 1wk after remission, then 1mg/kg PO qod x 1mo, then taper*

8.5   Polycycstic Kidney Disease

Cyst infection

	Fluoroquinolone	**Ciprofloxacin** (Cipro)	*250mg bid x 14d*
		Ofloxacin (Floxin)	*200mg bid x 14d*
or	**Folate + p–Aminobenzoic acid antagonist**	**Sulfamethoxazole + Trimethoprim** (Bactrim, Cotrim, Septra, Sulfatrim, Sulfamethoprim, Gens)	*800+160mg PO bid x 14d Avoid in last 2wk of preg. E coli resist. 18% in US.*

Hypertension

	ACE inhibitor	**Benazepril** (Lotensin)	*2.5-20mg PO qd.* **Caution:** *coughing Follow renal function*
		Lisinopril (Prinivil, Zestril)	
		Quinapril (Accupril)	
		Ramipril (Altace)	

	Angiotensin II receptor blocker	**Candesartan** (Atacand)	*16-32mg PO qd*
		Irbesartan (Avapro)	*75-200mg PO qd*
		Losartan (Cozaar)	*25-100mg PO qd*
		Valsartan (Diovan)	*80-320mg PO qd*

8.6 Diabetes Insipidus (DI)
8.6.1 Central DI

	Vasopressin	**Desmopressin** (DDAVP)	*0.05-0.5mg PO bid or 0.1-0.2ml (10-20µg) intranasally bid*

8.6.2 Nephrogenic DI

	Thiazide diuretic	**Hydrochlorothiazide/ HCTZ**	*25-50mg PO qd*
	K$^+$ sparing diuretic	**Amiloride**	*5-10mg PO qd*

8.7 Contrast Nephropathy

	Antioxidant	**N-Acetylcysteine** (Mucomyst)	*1000mg 1h before and 4h after*
or	Na-Bicarbonate	**Na-Bicarbonate**	*150meq/l, 3ml/kg over 1h before +1ml/kg/h x 6h*

8.8 Nephrolithiasis
8.8.1 Urate Stone

	Urine alkalinization (Litholysis)	**K$^+$ citrate** (Urocit K)	*10-20meq PO tid. Keep urine pH > 6.5*
plus	Xanthine oxidase inhibitor (uric acid synthesis ↓)	**Allopurinol** (Zyloprim, Gens)	*100-300mg PO qd*

Water intake >2l/d for all stones!

8.8.2 Cystine Stone

	Urine alkalinization (Litholysis)	**K$^+$ citrate** (Urocit K)	*20-30meq PO tid Keep urine pH >7.0*

poss. plus	**Disulfide formation with Cysteine** (cystine formation ↓)	**Captopril** (Capoten, Gens)	*25-75mg PO bid;* **Caution:** *↑ PO intake to avoid hypotension*
or		**Alpha-Mercapto-propionylglycine** (Tiopronin)	*0.5-4g qd*
final resort		**D-Penicillamine** (Cuprimine, Depen)	*150mg qid*

Water intake >2l/d for all stones!

8.8.3   Calcium Oxalate Stone

	Thiazide diuretic (Ca secretion ↓)	**Chlorthalidone** (Hygro-ton, Thalitone, Gens)	*25-50mg PO qd*
poss.	**K⁺ sparing diuretic** (Ca secretion ↓)	**Amiloride** (Midamor, Gens)	*5-10mg PO qd*
poss.	**Xanthine oxidase inhibitor** (uric acid synthesis ↓)	**Allopurinol** (Zyloprim, Gens)	*100-300mg PO qd*
poss.	**Citrate replacement** (litholysis)	**K⁺ citrate** (Urocit K)	*10-20meq PO tid. Keep urine citrate >320mg/d*

Water intake >2l/d for all stones!

8.8.4   Calcium Phosphate Stone (Associated with Renal Tubular Acidosis)

poss.	**Citrate replacement** (litholysis)	**K⁺ citrate** (Urocit K)	*10-20meq PO tid. Keep urine citrate >320mg/d*

Water intake >2l/d for all stones!

8.9   Renal Colic

8.9.1   Basic Therapy

	Non-steroid anti-inflammatory drug	**Ketorolac** (Acular PF, Toradol, Gens)	*60mg IV or IM, 100mg PR, then cont with PO NSAID. Stop 3d before lithotripsy.*
		Indomethacin (Indocin SR, Indocin, Gens)	*25-50mg tid*

Caution: Acute renal failure if dehydrated

or	Narcotic analgesic	Morphine sulfate	*4-10mg IV slowly or 5-20mg IM, q4h prn*
or	Narcotic analgesic	Hydrocodone/ Acetaminophen (Vicodin, Norco)	*5-10mg + 325-650mg PO q4-6h prn*

CT of kidney and pelvis without contrast to guide therapy

8.9.2 Renal Colic with UTI

	Fluoroquinolone	Ciprofloxacin (Cipro)	*250mg bid x 3d*
		Ofloxacin (Floxin)	*200mg bid x 3d 7d for preg and DM*
or	Folate + p-Aminobenzoic acid antagonist	Sulfamethoxazole + Trimethoprim (Bactrim, Cotrim, Septra, Sulfatrim, Sulfamethoprim, Gens)	*800+160mg PO bid x 3d. 7d for preg and DM. Avoid in last 2wk of preg. E coli resist. 18% in US.*

8.10 Cystitis

8.10.1 Acute Urinary Tract Infection (UTI, Cystitis-Urethritis)

	Fluoroquinolone	Ciprofloxacin (Cipro)	*250mg PO bid x 3d*
		Ofloxacin (Floxin)	*200mg PO bid x3 d 7d for preg and DM*
or	Folate + p-Aminobenzoic acid antagonist	Sulfamethoxazole + Trimethoprim (Bactrim, Cotrim, Septra, Sulfatrim, Sulfamethoprim, Gens)	*800+160mg PO bid x 3d. 7d for preg and DM. Avoid in last 2wk of preg. E coli resist. 18% in US.*
or	Macrolide	Azithromycin (Zithromax)	*1g PO qd (once) for possible STD (C. trachomatis)*

8.10.2 Recurrent Urinary Tract Infection

ini	Initial treatment as acute UTI		
then	Folate + p-Aminobenzoic acid antagonist	Sulfamethoxazole + Trimethoprim (Bactrim, Cotrim, Septra, Sulfatrim, Sulfamethoprim, Gens)	*400+80mg PO qd as longterm Tx*

8.11 Pyelonephritis

8.11.1 Outpatient. Mild Clinical Course, without Predisposing Factors

	Fluoroquinolone	**Ciprofloxacin** (Cipro)	*500mg PO bid x 7d*
		Ofloxacin (Floxin)	*400mg PO bid x 7d*
or	Aminopenicillin + β–lactamase inhibitor	**Amoxicillin + Clavulanic acid** (Augmentin)	*500+125mg PO tid x 14d*
or	Folate + p-Aminobenzoic acid antagonist	**Sulfamethoxazole + Trimethoprim** (Bactrim, Cotrim, Septra, Sulfatrim, Sulfamethoprim, Gens)	*800+160mg PO bid x 14d*
or	Cephalosporin 2nd generation	**Cefuroxime** (Ceftin)	*500mg PO bid x 14d*

8.11.2 Nosocomial. Severe Clinical Course with Predisposing Factors

Initial treatment (adjust antibiotics according to culture result; switch to PO 1–2d after defervescence)

	Fluoroquinolone	**Ciprofloxacin** (Cipro)	*400mg PO bid x 7d*
		Ofloxacin (Floxin)	
or	Cephalosporin 3rd generation	**Ceftriaxone** (Rocephin)	*2g IV qd. Do not use if suspect enterococcus*
or	Penicillin 4th generation	**Piperacillin** (Pipracil)	*3g IV q6h*

After defervescence, continue with PO antibiotics based on culture and sensitivity results to complete 2wk course

	Fluoroquinolone	**Ciprofloxacin** (Cipro)	*500mg PO bid*
		Ofloxacin (Floxin)	*400mg PO bid*
or	Aminopenicillin + β-lactamase inhibitor	**Amoxicillin + Clavulanic acid** (Augmentin)	*500+125mg PO tid*
or	Folate + p-Aminobenzoic acid antagonist	**Sulfamethoxazole + Trimethoprim** (Bactrim, Cotrim, Septra, Sulfatrim, Sulfamethoprim, Gens)	*800+160mg PO bid*

8.12 Urosepsis

Initial treatment (adjust antibiotics according to culture results)

	Cephalosporin 3rd gen.	Ceftriaxone (Rocephin)	2g IV q8h
plus	Aminoglycoside	Gentamicin (Garamycin, U-gencin, Gens)	5mg/kg IV qd;
	Caution: nephrotoxic, follow blood levels!		
Or			
	Fluoroquinolone	Ciprofloxacin (Cipro)	400mg IV q12h
Or			
	Penicillin 4th gen. + β-lactamase inhibitor	Piperacillin + Tazobactam (Zosyn)	4g+0.5g IV q8h
Or			
	Carbapenem	Imipenem (Primaxin)	0.5g IV q6h

8.13 Urethritis
8.13.1 Initial Treatment

	Fluoroquinolone	Ciprofloxacin (Cipro)	250mg bid x 3d
		Ofloxacin (Floxin)	200mg bid x 3d
or	Folate + p-Aminobenzoic acid antagonist	Sulfamethoxazole + Trimethoprim (Bactrim, Cotrim, Septra, Sulfatrim, Sulfamethoprim, Gens)	800+160mg PO bid x 3d

8.13.2 Mycoplasma

	Macrolide	Clarithromycin (Biaxin)	250mg PO bid x 7d
or		Azithromycin (Zithromax)	500mg PO qd x 3d
or	Tetracycline	Doxycycline (Doryx, Vibramycin)	100mg PO qd x 7d

8.13.3	Chlamydia Trachomatis		
	Macrolide	**Azithromycin** (Zithromax)	*1g PO qd (once)*
or	**Tetracycline**	**Doxycycline** (Doryx, Vibramycin)	*100mg PO qd x 7d*
8.13.4	**Candida**		
	Imidazole derivative (antimycotic)	**Fluconazole** (Diflucan)	*100-200mg PO qd x 10-14d*
8.13.5	**Trichomonas Vaginalis**		
	Nitroimidazole (antiparasitic)	**Metronidazole** (Flagyl, Metro, Metryl, Protostat, Gens)	*2g PO x 1d or 500mg PO bid x 7d*

8.14 Prostatitis

8.14.1	Acute Bacterial Prostatitis		
	Fluoroquinolone	**Ofloxacin** (Floxin)	*400mg PO x 1d, then 300mg bid x 10d*
or	**Cephalosporin 3rd gen.**	**Ceftriaxone** (Rocephin)	*250mg IM x 1d*
plus	**Tetracycline**	**Doxycycline** (Doryx, Vibramycin)	*100mg PO qd x 10d*
8.14.2	**Chronic Bacterial Prostatitis**		
	Fluoroquinolone	**Ciprofloxacin** (Cipro)	*500mg bid x 4wk*
		Ofloxacin (Floxin)	*300mg bid x 6wk*
or	**Folate + p-Aminobenzoic acid antagonist**	**Sulfamethoxazole + Trimethoprim** (Bactrim, Cotrim, Septra, Sulfatrim, Sulfamethoprim, Gens)	*800+160mg PO bid x 1-3mo*

8.14.3 Nonbacterial Prostatitis

	Tetracycline	**Doxycycline** (Doryx, Vibramycin)	*100mg PO qd x 10d*
poss. cont. with	Nitroimidazole (anti-protozoa drug)	**Metronidazole** (Flagyl, Metro, Metryl, Protostat, Gens)	*500mg PO bid x 10d*
or	Macrolide	**Erythromycin** (E-Base, E-Mycin, Eryc, Ery-Tab, Ilosone, Gens)	*500mg PO qid x 10d*

8.15 Epididymitis

	Fluoroquinolone	**Ofloxacin** (Floxin)	*300mg bid x 10d*
or	Cephalosporin 3rd gen.	**Ceftriaxone** (Rocephin)	*250mg IM x 1d*
plus	Tetracycline	**Doxycycline** (Doryx, Vibramycin)	*100mg qd x 10d*

8.16 Prostate Hyperplasia

	Alpha-1-blocker (makes urination easier)	**Doxazosin** (Cardura, Gens)	*Start 1mg PO hs, then incr to 2-5mg PO bid.* **Caution**: *orthostatic hypotension with ini Tx*
		Prazosin (Minipress, Minipress XL, Gens)	
		Terazosin (Hytrin, Gens)	
or	5-alpha-reductase inhibitor (hyperplasia↓)	**Finasteride** (Proscar)	*5mg PO qd (long-term Tx)*

8.17 Urinary Incontinence
8.17.1 Stress Incontinence

poss.	Estrogen	**Conjugated estrogen** (Premarin)	*0.3 -0.6mg PO qd or vaginal crm 2g topically qd*
poss.	Alpha-Sympathomim. (bladder neck toning)	**Midodrine** (ProAmatine)	*2.5-5mg PO bid* **Caution**: *hypertension*

8.17.2	Urge Incontinence		
poss.	**Antispasmodic** (parasympatholytic, spasmolytic)	**Oxybutynin** (Ditropan, Ditropan XL, Gens)	*5mg PO bid-tid*
or poss.		**Tolterodine** (Detrol, Detrol LA)	*1-2mg PO bid*
or poss.	**Spasmolytic** (detrusor hyperactivity↓)	**Flavoxate** (Urispas)	*200mg PO tid-qid*
poss.	**Tricycl. Anti-depressant** (modulation of urinary urgency feeling)	**Imipramine** (Tofranil, Gens)	*25-100mg PO qhs*

9. Infections

Helmut Albrecht, MD
Division of Infectious Diseases
Emory University, Atlanta, GA

9.1 Empiric Antimicrobial Therapy

Cardiovascular System
- Infective endocarditis →39
- Endocarditis prophylaxis →41

Respiratory System
- Chronic bronchitis, acute exacerbations →88
- Community-acquired pneumonia (CAP) →89
- Hospital-acquired pneumonia →95
- Pleural infections →97
- Infections in cystic fibrosis →102

Rheumatolgy
- Reactive arthritis/Reiter's syndrome (enteropathic form) →108

Gastroenterology
- Infectious esophagitis →141
- PUD, Helicobacter →142
- Diverticular disease →143
- Biliary/necrotizing pancreatitis →145
- Viral hepatitis →146

Nephrology, Urology
- Urinary tract infection (UTI) →161
- Pyelonephritis →162
- Urosepsis →163
- Acute post-streptococcal glomerulonephritis →155
- Urethritis →163
- Prostatitis →164
- Epididymitis →165

Neurology
- Meningitis →216
- Encephalitis →216

Ophthalmology
- Hordeolum, chalazion →241
- Blepharitis →241
- Infections of the eyelids →243
- Dacryoadenitis →244
- Dacryocystitis →246
- Conjunctivitis →246
- Keratitis →250

ENT
- Rhinosinusitis →275
- Furuncles of the nose →277
- Tonsillitis →278
- Pharyngitis →278
- Bacterial laryngitis, epiglottitis →279
- Perichondritis, external otitis →280
- Herpes zoster oticus →282
- Otitis media →282
- Mastoiditis →283
- Sialadenitis →284

Dermatology
- Abscess →285
- Acne vulgaris →285
- Lyme borreliosis →298
- Condyloma acuminata →289
- Eczema →292
- Scabies, pediculosis →298
- Erysipelas, erythrasma →293
- Folliculitis →294
- HSV infection →295
- Impetigo →296
- Tinea, tinea versicolor →303
- Rosacea →301
- Sexually transmitted diseases →302
- Pityriasis rosea →300

9.2 Specific Antibacterial Therapy
9.2.1 Organism – Antibiotic

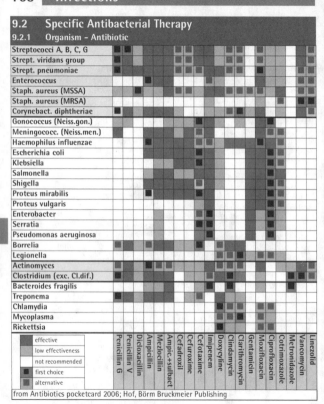

Organisms (rows):
- Streptococci A, B, C, G
- Strept. viridans group
- Strept. pneumoniae
- Enterococcus
- Staph. aureus (MSSA)
- Staph. aureus (MRSA)
- Corynebact. diphtheriae
- Gonococcus (Neiss.gon.)
- Meningococc. (Neiss.men.)
- Haemophilus influenzae
- Escherichia coli
- Klebsiella
- Salmonella
- Shigella
- Proteus mirabilis
- Proteus vulgaris
- Enterobacter
- Serratia
- Pseudomonas aeruginosa
- Borrelia
- Legionella
- Actinomyces
- Clostridium (exc. Cl.dif.)
- Bacteroides fragilis
- Treponema
- Chlamydia
- Mycoplasma
- Rickettsia

Antibiotics (columns):
Penicillin G, Penicillin V, Dicloxacillin, Ampicillin, Mezlocillin, Ampic.+sulbact, Cefadroxil, Cefuroxime, Cefotaxime, Imipenem, Doxycycline, Clindamycin, Clarithromycin, Gentamicin, Moxifloxacin, Ciprofloxacin, Cotrimoxazole, Metronidazole, Vancomycin, Linezolid

Legend:
- effective
- low effectiveness
- not recommended
- first choice
- alternative

from Antibiotics pocketcard 2006; Hof, Börm Bruckmeier Publishing

9.2.2 Acinetobacter Species

Empiric therapy

	Carbapenem	Imipenem–Cilastim (Primaxin)	0.5g IV q6h
		Meropenem (Merrem)	1g IV q8h

Alternatives

	Cephalosporin 3rd Gen.	Ceftazidime (Ceptaz, Fortaz, Tazicef, Tazidime, Gens)	1-2g IV q8-12h
or	Cephalosporin 4th Gen.	Cefepime (Maxipime)	1-2g IV q12h
or	Penicillin 4th Gen.	Piperacillin (Pipril)	3-4g IV/IM q4-6h
PLUS	Fluoroquinolone	Ciprofloxacin (Cipro)	400mg IV q8-12h
or	Aminoglycoside (often most sensitive to amikacin)	Amikacin (Amikin, Gens)	15mg/kg IV qd (check level in prolonged Tx)

Carbapenem-resistant isolates

	Acylaminopenicillin + lactamase inhibitor	Ampicillin + Sulbactam (Unasyn)	3g IV q6h
or	Polymxyin	Colistin (Coly-Mycin M)	5mg/kg qd (div bid-qid)

If hospital-acquired often multi-drug resistant, adjust empiric Tx according to local susceptibility pattern. Double coverage for serious infection until susceptibility tests available. Duration of Tx dependant on location and severity of infection.

9.2.3 Actinomyces Species

Empiric therapy

wk1 - wk4 (wk6)	Benzylpenicillin	Penicillin G (Pfizerpen, Gens)	10-20 M IU IV qd (div qid or cont Inf), for 4-6wk
then		Penicillin V (Beepen VK, Betapen VK, Ledercillin VK, Pen-vee K, Uticillin VK, V-cillin VK, Veetids, Gens)	0.5-1g qid PO for 2-6mo

Alternatives

or	Cephalosporin 3rd Gen.	Ceftriaxone (Rocephin)	*1-2g IV qd*
or	Lincosamide	Clindamycin (Cleocin, Gens)	*300-600mg IV tid-qid*
or	Chloramphenicol	Chloramphenicol (Chloromycetin)	*12.5-15mg/kg IV q6h*

In Penicillin allergic patients or Penicillin-resistant isolates

	Tetracycline	Doxycycline (Doryx, Monodox, Periostat, Vibramycin, Gens)	*0.1g IV/PO bid*

9.2.4 Alcaligenes xylosoxidans

	Carbapenem	Imipenem–Cilastim (Primaxin)	*0.5g q6h*
		Meropenem (Merrem)	*1g q8h*
or	Folate antagonist + p-Aminobenzoic acid antagonist	Sulfamethoxazole + Trimethoprim (Cotrimoxazole) (Bactrim, Cotrim, Septra, Sulfamethoprim, Sulfatrim, Gens)	*8-10mg trimethoprim equivalent/kg IV (div bid-qid) or 800+160mg PO bid*

Alcaligenes xylosoxidans are usually resistant to penicillins, cephalosporins (some sensitive to ceftazidime), FQ, aztreonam. Duration of Tx dependant on location and severity of infection.

9.2.5 Bacillus anthracis (Anthrax)

	Fluoroquinolone	Ciprofloxacin (Cipro)	*500-750mg PO bid, or 400mg IV bid, max 400mg IV tid for 100d*
or	Tetracycline	Doxycycline (Doryx, Monodox, Periostat, Vibramycin, Gens)	*d1: 200mg PO/IV qd, then 100mg PO/IV qd*

Note: Severe infections (pulmonary, bacteremia, meningitis) usually require multi-drug and intensive supportive Tx. Immediately notify local/federal authorities.

9.2.6	Bacteroides fragilis		
Infection below diaphragm			
	Antiprotozoal (nitroimidazole)	**Metronidazole** (Flagyl, Metro, Metryl, Protostat, Gens)	250-500mg PO bid-qid, 500mg IV bid-qid
Infection above diaphragm			
	Lincosamide	**Clindamycin** (Cleocin, Gens)	150-450mg PO bid-tid, 200-600mg IV tid-qid

Also effective: carpapenems, moxifloxacin, beta-lactams/beta-lactamase inhibitor combinations, chloramphenicol. Duration of Tx depends on location/severity of infection

9.2.7	Bordetella pertussis		
1st choice			
	Macrolide	**Clarithromycin** (Biaxin)	250mg PO bid for 2wk
In intolerance			
	Folate antagonist + p-Aminobenzoic acid antagonist	**Sulfamethoxazole + Trimethoprim (Cotrimoxazole)** (Bactrim, Cotrim, Septra, Sulfamethoprim, Sulfatrim, Gens)	8-10mg trimethoprim equivalent/kg IV (div bid-qid for 14d), 800+160mg PO bid

9.2.8	Borrelia burgdorferi		
1st choice			
	Tetracycline	**Doxycycline** (Doryx, Monodox, Periostat, Vibramycin, Gens)	d1: 200mg PO/IV qd, then 100mg PO/IV qd
In children			
	Benzylpenicillin	**Penicillin V** (Beepen VK, Betapen VK, Ledercillin VK, Pen-vee K, Uticillin VK, V-cillin VK, Veetids, Gens)	0.6-1.5 M IU PO tid for 21d

In neuroborreliosis			
	Cephalosporin 3rd Gen.	**Ceftriaxone** (Rocephin)	*1-2g IV qd for 2-4wk*

9.2.9	Borrelia recurrentis		
1st choice	Tetracycline	**Doxycycline** (Doryx, Monodox, Periostat, Vibramycin, Gens)	*0.2g IV once*
or	Benzylpenicillin	**Penicillin G** (Pfizerpen, Gens)	*0.5-10 M IU IV qid-6x/d*

9.2.10	Brucella abortus, melitensis, suis, canis		
1st choice			
	Tetracycline	**Doxycycline** (Doryx, Monodox, Periostat, Vibramycin, Gens)	*200mg PO qd for 6wk*
Plus	Antimycobacterial	**Rifampin** (Rifadin, Rimactane, Generic)	*10mg/kg PO qd for 6wk*
or	Aminoglycoside	**Gentamicin** (Garamycin, U-gencin, Gens)	*2-5mg/kg IV/IM qd (monitor drug level)*
CH < 8 years			
	Folate antagonist + p-Aminobenzoic acid antagonist	**Sulfamethoxazole + Trimethoprim (Cotrimoxazole)** (Bactrim, Cotrim, Septra, Sulfamethoprim, Sulfatrim, Gens)	*800+160mg PO/IV bid*
Plus	Antimycobacterial	**Rifampin** (Rifadin, Rimactane, Generic)	*10mg/kg PO qd*
or	Aminoglycoside	**Gentamicin** (Garamycin, U-gencin, Generic)	*2-5mg/kg IV/IM qd (monitor drug level)*

Endocarditis, meningoencephalitis, relapses

	Tetracycline	**Doxycycline** (Doryx, Monodox, Periostat, Vibramycin, Gens)	*500mg PO qd-tid*
plus	Aminoglycoside	**Gentamicin** (Garamycin, U-gencin, Gens)	*2-5mg/kg IV/IM qd (monitor drug level)*
plus	Antimycobacterial	**Rifampin** (Rifadin, Rimactane, Generic)	*10mg/kg PO qd*

Chronic disease, osteomyelitis

1st choice	Aminoglycoside	**Gentamicin** (Garamycin, U-gencin, Gens)	*2-5mg/kg IV/IM qd (monitor drug level)*
plus	Antimycobacterial	**Rifampin** (Rifadin, Rimactane, Generic)	*10mg/kg PO qd*
plus	Tetracycline	**Doxycycline** (Doryx, Monodox, Periostat, Vibramycin, Gens)	*500mg PO qd-tid for 5mo*
OR	Antimycobacterial	**Rifampin** (Rifadin, Rimactane, Generic)	*10mg/kg PO qd*
plus	Folate antagonist + p-Aminobenzoic acid antagonist	**Sulfamethoxazole + Trimethoprim (Cotrimoxazole)** (Bactrim, Cotrim, Septra, Sulfamethoprim, Sulfatrim, Gens)	*800+160mg PO/IV bid*

9.2.11   Campylobacter

Enteritis (Campylobacter jejuni)

	Macrolide	**Clarithromycin** (Biaxin)	*250mg PO bid for 3d*
or	Fluoroquinolone	**Ciprofloxacin** (Cipro)	*250-750mg PO bid for 3d*

Note: resistance to fluoroquinolones rising

Sepsis (Campylobacter fetus)

	Fluoroquinolone	**Ciprofloxacin** (Cipro)	*400mg IV bid*
plus	Aminoglycoside	**Gentamicin** (Garamycin, U-gencin, Gens)	*2-5mg/kg IV/IM qd (monitor drug level)*

9.2.12   Chlamydia

Psittacosis (Chlamydia psittaci)

	Tetracycline	**Doxycycline** (Doryx, Monodox, Periostat, Vibramycin, Gens)	*200mg PO/IV bid*
or	Macrolide	**Azithromycin** (Zithromax)	*500mg PO qd*
		Clarithromycin (Biaxin)	*500mg PO bid*

Urethritis (Chlamydia trachomatis)

	Macrolide	**Azithromycin** (Zithromax)	*500mg PO qd (once)*
or	Tetracycline	**Doxycycline** (Doryx, Monodox, Periostat, Vibramycin, Gens)	*100mg PO bid for 7-20d*

Lymphogranuloma venereum (Chlamydia trachomatis)

	Tetracycline	**Doxycycline** (Doryx, Monodox, Periostat, Vibramycin, Gens)	*200mg PO/IV qd for 3wk*
or	Macrolide	**Clarithromycin** (Biaxin)	*250mg PO bid*

9.2.13   Clostridium perfringens (Gas Gangrene)

Primary Tx: surgical debridement

plus	Benzylpenicillin	**Penicillin G** (Pfizerpen, Gens)	*24 M IU IV qd (div qid-6x/d)*
plus	Lincosamide	**Clindamycin** (Cleocin, Gens)	*900mg IV tid*

In penicillin allergy

	Macrolide	**Erythromycin** (Erythrocin, Gens)	*1g IV q6h*
or	Tetracycline	**Doxycycline** (Vibramycin, Gens)	*200mg IV bid*

9.2.14 Clostridium botulinum (Botulism)

Specific antidote (toxin binding ⇒ toxin effects ↓)	**Botulinin Antitoxin (ABE)** (CDC)	*1-2 vials IV q4h for 4-5 doses, duration depends on response; not indicated in infants*

Comment: Consider use as bioweapon if no reasonable exposure history. Prolonged supportive therapy (irreversible binding of toxin).

9.2.15 Clostridium tetani (Tetanus)

Antibiotic

	Benzylpenicillin	**Penicillin G** (Pfizerpen, Gens)	*12-24 M IU IV qd (div qid-6x/d) for >30d*
or	**Tetracycline**	**Doxycycline** (Vibramycin, Gens)	*200mg IV bid for >30d*

Symptomatic

	Benzodiazepine (sedation)	**Diazepam** (Diastat, Diazepam Intensol, Valium, Gens)	*5-15mg IV/PR*
plus	**Non-depolarising muscle relaxant** (compet. ACH-antagonism)	**Pancuronium bromide** (Pavulon)	*Ini 0.008-0.01mg/kg IV, then 0.02-0.04mg/kg IV*
plus	**Beta-1-selective blocker** (CO ↓, neg. chronotropic, neg. inotropic, central sympathetic activity ↓)	**Metoprolol** (Lopressor, Toprol-xl, Gens)	*50-100mg PO qd-bid; 5-10mg slowly IV qd, max 15mg IV*
plus	**Immunoglobulin serum** (toxin neutralization)	**Tetanus Immune Globulin** (BayTet)	*6000 IU IM*

9.2.16 Clostridium difficile (Pseudomembranous Colitis)

	Antiprotozoal (nitroimidazole)	**Metronidazole** (Flagyl, Protostat, Gens)	*500mg PO tid for 10-14d*
or	**Glycopeptide**	**Vancomycin** (Vancocin, Vancoled, Gens)	*250mg PO qid for 10d*

9.2.17 Corynebacterium diphtheriae

	Immunoglobulin serum (toxin neutralisation)	**Diphtheria antitoxin**	*30,000–50,000 IU IV Inf over 1h, up to 120.000 IU*
plus	**Macrolide**	**Clarithromycin** (Biaxin)	*250mg PO bid for 10d*

9.2.18 Coxiella burnetti

Acute Q fever

	Tetracycline	**Doxycycline** (Doryx, Monodox, Periostat, Vibramycin, Gens)	*d1: 200mg PO/IV qd, then 100mg PO/IV qd for 10–12d or 3d after defervescence*
or	**Macrolide**	**Clarithromycin** (Biaxin)	*250–500mg PO bid*

Endocarditis, chronic disease

	Tetracycline	**Doxycycline** (Doryx, Monodox, Periostat, Vibramycin, Gens)	*d1: 200mg PO/IV qd, then 100mg PO/IV qd (>12mo)*
plus	**Antimycobacterial**	**Rifampin** (Rifadin, Rimactane, Gens)	*10mg/kg PO/IV qd, max 750mg*
Or	**Fluoroquinolone**	**Ciprofloxacin** (Cipro)	*500–750mg PO bid, or 200–400mg IV bid*
plus	**Antimycobacterial**	**Rifampin** (Rifadin, Rimactane, Gens)	*10mg/kg PO/IV qd, max 750mg*

9.2.19 Enterobacter

If hospital acquired, often beta-lactamase producers

	Carbapenem	**Imipenem–Cilastim** (Primaxin)	*0.5g IV q6h*
		Meropenem (Merrem)	*1g IV q8h*
or	**Fluoroquinolone**	**Ciprofloxacin** (Cipro)	*400mg IV bid*

9.2.20 Enterococci

Ampicillin-sensitive isolates

	Aminopenicillin	**Ampicillin** (Omnipen, Principen, Totacillin, Gens)	*2g IV qid-6x/d*
plus	Aminoglycoside	**Gentamicin** (Garamycin, U-gencin, Gens)	*1-1.5mg/kg IV/IM q8h (monitor drug level)*

In Penicillin allergy or resistance

	Glycopeptide	**Vancomycin** (Vancocin, Vancoled, Gens)	*1g IV bid as short Inf (monitor drug level)*
plus	Aminoglycoside	**Gentamicin** (Garamycin, U-gencin, Gens)	*1-1.5mg/kg IV/IM q8h (monitor drug level)*

Vancomycin-resistant E. faecium

	Oxazolidinone	**Linezolid** (Zyvox)	*600mg IV bid*
or	Streptogramine	**Dalfopristin + Quinupristin** (Synercid)	*7.5mg/kg IV q8h*

9.2.21 Escherichia coli

Community acquired

	Fluoroquinolone	**Ciprofloxacin** (Cipro)	*250-750mg PO bid*

Hospital acquired

Hospital acquired strains may become multi-drug resistant and require alternative antibiotics. Choice based on local susceptability pattern.

9.2.22 Francisella tularensis (Tularemia)

	Aminoglycoside	**Gentamicin** (Garamycin, U-gencin, Gens)	*1-1.5mg/kg IV/IM q8h for 7-14d (monitor drug level)*

9.2.23 Gonococci

Note: always treat patient and partner for Gonococci and Chlamydia!

Urethritis, cervicitis, proctitis (uncomplicated)

	Cephalosporin 3rd Gen.	Ceftriaxone (Rocephin)	0.125g IV qd (once)
or	Fluoroquinolone	Ciprofloxacin (Cipro)	500mg PO qd (once)
Plus	Tetracycline	Doxycycline (Doryx, Monodox, Periostat, Vibramycin, Gens)	200mg PO qd for 7d
or	Macrolide	Azithromycin (Zithromax)	1g PO once

Complicated (salpingitis, endometritis, epididymitis, ...)

	Cephalosporin 3rd Gen.	Ceftriaxone (Rocephin)	1g IV qd for 10d
Plus	Tetracycline	Doxycycline (Doryx, Monodox, Periostat, Vibramycin, Gens)	200mg PO/IV qd for 7d
or	Macrolide	Azithromycin (Zithromax)	1g PO once

Sepsis, arthritis, meningitis, endocarditis

	Cephalosporin 3rd Gen.	Ceftriaxone (Rocephin)	1g IV qd for 2-4wk

Generalized disease in newborns

After amniotic fliud infection and gonorrhea of the mother

	Cephalosporin 2nd Gen.	Cefuroxime (Kefurox, Zinacef, Gens)	100mg/kg IV qd

9.2.24 Haemophilus ducreyi (soft chancre)

In general

	Cephalosporin 3rd Gen.	Ceftriaxone (Rocephin)	0.25g IV qd (once)
or	Fluoroquinolone	Ciprofloxacin (Cipro)	1g PO qd for 3d

9.2.25 Haemophilus influenza

Sepsis

	Cephalosporin 3rd Gen.	Ceftriaxone (Rocephin)	1–2g IV qd
or	Fluoroquinolone	Ciprofloxacin (Cipro)	200–400mg IV bid

Epiglottitis in children

	Cephalosporin 2nd Gen.	Cefuroxime (Kefurox, Zinacef, Gens)	0.75–1.5g IV tid for 1wk

Pneumonia

	Cephalosporin 3rd Gen.	Ceftriaxone (Rocephin)	1g IV q12h for 10–14d

Meningitis

	Cephalosporin 3rd Gen.	Ceftriaxone (Rocephin)	2g IV q12h for 10–14d

In children additionally to prevent hearing damage

	Glucocorticoid (anti-inflammatory)	Dexamethasone (Decadron, Hexadrol, Mymethasone, Gens)	0.15mg/kg IV q6h for 4d

Prophylaxis following exposure to patient with meningitis

	Antimycobacterial	Rifampin (Rifadin, Rimactane, Generic)	10mg/kg PO bid for 4d

9.2.26 Klebsiella

	Cephalosporin 3. Gen.	Ceftriaxone (Rocephin)	1g IV q12h
plus	Fluoroquinolone	Ciprofloxacin (Cipro)	250–750mg PO bid, 100–200mg IV bid

In severe infection

plus	Aminoglycoside	Gentamicin (Garamycin, U-gencin, Gens)	2–5mg/kg IV/IM qd (monitor drug level)

Duration depending on location and severity. Hospital acquired strains may become multi-drug resistant + require modified Tx depending on local susceptibility patterns.

9.2.27 Legionella

	Fluoroquinolone	**Ciprofloxacin** (Cipro)	*400mg IV bid*
or	Macrolide	**Azithromycin** (Zithromax)	*500mg IV qd*
In severe infection			
plus	Antimycobacterial	**Rifampin** (Rifadin, Rimactane, Generic)	*0.6g IV qd;* **Ped** *6-10mg/kg IV qd*
Following defervescence			
	Macrolide	**Clarithromycin** (Biaxin)	*250-500mg PO bid for 1-3wk*

9.2.28 Leptospira

In mild infection			
	Tetracycline	**Doxycycline** (Doryx, Monodox, Periostat, Vibramycin, Gens)	*200mg PO qd for 7d*
In severe infection			
	Benzylpenicillin	**Penicillin G** (Pfizerpen, Gens)	*1.5 M IU IV qid for 7d*
or	Aminopenicillin	**Ampicillin** (Omnipen, Principen, Totacillin, Gens)	*0.5-2g IV qid*

9.2.29 Listeria

Sepsis, endocarditis, meningoencephalitis			
	Aminopenicillin	**Ampicillin** (Omnipen, Principen, Totacillin, Gens)	*2g IV q4h,* **Ped** *400mg/kg IV qd for >4-6wk*
poss. plus	Aminoglycoside	**Gentamicin** (Garamycin, U-gencin, Gens)	*2-5mg/kg IV/IM qd (monitor drug level)*

Comment: Ampicillin plus Sulfamethoxazole + Trimethoprim may become preferred Tx for patients with meningitis

Penicillin allergy			
	Folate antagonist + **p-Aminobenzoic acid** **antagonist**	**Sulfamethoxazole +** **Trimethoprim** **(Cotrimoxazole)** (Bactrim, Cotrim, Septra, Sulfamethoprim, Sulfatrim, Gens)	*800+160mg IV bid*
poss. plus	**Aminoglycoside**	**Gentamicin** (Garamycin, U-gencin, Gens)	*2-5mg/kg IV/IM qd* *(monitor drug level)*

9.2.30	Meningococci – Meningitis, Sepsis		
1st choice	**Benzylpenicillin**	**Penicillin G** (Pfizerpen, Gens)	*0.1-4 M IU IV qid-6x/d* *(until 7-10d after* *defervescence)*
or	**Cephalosporin 3rd Gen.**	**Ceftriaxone** (Rocephin)	*4g IV qd,* **Ped** *50-80mg/kg IV qd*
	Cephalosporin in Penicillin allergy		

9.2.31	Meningococci – Prophylaxis after Exposure to Meningococcal Carrier		
1st choice	**Antimycobacterial**	**Rifampin** (Rifadin, Rimactane, Generic)	*0.6g PO bid,* **Ped** *10mg/kg PO* *bid for 2d*
or	**Fluoroquinolone**	**Ciprofloxacin** (Cipro)	*500mg Tab qd (once)*
Or	**Cephalosporin 3rd Gen.**	**Ceftriaxone** (Rocephin)	*1g IV qd (once)*
	Cephalosporin in pregnancy		

9.2.32	Mycobacterium tuberculosis		
Treatment of latent tuberculosis (prophylaxis)			
	Antimycobacterial	**Isoniazid** (Laniazid, Gens)	*5mg/kg PO qd (max* *300mg);* **Ped** *10mg/kg* *PO qd for 6-9mo*
plus	**Vitamin** (for prevention of INH- associated neuropathy)	**Vitamin B6 =** **Pyridoxine** (Gens)	*25-50mg PO qd for* *6-9mo*

Pulmonary tuberculosis

	Antimycobacterial	**Rifampin** (Rifadin, Rimactane, Generic)	10mg/kg PO qd for 6mo
plus	Antimycobacterial	**Isoniazid** (Laniazid, Gens)	5mg/kg PO qd for 6mo
plus	Vitamin (for prevention of INH-associated neuropathy)	**Vitamin B6 = Pyridoxine** (Gens)	25-50mg PO qd for 6mo
plus	Antimycobacterial	**Ethambutol** (Myambutol, Gens)	15mg/kg PO qd for 2mo
plus	Antimycobacterial	**Pyrazinamide** (Gens)	25-30mg/kg PO qd for 2mo

Extrapulmonary tuberculosis

	Antimycobacterial	**Rifampin** (Rifadin, Rimactane, Generic)	10mg/kg PO qd for 1-2yr
plus	Antimycobacterial	**Isoniazid** (Laniazid, Gens)	5mg/kg PO qd for 1-2yr
plus	Vitamin (for prevention of INH-associated neuropathy)	**Vitamin B6 = Pyridoxine** (Gens)	25-50mg PO qd for 1-2yr
plus	Antimycobacterial	**Ethambutol** (Myambutol, Gens)	15mg/kg PO qd for 2mo
plus	Antimycobacterial	**Pyrazinamide** (Gens)	25-30mg/kg PO qd for 2mo

Miliary tuberculosis, TB meningitis, and TB suppurative pleuritis

	Glucocorticoid (anti-inflammatory, sensitivity of β-recept. ↑)	**Prednisone** (Deltasone, Meticorten, Prednisone Intensol, Gens)	Ini 30-50mg PO qd, taper to 10-20mg PO qd for 1-4wk

Some experts recommend addition of glucocorticoids for miliary tuberculosis, TB meningitis, and TB suppurative pleuritis

9.2.33 Mycoplasma

	Macrolide	**Clarithromycin** (Biaxin)	250mg PO bid
or	Tetracycline	**Doxycycline** (Doryx, Monodox, Periostat, Vibramycin, Gens)	d1: 200mg PO/IV, then 100mg PO qd

9.2.34 Nocardia

1st choice

	Folate antagonist + p-Aminobenzoic acid antagonist	Sulfamethoxazole + Trimethoprim (Cotrimoxazole) (Bactrim, Cotrim, Septra, Sulfamethoprim, Sulfatrim, Gens)	800+160mg PO/IV bid for 6mo (longer in CNS disease or immuno-compromised)
or	Tetracycline	Minocycline (Dynacin, Minocin, Vectrin, Gens)	200mg PO/IV bid for 6mo

In severe cases, until stabilization

	Carbapenem	Imipenem–Cilastatin (Primaxin)	0.5-1g IV tid-qid, max 50mg/kg/d or 4g/d
plus	Cephalosporin 3. Gen.	Cefotaxime (Claforan, Gens)	1g IV tid
then	After stabilization: Cotrimoxazole or Tetracycline (see 1st choice)		

9.2.35 Pneumococci – Pneumonia (usually lobar-/segmental pneumonia)

1st choice

	Benzylpenicillin	Penicillin G (Pfizerpen, Gens)	0.5-10 M IU IV qid-6x/d for 8-10d
or	Cephalosporin 3rd Gen.	Ceftriaxone (Rocephin)	1g IV qd, Ped 50mg/kg qd for 8-10d

In penicillin or cephalosporin allergy

	Macrolide	Clarithromycin (Biaxin)	250mg PO bid

In areas or patients with increased risk of penicillin resistance

	Fluoroquinolone	Moxifloxacin (Avelox)	400mg IV/PO qd
		Levofloxacin (Levaquin)	500mg IV/PO qd
		Gatifloxacin (Tequin)	400mg IV/PO qd

9.2.36 Pneumococci – Meningitis

	Glycopeptide	**Vancomycin** (Vancocin, Vancoled, Gens)	*1g IV bid as short Inf,* **Ped** *50mg/kg IV qd for 10-14d*
Plus	Benzylpenicillin	**Penicillin G** (Pfizerpen, Gens)	*1-2 M IU IV qid,* **Ped** *0.5 M IU/kg qd for 10-14d*
or	Cephalosporin 3rd Gen.	**Ceftriaxone** (Rocephin)	*2g IV bid,* **Ped** *50mg/kg IV bid for 10-14d*

9.2.37 Proteus mirabilis (especially UTI)

Aminopenicillin	**Ampicillin** (Omnipen, Principen, Totacillin, Gens)	*1g PO tid-qid; 0.5-2g IV tid-qid, max 5g IV tid*

9.2.38 Proteus vulgaris

Cephalosporin 3. Gen.	**Cefotaxime** (Claforan, Gens)	*1-2g IV bid*

9.2.39 Pseudomonas aeruginosa

Sepsis, pneumonia

	Carbapenem	**Imipenem–Cilastatin** (Primaxin)	*1g IV tid-qid, max 50mg/kg/d or 4g/d*
or	Cephalosporin 3rd Gen.	**Ceftazidime** (Ceptaz, Fortaz, Tazicef, Tazidime, Gens)	*2g IV tid,* **Ped** *100-200mg/kg IV qd*
or	Acylaminopenicillin	**Piperacillin** (Pipracil)	*4g IV tid*
Plus	Fluoroquinolone	**Ciprofloxacin** (Cipro)	*400mg IV q8h*
or	Aminoglycoside	**Gentamicin** (Garamycin, U-gencin, Gens)	*2-5mg/kg IV/IM qd (monitor drug level)*

UTI

Fluoroquinolone	**Ciprofloxacin** (Cipro)	*250-750mg PO bid*

9.2.40 Rickettsia

	Tetracycline	**Doxycycline** (Doryx, Monodox, Periostat, Vibramycin, Gens)	*200mg IV/PO qd (until 6d after defervescence)*

Rickettsia prowazeki (typhus), R. rickettsii (Rocky Mountain spotted fever), R. tsutsugamushi (scrub typhus)

9.2.41 Salmonella

	Fluoroquinolone	**Ciprofloxacin** (Cipro)	*500-750mg PO bid for 2wk*
or	Cephalosporin 3rd Gen.	**Ceftriaxone** (Rocephin)	*1-2 g IV qd,* **Ped:** *50mg/kg IV qd for 2wk*

Chronic Carriers

	Fluoroquinolone	**Ciprofloxacin** (Cipro)	*500mg PO bid for 4wk*

9.2.42 Serratia

	Aminoglycoside	**Amikacin** (Amikin, Gens)	*10-15mg/kg/d IV/IM qd*
Plus	Cephalosporin 3rd Gen.	**Ceftazidime** (Ceptaz, Fortaz, Tazicef, Tazidime)	*2g IV tid*
or	Fluoroquinolone	**Ciprofloxacin** (Cipro)	*400-750mg PO/IV bid*
or	Carbapenem	**Imipenem–Cilastatin** (Primaxin)	*0.5-1g IV tid-qid, max 50mg/kg/d or 4g/d*

9.2.43 Shigella

Adults

	Fluoroquinolone	**Ciprofloxacin** (Cipro)	*500mg PO bid for 1-3d*

Children

	Folate antagonist + p-Aminobenzoic acid antagonist	**Sulfamethoxazole + Trimethoprim (Cotrimoxazole)** (Bactrim, Cotrim, Septra, Sulfamethoprim, Sulfatrim, Gens)	*10-15mg TMP eyuivalent/kg PO/IV bid for 5-7d*

9.2.44 Staphylococcus, Methicillin-sensitive (MSSA)

Naphthylpenicillin	**Nafcillin** (Nallpen, Unipen, Gens)	*2g IV tid-6x/d*

In Penicillin-allergy

Cephalosporin 1st Gen.	**Cefazolin** (Ancef, Kefzol, Gens)	*0.5-2g IV bid-tid (until defervescence)*

9.2.45 Staphylococcus aureus, Methicillin-resistant (MRSA) and Coagulase-negative Staphylococcus species

	Glycopeptide	**Vancomycin** (Vancocin, Vancoled, Gens)	*1g IV bid as short Inf for 7-28d;* **Ped** *50mg/kg IV qd*
or	Oxazolidinone	**Linezolid** (Zyvox)	*600mg IV bid for 7-28d*

152. Stevens DL, Herr D, Lampiris H, Hunt JL, Batts DH, Hafkin B. Linezolid versus Vancomycin for the Treatment of Methicillin-Resistant Staphylococcus aureus Infections. Clin Infect Dis 2002; 34: 1481-90

Sepsis, endocarditis

add	Aminoglycoside	**Gentamicin** (Garamycin, U-gencin, Gens)	*1-1.5mg/kg IV/IM tid for 3d*

In infection involving bones or prosthetic material

add	Antimycobacterial	**Rifampin** (Rifadin, Rimactane, Generic)	*10mg/kg PO qd*

9.2.46 Streptococci, Group A

Strep throat, scarlet fever

Benzylpenicillin	**Penicillin V** (Beepen VK, Betapen VK, Ledercillin VK, Pen-vee K, Uticillin VK, V-cillin VK, Veetids, Gens)	*0.6-1.5 M IU PO tid for 2wk*

In penicillin allergy

Macrolide	**Clarithromycin** (Biaxin)	*250mg PO bid,* **Ped** *12mg/kg qd*

Sepsis			
	Benzylpenicillin	**Penicillin G** (Pfizerpen, Gens)	*10-20 M IU IV qd for 1-2 wk*
then		**Penicillin V** (Beepen VK, Betapen VK, Ledercillin VK, Pen-vee K, Uticillin VK, V-cillin VK, Veetids, Gens)	*1.5-3 M IU PO qd for 2wk*

In penicillin allergy			
	Cephalosporin 1st Gen.	**Cefazolin** (Ancef, Kefzol, Gens)	*0.5-2g IV bid-tid*

9.2.47 Streptococci, Beta-hemolytic

Subacute bacterial endocarditis			
	Benzylpenicillin	**Penicillin G** (Pfizerpen, Gens)	*20-30 M IU IV qd (div in 2-3 short Inf) for 3wk*
plus	Aminoglycoside	**Gentamicin** (Garamycin, U-gencin, Gens)	*1-1.5mg/kg IV/IM tid (monitor drug level)*

In penicillin allergy			
	Cephalosporin 1st Gen.	**Cefazolin** (Ancef, Kefzol, Gens)	*0.5-2g IV bid-tid for 3wk*
plus	Aminoglycoside	**Gentamicin** (Garamycin, U-gencin, Gens)	*2-5mg/kg IV/IM qd (monitor drug level)*

9.2.48 Treponema pallidum, Aquired Syphilis

Primary/secondary syphilis			
	Depot Benzylpenicillin	**Procaine Penicillin** (Pfizerpen-as, Wycillin, Gens)	*1.2 M IU IM once*

Late latent syphilis			
	Depot Benzylpenicillin	**Procaine Penicillin** (Pfizerpen-as, Wycillin, Gens)	*1.2 M IU IM qwk for 3wk*

2

Tertiary syphilis, neurosyphilis

	Benzylpenicillin	**Penicillin G** (Pfizerpen, Gens)	*10-20 M IU IV Inf qd (div qid-6x/d or cont Inf) for 14d*

In penicillin allergy

	Cephalosporin 3rd Gen.	**Ceftriaxone** (Rocephin)	*1g IV qd for 14d*
or	Tetracycline	**Doxycycline** (Vibramycin, Gens)	*200mg IV qd for 3wk*

9.2.49 Vibrio cholerae (Cholera)

Antibiotic Therapy

	Folate antagonist + p-Aminobenzoic acid antagonist	**Sulfamethoxazole + Trimethoprim** (Bactrim, Cotrim, Septra, Sulfamethoprim, Sulfatrim, Gens)	*800+160mg PO/IV bid for 3d*
or	Tetracycline	**Doxycycline** (Doryx, Monodox, Periostat, Vibramycin, Gens)	*300mg PO/IV qd once*
or	Fluoroquinolone	**Ciprofloxacin** (Cipro)	*500mg PO bid for 3d*

Adjuvant Therapy

poss.	Glucose electrolyte solution (volume substitution)	**WHO „Oral rehydration formula"** (Glucose, Na^+Cl^-, $Na^+HCO_3^-$, K^+Cl^-)	*20g Glucose + 3.5g Na^+Cl^- + 2.5g $NaHCO_3^-$ + 1.5g K^+Cl^- in 1 l H_2O PO prn*
poss.	Glucose solution (nutrition substitution)	**Glucose 20%**	*Ca. 2000 kcal qd prn*
poss.	Isotonic saline solution (volume + electrolyte substitution)	**Saline 0.9%**	*IV after CVP and elecrolytes prn*
poss.	Cristalloid plasma expander (volume + electrolyte substitution)	**Ringer's solution**	*prn*

9.2.50   Vibrio parahaemolyticus

poss.	**Folate antagonist + p-Aminobenzoic acid antagonist**	**Sulfamethoxazole + Trimethoprim** (Cotrimoxazole) (Bactrim, Cotrim, Septra, Sulfamethoprim, Sulfatrim, Gens)	*800+160mg PO/IV bid for 5-7d*
or	**Tetracycline**	**Doxycycline** (Doryx, Monodox, Periostat, Vibramycin, Gens)	*200mg PO/IV qd for 5-7d*

9.2.51   Yersinia

	Folate antagonist + p-Aminobenzoic acid antagonist	**Sulfamethoxazole + Trimethoprim (Cotrimoxazole)** (Bactrim, Cotrim, Septra, Sulfamethoprim, Sulfatrim, Gens)	*800+160mg PO/IV bid*
or	**Fluoroquinolone**	**Ciprofloxacin** (Cipro)	*500mg PO bid*

9.3   Specific Antiviral Therapy
9.3.1   Cytomegalovirus

In retinitis, pneumonia in Non-HIV

	Virostatic (purine antagonist, inhibits DNA polymerase)	**Ganciclovir** (Cytovene)	*5-10mg/kg IV over 1h qd for 2-4wk*
or	**Virostatic** (pyrophosphate analogue, then polymerase inhibitor)	**Foscarnet** (Foscavir)	*wk1-3: 90mg/kg IV bid, then 90-120mg/kg IV qd for 2-4wk*

Prevention in transplant recipients

	Virostatic (purine antagonist, inhibits DNA polymerase)	**Ganciclovir** (Cytovene, Valcyte)	*500-1000mg PO tid (up to 120d after transplantation)*

9.3.2   Ebstein-Barr Virus (Inf. Mononucleosis)

General measures

poss.	**Aniline derivative** (analgesic, antipyretic)	**Acetaminophen** (Acephen, Neopap, Tylenol, Gens)	*500-1000mg PO/PR tid-qid prn*

In severe infection

	Virostatic (purine antagonist, DNA polymerase inhibitor)	**Acyclovir** (Zovirax, Gens)	*10mg/kg IV tid or 800mg 5x/d PO for 2-3wk*

9.3.3   Herpes Simplex Virus

Meningoencephalitis, systemic infection

	Virostatic (purine antagonist, inhibits DNA polymerase)	**Acyclovir** (Zovirax, Gens)	*10mg/kg IV tid for 2-3wk*

Primary genital infection

	Virostatic (purine antagonist, inhibits DNA polymerase)	**Valacyclovir** (Valtrex)	*400mg PO tid*

Recurring genital infection

	Virostatic (purine antagonist, inhibits DNA polymerase)	**Acyclovir** (Zovirax, Gens)	*Ini 400mg PO tid, then 200mg PO bid*

Keratitis

	Virostatic (pyrimidine antagonist ⇒ transcription errors)	**Trifluridine solution (oph)** (Viroptic)	*Admin q4h*

Herpes labialis

	Virostatic (purine antagonist, inhibits DNA polymerase)	**Acyclovir 0.5%** (Zovirax)	*Admin q4h for ca. 5d*

9.3.4 Human Immunodeficiency Virus, Anti-HIV Therapy

Note: HIV expertise required

Combination of 2 nucleoside/nucleotide reverse transcriptase inhibitors (NRTIs)

NRTI (nucleoside reverse transcriptase inhibitor ⇒ virostatic)	**Zidovudine (AZT)** (Retrovir)	250-300mg PO bid (not azt + d4T)
	Zalcitabine (ddC) (Hivid)	0.75mg PO tid (not ddl + ddC)
	Didanosine (ddl) (Videx, Videx EC)	<60kg: 250mg PO qd, >60kg: 400mg PO qd (not ddl + ddC)
	Lamivudine (3TC) (Epivir, Epivir-HBV)	150mg PO bid
	Stavudine (d4T) (Zerit)	<60kg: 30mg PO bid, >60kg: 40mg PO bid (not azt + d4T)
	Abacavir (ABC) (Ziagen)	300mg PO bid (Caution: hypersensitivity)
NRTI (nucleotide RTI ⇒ virostatic)	**Tenofovir Disoproxil Fumarate (TDF)** (Viread)	300mg PO qd

With either a protease inhibitor

Plus	Protease inhibitor (production of immature, non-infectious viral hulls, virostatic)	**Amprenavir (APV)** (Agenerase)	1200mg PO bid
		Indinavir (IDV) (Crixivan)	800mg PO tid or 800mg PO bid in combination with ritonavir
		Nelfinavir (NFV) (Viracept)	1250mg PO bid
		Ritonavir (RTV) (Norvir)	600mg PO bid
		Ritonavir (RTV) + Lopinavir (LPV) (Kaletra)	400/100mg PO bid
		Saquinavir (SQV) (Fortovase, Invirase)	600mg PO tid or 400mg PO bid in combination with ritonavir

Or a non-nucleoside reverse transcriptase inhibitor (NNRTIs)

or	NNRTI (non-nucleoside reverse-transcriptse inhibitor ⇒ virostatic)	Delavirdine (DLV) (Rescriptor)	400mg PO tid
		Efavirenz (EFV) (Sustiva)	600mg PO qd
		Nevirapine (NVP) (Viramune)	200mg PO qd for 14d, then 200mg PO bid

9.3.5   HIV, Opportunistic Infections

Pneumocystis carinii, 1st choice

	Folate antagonist + p-Aminobenzoic acid antagonist	Sulfamethoxazole + Trimethoprim (Cotrimoxazole) (Bactrim, Cotrim, Septra, Sulfamethoprim, Sulfatrim, Gens)	5mg TMP equivalent/kg IV tid for 21d

Pneumocystis carinii, in moderate/severe pneumonia (pO₂ <70 mm Hg)

plus	Glucocorticoid (anti-inflammatory, sensitivity of β-recept. ↑)	Prednisone (Deltasone, Meticorten, Prednisone Intensol, Gens)	40mg bid for 5d, then 40mg qd for 5d, then 20mg qd for 11d

Pneumocystis carinii, in Cotrimoxazole failure/intolerance

	Antiparasitic (diamidine derivative)	Pentamidine (Pentam, Gens)	4mg/kg IV qd for 14-21d
or	Hydroxy-naphthochinone	Atovaquone (Mepron)	1500mg PO qd for 21d
or	Lincosamide	Clindamycin (Cleocin, Gens)	600mg PO/IV tid
plus	Anti-malarial	Primaquine (Gens)	30mg base PO qd

Pneumocystis carinii, primary prophylaxis

	Folate antagonist + p-Aminobenzoic acid antagonist	Sulfamethoxazole + Trimethoprim (Cotrimoxazole) (Bactrim, Septra, Gens)	800+160mg IV tiw
or	Hydroxy-naphthochinone	Atovaquone (Mepron)	1500mg PO qd
or	Antimycobacterial	Dapsone (Gens)	100mg PO qd

Toxoplasma gondii, 1st choice →201

	Dihydrofolate reductase inhibitor	Pyrimethamine (Daraprim, Gens)	100-200 mg PO qd for 3d, then 50-75 mg (until >3wk after resolution)
plus	Sulfonamide (folate antagonist)	Sulfadiazine (Gens)	4-8g PO qd
plus	Folic acid derivative (thrombocytopenia Pro)	Folinic acid (Leucovorin, Gens)	15mg PO qd

Toxoplasma gondii, alternative →201

	Dihydrofolate reductase inhibitor	Pyrimethamine (Daraprim, Gens)	100-200 mg PO qd for 3d then 50-75 mg (until 3wk after resolution)
plus	Lincosamide	Clindamycin (Cleocin, Gens)	600mg PO/IV qid
plus	Folic acid derivative (thrombocytopenia Pro)	Folinic acid (Leucovorin, Gens)	15mg PO qd

Toxoplasma gondii, primary prophylaxis →201

	Folate antagonist + p-Aminobenzoic acid antagonist	Sulfamethoxazole + Trimethoprim (Cotrimoxazole) (Bactrim, Cotrim, Septra, Sulfamethoprim, Sulfatrim, Gens)	800+160mg PO qd
or	Hydroxy-naphthochinone	Atovaquone (Mepron)	1500-2250mg PO qd
or	Sulfone derivative	Dapsone (Gens)	0.1g PO qd
Plus	Dihydrofolate reductase inhibitor	Pyrimethamine (Daraprim, Gens)	25mg PO biw
Plus	Folic acid derivative (thrombocytopenia Pro)	Folinic acid (Leucovorin, Gens)	15mg PO biw

Mycobacterium tuberculosis →181

	Antimycobacterial	Rifampin (Rifadin, Rimactane, Generic)	10mg/kg PO qd for 6mo
plus	Antimycobacterial	Isoniazid (Laniazid, Gens)	5mg/kg PO qd for 6mo

plus	**Vitamin** (prevention of INH-associated neuropathy)	**Vitamin B6 = Pyridoxine** (Gens)	*25-50mg PO qd for 6mo*
plus	**Antimycobacterial**	**Ethambutol** (Myambutol, Gens)	*15mg/kg PO qd for 2mo*
plus	**Antimycobacterial**	**Pyrazinamide** (Gens)	*25-30mg/kg PO qd for 2mo*
Mycobacterium avium			
	Macrolide	**Clarithromycin** (Biaxin)	*500mg PO bid*
plus	**Antimycobacterial**	**Ethambutol** (Myambutol, Gens)	*15mg/kg PO qd*
poss. plus	**Antimycobacterial**	**Rifabutin** (Mycobutin)	*300-450mg PO qd*
Varizella-Zoster virus →196			
1sr choice	**Virostatic** (purine antagonist, DNA polymerase inhibitor)	**Acyclovir** (Zovirax, Gens)	*10mg/kg IV tid*
Cytomegalovirus (CMV: retinitis, colitis, →189)			
	Virostatic (purine antagonist, DNA polymerase inhibitor)	**Ganciclovir** (Cytovene, Valcyte)	*5mg/kg IV bid for 14-21d, then 5mg/kg IV qd (5-7d/wk) or 1g PO tid*
or	**Virostatic** (pyrophosphate analogue, DNA polymerase inhibitor)	**Foscarnet** (Foscavir)	*90mg/kg IV bid over >1h for 14-21d, then 90-120mg/kg qd over >2h*
Cryptococcus neoformans →203			
	Antifungal – polyene (antimycotic, membrane deposition)	**Amphotericin B** (Fungizone, Gens)	*Test dose 1mg slow IV, if tolerated: 0.7mg/kg IV qd over 2-6h*
plus	**Antimetabolite** (antimycotic)	**Flucytosine** (Ancobon)	*25mg/kg PO qid*
Or in mild cases	**Antifungal – azole**	**Fluconazole** (Diflucan)	*400mg IV qd*

Cryptosporidium

No established effective therapy! Symptomatic control of diarrhea and amelioration of immune deficiency mainstay of therapy!

poss.	**Antiparasitic** (benzimidazole derivative)	**Albendazole** (Albenza)	*400mg PO bid*
poss.	**Aminoglycoside**	**Paromomycin** (Humatin)	*500mg PO tid for 2-4wk*
poss.	**Macrolide**	**Azithromycin** (Zithromax)	*1200mg PO qd for 4wk*

Microsporida

	Antiparasitic (benzimidazole derivative)	**Albendazole** (Albenza)	*400mg PO bid*

Candidiasis, mucosal →202

	Antifungal – azole	**Fluconazole** (Diflucan)	*100-200mg PO qd*

Candidiasis, severe →202

	Imidazole derivative (antimycotic)	**Fluconazole** (Diflucan)	*Up to 800mg IV qd*
or	**Antifungal – polyene** (antimycotic, membrane deposition)	**Amphotericin B** (Fungizone, Gens)	*Test dose 1mg slow IV, if tolerated: 0.3-0.6mg/kg IV qd over 2-6h* **Caution:** *toxicity*
poss. plus	**Antimetabolite** (antimycotic)	**Flucytosine** (Ancobon)	*25-30mg/kg IV tid*

9.3.6   Influenza Virus

Uncomplicated

poss.	**Opioid** (antitussive)	**Codeine** (Gens)	*30-50mg PO bid, max 150mg qd prn*
poss.	**Aniline derivative** (analgesic, antipyretic)	**Acetaminophen** (Acephen, Infants' feverall, Neopap, Tylenol, Gens)	*500-1000mg PO/PR tid-qid prn*

Severe			
or	**Virostatic** (neuroaminidase inhib.)	**Zanamivir** (Relenza)	*Inhal 10mg bid for 5d*
		Oseltamivir (Tamiflu)	*75mg PO bid for 5d*

Also effective in Influenza A			
or	**Virostatic**	**Amantadine** (Symmetrel)	*100mg PO bid (qd if >65yr) for 3-7d*
		Rimantadine (Flumadine)	*100mg PO bid (qd if >65yr) for 3-7d*

9.3.7	Measles Virus		
poss.	**Aniline derivative** (analgesic, antipyretic)	**Acetaminophen** (Acephen, Infants' feverall, Neopap, Tylenol, Gens)	*10-15mg/kg PO/PR q4-6h prn, max 5 doses/d*

9.3.8	Mumps Virus		
poss.	**Aniline derivative** (analgesic, antipyretic)	**Acetaminophen** (Acephen,Neopap,Tylenol, Infants' feverall, Gens)	*10-15mg/kg PO/PR q4-6h prn, max 5 doses/d*

9.3.9	Respiratory Syncytial Virus (RVS)		
	Virostatic (purine antagonist)	**Ribavirin** (Rebetol, Virazole)	*Dissolve 6g in 300ml, as aerosol over 12-18h for 3-7d*

9.3.10	Varicella–Zoster Virus		

Varicella (in immunosuppressed patient or pneumonia)			
	Virostatic (purine antagonist, inhibits DNA polymerase)	**Acyclovir** (Zovirax, Gens)	*10mg/kg IV tid for 10d*

Shingles			
	Virostatic (purine antagonist, inhibits DNA polymerase)	**Valacyclovir** (Valtrex)	*500-1000mg PO tid*

9.4 Specific Antiparasitic Therapy
9.4.1 Ascaris lumbricoides (roundworm)

	Anthelmintic (tubulin binding, glucose uptake ↓)	Mebendazole (Vermox)	100mg PO bid x 6 doses or 500mg PO once
poss.	Anthelmintic (benzimidazole)	Albendazole (Albenza)	400mg PO (once)
or	Anthelmintic (inhibits choline esterase)	Pyrantel (Combantrin, Pin-X)	10mg/kg PO to max 1g (once)

9.4.2 Echinococci

| | Antiparasitic (benzimidazole) | Albendazole (Albenza) | 400mg PO bid for 28d |

Effective in E. granulosus = dog tapeworm infection, E. multilocularis = fox tapeworm infection usually requires surgical intervention

9.4.3 Entamoeba histolytica
Hepatic abscess, enteritis

| | Antiprotozoal (nitroimidazole) | Metronidazole (Flagyl, Metro, Metryl, Protostat, Gens) | 750mg PO/IV tid for 10d |
| then | Aminoglycoside | Paromomycin (Humatin) | 500mg PO tid for 7d |

9.4.4 Enterobius vermicularis (pinworm, oxyuriasis)

	Anthelmintic (inhibits choline esterase)	Pyrantel (Combantrin, Pin-X)	10mg/kg PO once, rep after 14d
or	Anthelmintic (benzimidazole)	Albendazole (Albenza)	400mg PO once, rep after 14d
or	Anthelmintic (tubulin binding, glucose uptake ↓)	Mebendazole (Vermox)	100mg PO once, rep after 14d

9.4.5 Lamblia intestinalis (Giardiasis)

	Antiprotozoal (Nitroimidazole)	Metronidazole (Flagyl, Protostat, Gens)	*250mg PO tid for 5d*
or	Nitroimidazole (antiprotozoal)	Tinidazole (Fasigyn)	*2g PO qd (once)*
or	Antiparasitic (benzimidazole)	Albendazole (Albenza)	*400mg PO qd for 5d*

9.4.6 Leishmaniasis

1st choice

	Antiprotozoal (pentavalent organic antimon connection)	Stibogluconate (Pentostam)	*20mg/kg IV/IM qd for 3-4wk*

In resistance

	Diamidine derivative	Pentamidine (Pentam, Gens)	*2-4mg/kg IV qd for 14d*
or	Antifungal – polyene (antimycotic, membrane deposition)	Amphotericin B (Fungizone, Gens)	*Test dose 1mg slow IV, if tolerated: 1mg/kg IV qd over 2-6h for 20d or 0.5 mg/kg IV qod for 8wk* **Caution:** *toxicity*
or	Antifungal (polyene derivative, membrane deposition)	Liposomal Amphotericin B (Ambisome)	*3-5mg/kg IV qd on d1-5, d14*

9.4.7 Plasmodium (Malaria), Prophylaxis

Individualized decision based on risk and travel destination recommended!
1st prophylaxis: protection from mosquito bites!

Zone A = no chloroquine resistance

	Antimalarial (DNA intercalation; Hb utilization disturbance; schizonticide)	Chloroquine (Aralen, Gens)	*300mg base qwk (1wk before until 4wk after trip)*

Zone B = moderate chloroquine resistance
Zone C = multiresistance areas

	Antimalarial (DNA intercalation, Hb utilization disturbance; schizonticide)	Mefloquine (Lariam)	1 Tab qwk (1wk before until 4wk after trip)
or	Tetracycline	Doxycycline (Doryx, Monodox, Periostat, Vibramycin, Gens)	100 mg PO qd

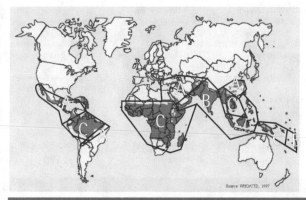

Source: WHO/CTD, 1997

9.4.8 Plasmodium, Therapy

P. malariae, P. ovale, chloroquine sensitive P. vivax and P. falciparum

	Antimalarial (DNA intercalation, Hb utilization disturbance; schizonticide)	Chloroquine (Aralen, Gens)	Ini 600mg base PO, then 300mg base after 6, 24, and 48h

Additionally for P. vivax and P. ovale (relapse prophylaxis)

	Antimalarial	Primaquine (Gens)	15mg base PO qd for 14d

Chloroquine–resistant P. falciparum or P. vivax

	Antimalarial	Quinine (Gens)	*Ini 20mg/kg IV over 4h, then 10mg/kg IV tid for 3-7d*
plus	Tetracycline	Doxycycline (Doryx, Monodox, Periostat, Vibramycin, Gens)	*100mg PO bid for 7d*
Or	Antimalarial	Quinine (Gens)	*Ini 20mg/kg IV over 4h, then 10mg/kg IV tid for 3-7d*
plus	Antimalarial combination	Pyrimethamine + Sulfadoxine (Fansidar)	*3 Tab qd, once on last day of quinine admin*
Or	Antimalarial	Mefloquine (Lariam)	*Ini 750mg base, at 6h 500mg, at 12h: 250mg*
Or	Antimalarial	Halofantrine (Halfan)	*500mg q6h x 3 doses, rep after 1wk*
Or	Antimalarial	Artesunate (experimental drug)	*Ini 20mg/kg over 4h, then 10mg/kg IV tid*
plus	Antimalarial	Mefloquine (Lariam)	*Ini 750mg base, at 6h 500mg*
Or	Antimalarial combination	Atovaquone + Proguanil (Malarone)	*4 Tabs qd PO with food for 3d*

Additionally for P. vivax (relapse prophylaxis)

	Antimalarial	Primaquine (Gens)	*15mg base PO qd for 14d*

9.4.9   Schistosoma

S. haematobium, S. mansoni, S. mekongi, S. japonicum

	Anthelmintic (tetanic contracture, worm paralysis)	Praziquantel (Biltricide)	*20mg/kg PO bid (4-6h apart) for 1d*

9.4.10   Taenia (tapeworm)

	Anthelmintic (tetanic contracture, worm paralysis)	Praziquantel (Biltricide)	10mg/kg PO once

T. saginata = cattle tapeworm, T. solium = pork tapeworm

9.4.11   Toxoplasma gondii, Pregnancy Toxoplasmosis

Before 16th week of pregnancy

	Macrolide	Spiramycin (available from FDA)	1g PO tid

After 16th week of pregnancy

	Dihydrofolate reductase inhibitor	Pyrimethamine (Daraprim, Gens)	25mg PO qd
plus	Sulfonamide (folate antagonist)	Sulfadiazine (Gens)	1g PO qid
plus	Folic acid derivative (thrombocytopenia Pro)	Folinic acid (Leucovorin, Gens)	10mg PO qd

9.4.12   Toxoplasma gondii, Chorioretinitis

	Dihydrofolate reductase inhibitor	Pyrimethamine (Daraprim, Gens)	25mg PO qd (until >1-2wk after resolution)
plus	Sulfonamide (folate antagonist)	Sulfadiazine (Gens)	1g PO qid (until >1-2wk after resolution)
plus	Folic acid derivative (thrombocytopenia Pro)	Folinic acid (Leucovorin, Gens)	10-15mg PO qd

In congenital toxoplasmosis, sight-threatening chorioretinitis, and meningitis in adults

plus	Glucocorticoid (anti-inflammatory, sensitivity of β-recept. ↑)	Prednisone (Deltasone, Meticorten, Prednisone Intensol, Gens)	0.5 mg/kg PO bid until CSF protein lower or inflammatory activity controlled

9.4.13   Trichomonas vaginalis

	Antiprotozoal (nitroimidazole)	Metronidazole (Flagyl, Protostat, Gens)	500mg PO bid for 7d or 2g PO once

9.5   Specific Antifungal Therapy

9.5.1   Aspergillus

	Antifungal – polyene (antimycotic, membrane deposition)	Amphotericin B (Fungizone, Generic)	*Test dose 1mg slow IV, if tolerated: 1mg/kg IV qd over 2-6h for 10-21d* **Caution:** *toxicity*
In mild cases or following initial Amphotericin Tx			
	Antifungal – azole	Itraconazole (Sporanox)	*200mg IV PO qd-tid (for up to 2-5mo)*

9.5.2   Candida

Candidemia			
	Antifungal – azole	Fluconazole (Diflucan)	*1.d: 400-800 mg IV/PO, then 200-400mg IV/PO qd*
Endocarditis, unstable patient			
	Antifungal – polyene (antimycotic, membrane deposition)	Amphotericin B (Fungizone, Gens)	*Test dose 1mg slow IV, if tolerated: 1mg/kg IV qd over 2-6h* **Caution:** *toxicity*
plus	Antimetabolite (antimycotic)	Flucytosine (Ancobon)	*25-37.5mg/kg PO qid*
UTI			
	Antifungal – azole	Fluconazole (Diflucan)	*100-200mg PO qd for 1-5d*
Dermal infection			
or	Antifungal – azole	Clotrimazole cream (Lotrimin, Mycelex, Gens)	*Admin bid*
90% C. albicans			

9.5.3   Coccidioides immitis

	Antifungal – azole	Itraconazole (Sporanox)	*200-400mg PO qd-bid for 3-12mo*

or	**Antifungal – polyene** (antimycotic, membrane deposition)	**Amphotericin B** (Fungizone, Gens)	*Test dose 1mg slow IV, if tolerated: 0.6-1mg/kg IV qd over 2-6h (until 2-3g total dose, followed by prolonged itra/fluco Tx)*

Meningitis

	Antifungal – azole	**Fluconazole** (Diflucan)	*400-800mg IV/PO qd (indefinitely)*

9.5.4   Cryptococcus neoformans

Mild cases

	Antifungal – azole	**Fluconazole** (Diflucan)	*d1: 400mg IV/PO then 200-400mg PO qd for 8wk-6mo*

Severe cases

	Antifungal – polyene (antimycotic, membrane deposition)	**Amphotericin B** (Fungizone, Gens)	*Test dose 1mg slow IV, if tolerated: 0.5-1mg/kg IV qd over 2-6h for 3wk, followed by prolonged fluconazole (see above)*
plus	**Antimetabolite** (antimycotic)	**Flucytosine** (Ancobon)	*25mg/kg PO qid for 3wk*

9.5.5   Dermatophytes

Onychomycosis (usually dermatophytes, also mixed infections)

	Antifungal – azole	**Itraconazole** (Sporanox)	*100-200mg PO qd (up to 3-6mo; as cure: admin for 1wk, 3wk pause, 3-6 cycles)*
or	**Antifungal – allylamine**	**Terbinafine** (Lamisil)	*250mg PO qd for 6wk*

Tinea

	Antifungal – azole	**Clotrimazole cream** (Lotrimin, Mycelex, Gens)	*Admin bid*

In refractory tinea capitis (ringworm)

	Antifungal – allylamine	**Terbinafine** (Lamisil)	*250 mg PO qd for 4-8wk*

9.5.6   Histoplasma capsulatum

Moderate disease

	Antifungal – azole	Itraconazole (Sporanox)	*200mg PO qd for 9mo*

Severe disease

d1–d10 (d20)	Antifungal – polyene (antimycotic, membrane deposition)	Amphotericin B (Fungizone, Gens)	*Test dose 1mg slow IV, if tolerated: 1mg/kg IV qd over 2-6h for 10-20d, then Itraconazole*
then	Antifungal – azole	Itraconazole (Sporanox)	*100-200mg PO qd (long term)*

Meningitis

d1–d10 (d20)	Antifungal – polyene (antimycotic, membrane deposition)	Amphotericin B (Fungizone, Gens)	*Test dose 1mg slow IV, if tolerated: 1mg/kg IV qd over 2-6h for 10-20d, then Fluconazole*
then	Antifungal – azole	Fluconazole (Diflucan)	*400-800mg IV/PO qd indefinitely*

9.5.7   Mucor

	Antifungal – polyene (antimycotic, membrane deposition)	Amphotericin B (Fungizone, Gens)	*Test dose 1mg slow IV, if tolerated: 0.8-1.5 mg/kg IV qd over 2-6h (total dose 2.5-3g)*

9.5.8   Pityriasis versicolor

	Antifungal – azole	Ketoconazole (Nizoral)	*2% cream/shampoo apply to affected areas qd for 2wk*
or	Selenium sulfate	Selenium sulfate (Selsun, several "dandruff shampoos")	*Apply to affected areas qd for 2wk*
or	Antifungal – azole	Ketoconazole (Nizoral)	*400mg PO once*

10. Neurology

Paul B. Pritchard, III, MD, Professor
Aljoeson Walker, MD, Assistant Professor
William R. Tyor, MD, Professor
Timothy D. Carter, MD, Associate Professor
Zoltan Kaliszky, MD
Department of Neuroscience,
Division of Neurology,
Medical University of South Carolina, Charleston, SC

10.1 Pain Control

A.	NSAID – nonsteroidal anti-inflammatory drug (exact mechanism of action unknown, inhibition of cyclooxygenase and lipoxygenase; reduction of prostaglandin synthesis)	Aspirin – ASA (Ascriptin, Asprimox, Bayer Aspirin, Bufferin, Easprin, Ecotrin, Empirin, Genprin, Halfprin, Zorprin, Gens)	325-650mg PO q4-6h
		Diclofenac (Voltaren, Voltaren-XR, Gens)	75mg PO bid
		Etodolac (Lodine, Lodine XL, Gens)	200-400mgH PO bid-tid, ext.rel 400mg-1g PO qd
		Ibuprofen (Advil, Children's advil, Motrin, Gens)	200-800mg PO tid-qid
		Ketoprofen (Orudis, Oruvail, Gens)	25-75mg PO tid-qid, ext.rel 100-200mg PO qd
		Nabumetone (Relafen, Gens)	1000mg PO qd/bid
		Naproxen (Anaprox, Naprelan, Naprosyn, Gens)	250-500mg PO bid, ext.rel 750-1000mg PO qd
		Oxaprozin (Daypro, Gens)	1200mg PO qd
		Piroxicam (Feldene, Gens)	20mg PO qd
		Salsalate (Salflex, Disalcid)	3000mg PO qd (div q8-12h)
		Sulindac (Clinoril, Gens)	150-200mg PO bid

B.	Narcotic analgesic – Opioid agonist (act at opiate receptors)	**Codeine** (Gens)	*15-60mg PO q4-6h, short acting*
		Meperidine (Demerol, Gens)	*50-150mg q3-4h PO/IM/ IV; **Note**: lowers seizure threshold, avoid ext. use*
		Oxycodone (Oxy Contin, Roxicodone)	*5-30mg PO q6h prn, short acting; ext.rel 10-160mg PO q12h, longer acting; **Note**: severe abuse potential*
		Propoxyphene (Darvon, Darvon-N, Dolene, Kesso-gesic, Gens)	*65-100mg PO q4h prn*
		Fentanyl (Actiq/PO, Duragesic patch, Fentanyl Oralet/PO, Sublimaze/Inj, Gens)	*50-100μg IV/IM, typically given prior to OP; transdermal patch with 25, 50, 75 or 100μg/h, change patch q3d, good for chronic use; 1 U PO prn episode, max 4 U/d*
		Morphine sulfate (Astramorph, Avinza, Duramorph, Infumorph, Kadian, MS Contin, MSIR, Numorphan, Oramorph, Roxanol, Gens)	*10-30mg PO q4h, short acting, poor absorption; ext.rel 15-30mg PO q8-12h, longer acting, good for chronic use; 0.1-0.2mg/kg IV/IM/SC up to 15mg q4h*
		Hydromorphone (Dilaudid, Gens)	*2-4mg PO q4-6h, 1-4mg IM/SC/IV q4-6h; **Note**: severe abuse potential*
		Methadone (Dolophine, Methadose, Gens)	*2.5-10mg q3-4h PO prn Pain long acting, good for chronic use*
C.	Narcotic analgesic – Opioid agonist/ antagonist (act at opiate receptors)	**Nalbuphine** (Nubain, Gens)	*10-20mg IV/IM/SC q3-6h*
		Butorphanol (Stadol nasal spray, Gens)	*1 spray q3-4h (=1mg/spray); **Note**: frequently abused drug*

D.	Narcotic combinations (short acting narcotic analgesics combined with non–narcotic drugs)	Hydrocodone 5mg + Acetaminophen 500mg (Allay, Anexsia, Co-gesic, Hydrocet, Hy-phen, Lorcet, Vicodin, Gens)	1-2 Tab PO q4-6h prn
		Hydrocodone 7.5mg + Ibuprofen 200mg (Vicoprofen)	1-2 Tab PO q4-6h prn
		Oxycodone/ Acetaminophen 5mg + 325mg (Oxycet, Percocet, Roxicet, Gens) 5mg + 500mg (Roxilox, Roxicet, Tylox, GensGens)	1 Tab PO q6h prn
		Oxycodone 5mg + ASA 325mg (Percodan)	1 Tab PO q6h prn
		Propoxyphene 100mg + Acetaminophen 650mg (Darvocet, Gens)	1 Tab PO q4h prn
E.	Tricyclic antidepressant (inhibit norepinephrine and serotonin reuptake)	Amitriptyline (Clavil, Elavil, Endep, Gens)	Ini 10-25mg PO qhs, incr slowly, usual dose 50-100mg/d
F.	Antiepileptic (in neuropathic pain, see also seizures, →217)	Gabapentin (Neurontin)	Ini 100mg PO tid, incr grad, max 3600mg/d
		Carbamazepine (Carbatrol, Epitol, Mazepine, Tegretol/-XR, Trileptal, Gens)	Ini 200mg PO bid, then tid, incr grad, max 1600mg/d; ext.rel 400-600mg PO bid
		Topiramate (Topamax)	Ini 10-25mg PO qpm, in wk2 incr to bid, then incr slowly, max 1600mg/d
G.	Topical agent (ionic influx ↓, depolariz. threshold ↑)	Lidocaine (Lidoderm)	Patch topically, max 3 at once up to 12h/d; jelly 2.5-5%, topically as dir.
H.	Others	Tramadol (Ultram)	50-100mg PO q4-6h prn
		Note: red in renal/hepatic impairment or elderly	

Kaliszky, 2003

10.2 Lower Back Pain

1.	**NSAID**	See Pain Control, →205
2.	**NSAID, COX-2 inhibitor** (inhib. cyclooxygenase-2 ⇒ prostaglandins ↓ ⇒ anti-inflammatory, analgesic)	Celecoxib (Celebrex) — *100-200mg PO qd-bid, max. 400mg/d*
3. Plus	**Centrally acting muscle relaxants**	Baclofen (Lioresal, Gens) — *Ini 5mg PO tid; max dose 20mg PO qid*
		Carisoprodol (Soma, Gens) — *350mg PO tid-qid; Note: frequently abused!*
		Chlorzoxazone (Parafon Forte, Strifon Forte, Gens) — *Ini 500-750mg PO tid-qid, then decr to 250mg PO tid/qid*
		Cyclobenzaprine (Flexeril, Gens) — *Ini 10mg PO tid, max 60mg/d*
		Metaxalone (Skelaxin) — *800mg PO tid-qid*
		Methocarbamol (Robaxin, Gens) — *For acute pain: 1500mg PO qid, maint 1000mg PO qid or 750mg PO q4h*
		Orphenadrine (Norflex, Gens) — *100mg PO bid; 60mg IV/IM q12h*
		Tizanidine (Zanaflex) — *Ini 4-8mg PO q6-8h, incr according to guideline, max 36mg/d*
	Benzodiazepine (Bind to benzodiazepine receptors, enhance GABA effects)	Clonazepam (Klonopin, Gens) — *Ini 0.5mg PO bid; incr up to 3mg PO tid*
		Diazepam (Valium, Gens) — *Ini 2mg PO tid; max 10mg PO tid-qid*
		**Note:** Use benzodiazepines carefully – frequently abused!
4.	**Other analgesic** (non narcotic, centrally acting analgesic, similar effect to opioids)	Tramadol (Ultram) — *50-100mg PO q4-6h prn; Note: red in renal/hepatic impairment or elderly*

5.	**Tricyclic antidepressant** (norepinephrine and serotonin reuptake inhibition)	**Amitriptyline** (Clavil, Elavil, Endep, Gens)	*Ini 10-25mg PO qhs; grad incr by 25mg, >100mg/d rarely necessary*

Note: Many different antidepressants are used for neuropathic pain, off-label.

Important note: In general, avoid the use of narcotic analgesics! For acute relapses may use narcotic analgesics for short periods of time (see pain section, →205).

6.	**Local Tx**: blocks release the substance P and other neuropeptides		
	Dermatologic agent	**Capsaicin** (Zostrix, Gens)	*0.025% cream: apply up to tid-qid locally*

Surgical Interventions: should be determined by an expert in pain Tx:
- **Intrathecal Narcotic Pump**

Kaliszky, 2003

10.3 Cluster Headaches
10.3.1 Acute Treatment

	Oxygen inhalation (blood oxygenation)	**Oxygen 100%**	*7 l/min nasal cannula (up to 15min)*
Poss	**Serotonin receptor agonist** (through 5-HT$_1$-receptor ⇒ vasoconstriction)	**Sumatriptan** (Imitrex)	*6mg SC, may rep once/ 24h (statpak)*
		Zolmitriptan (Zomig)	*10mg PO/24h*
or	**Ergot derivative** (serotonine receptor agonism ⇒ vasocon- striction, pro-inflam. neuropeptide release ↓)	**Dihydroergotamine** (D.H.E. 45, Migranal)	*1mg IV or IM qh up to 3mg/d; 2mg nasal spray (5mg both nostrils, rep at 15min)*

10.3.2 Prophylaxis in > 1 Attack Daily

	Glucocorticoid (anti-inflammatory)	**Methylprednisolone** (Medrol, Depo-Medrol, Solu-Medrol, Gens)	*40-80mg qd for 5d, then taper quickly, disc in <3wk*
	Calcium channel blocker (affects release of substance P, vasodilation)	**Verapamil** (Calan, Calan SR, Covera-HS, Isoptin, Isoptin SR, Riva-Verapamil SR, Tarka Verelan, -PM, Gens)	*80-120mg PO tid-qid, max 480mg/d*

or	**Mood stabilizer** (mechanism of action unclear, alteration of electrical conductivity, arterial relaxation)	**Lithium carbonate** (Eskalith, Eskalith-CR, Lithane, Lithobid, Gens)	*600-1800 mg/d PO*
	Caution: need to monitor liver function test		
or	**Anticonvulsive** (GABAergic effects, blocks Na^+ channels)	**Valproic acid** (Depacon, Depakene, Depakote, Gens)	*Ini 125-250mg/d*
or	**Anticonvulsive** (blocks voltage-dependent sodium channels + activ. of AMP, affects GABA mediated chloride currents)	**Topiramate** (Topamax)	*50-150mg PO bid*

Walker, 2005

10.4 Migraine
10.4.1 Acute Treatment

NSAID – nonsteroidal anti-inflammatory drug	**Ibuprofen** (Advil, Advil Migraine, Motrin, Motrin Migraine, Gens)	*200mg PO bid*
	See Lower Back Pain section for **other NSAID**, →208	
NSAID + Caffeine	**Acetaminophen 250mg, Aspirin 250mg + Caffeine 65mg** (Excedrin, Excedrin Migraine)	*2 tab PO prn q6h, max 8 tab/d*
Isometheptene (sympathomimetic → constricting dilated cerebral vessels)	**Isometheptene Mucate** (Midrin)	*Ini 2 Cap PO, then 1 Cap/h, max 10 Cap/d (1Cap=65mg)*
Ergot derivative (cerebral vessel regulation)	**Dihydroergotamine** (D.H.E. 45, Migranal)	*2mg PR; 1-2mg IM/IV* **(Caution: vomiting);** *2mg nasal spray/d*
Caution in angina pectoris, myocardial-/cerebral infarct: need 24h between administrations of dihydroergotamine!		

Serotonin receptor agonist (serotonin agonism through 5-HT$_1$-receptor $\Rightarrow$ vasoconstriction)	Almotriptan (Axert)	6.25-12.5mg PO
	Frovatriptan (Frova)	2.5mg PO
	Naratriptan (Amerge)	1-2.5mg PO
	Rizatriptan benzoate (Maxalt, Maxalt-MLT)	5-10mg PO, max 30mg/d; **Caution:** under propranolol Tx max 5mg PO tid
	Sumatriptan (Imitrex)	25-100mg PO, 6mg SC, 20mg nasal spray
	Zolmitriptan (Zomig, Zomig ZMT)	2.5-5mg PO
	Eletriptan (Relpax)	20-40mg PO, max dose 80mg/d

Walker, 2005

10.4.2 Prophylaxis in > 2 Attacks/mo

Betablocker (vascular tone sympathetic)	Propranolol (Inderal, Inderal LA, Gens)	Ini 60 mg PO qd (div bid, ext.rel qd), titrate prn, max 320 mg/d; long-term admin
	Timolol (Blocadren, Gens)	10mg PO bid-tid
Anticonvulsive (GABAergic effects↑, blocks Na$^+$ channel)	Valproic acid (Depacon, Depakene, Depakote, Myproic Acid, Gens)	Ini 125-250 mg/d PO, titrate prn, max 1500 mg/d
Anticonvulsive (blocks voltage-dependent Na$^+$ channels and activity of AMP, affects GABA mediated chloride currents)	Topiramate (Topamax)	25-100mg/d PO

Walker, 2005

10.5 Trigeminal Neuralgia

	Anticonvulsive (repeated stimulation of afferences ⇒ increased response to stimuli ↓)	**Carbamazepine** (Epitol, Mazepine, Tegretol/-XR, Trileptal, Gens)	*Ini 200mg PO tid, incr to max 1200mg/d PO (div 6x/d; after plasma level)*
or	**Anticonvulsive** (ion permeability ↓ ⇒ membrane stabilization)	**Phenytoin** (Dilantin, Gens)	*Slowly incr to 100mg PO tid-5 times/d (after plasma level)*
	Anticonvulsive (GABAergic effects, blocks Na⁺ channel)	**Valproic acid** (Depacon, Depakene, Depakote, Myproic Acid, Gens)	*Ini 5-10mg/kg, incr by 5-10mg/kg/d qwk, max 60mg/kg*
	Anticonvulsive (brain GABA concentration↑)	**Gabapentin** (Neurontin)	*Ini 300mg PO, dose up by 1 Tab over 3d; then incr according to symptoms*
or	**Antipsychotic – D₂ antagonist** (antagonism at central dopamine receptors)	**Pimozide** (Orap)	*Slowly incr to 4-12mg/d PO; cholinergic AE*
or	**Myotonolytic** (antispastic)	**Baclofen** (Lioresal, Gens)	*10-20mg qid*

Walker, 2005

10.6 Cerebrovascular Disease
10.6.1 Acute Ischemic Stroke

Thrombolytic Tx

Intravenous thrombolytic Tx (plasminogen activation ⇒ fibrin proteolysis)	**rt-PA – Alteplase** (Activase I.V.)	*0.9mg/kg, max 90mg, over 60min IV, start with 10% of total dose as IV bolus over 1min; Only to carefully selected patients meeting all in-/ exclusion criteria*

Note: Decision must be made on an individual basis following NINDS guidelines. Patients treated with IV tPA must not receive any other anticoagulant, antiplatelet agent, or thrombolytic for 24h after initial tPA Tx.

Intraarterial thrombolytic Tx (plasminogen activation ⇒ fibrin proteolysis)	rt-PA – Alteplase (Activase I.V.)	

May be useful for carefully selected patients, who are not candidates for IV tPA. At centers with appropriate expertise.

Antiplatelet drug Tx

poss	Antiplatelet drug (phosphodiesterase/ platelet aggregation-adhesion inhibition)	Aspirin – ASA (Ascriptin, Asprimox, Bayer Aspirin, Bufferin, Easprin, Ecotrin, Empirin, Genprin, Halfprin, St. Joseph Pain Reliever, Zorprin, Gens)	325mg PO qd started within 48h of symptom onset

For patients who are not candidates for thrombolytic Tx. Has been associated with improved outcome.

	Antiplatelet drug (inhibition of adenosine diphosphate-mediated platelet aggregation)	Clopidogrel (Plavix)	75mg PO qd
		Ticlopidine (Ticlid)	250mg PO bid
	Antiplatelet drug (Dipyridamole: inhibition of cAMP-mediated platelet aggregation)	Aspirin + Dipyridamole–ER (Aggrenox)	1 Cap (25+200mg ext.rel) PO bid

Clopidogrel, Ticlopidine, Dipyridamole for patients with acute stroke who are not candidates for thrombolytic Tx and cannot take ASA

Anticoagulant Tx

poss	Heparin, unfractionated (inhibition of thrombin and Factor Xa ⇒ conversion of fibrinogen to fibrin ↓)	Heparin (Gens)	5000 U SC q8-12h, or adj dose based on PTT for IV administered heparin

While conclusive evidence regarding its utility is unavailable, many practitioners use dose adjusted IV heparin, especially for stroke of presumed embolic origin or secondary to large artery disease.

General Measures

- BP monitoring (avoid even relative hypotension)
- Check ECG
- Supplemental O_2 (if hypoxic)
- Normoglycemia
- Normothermia
- Maintain fluid and electrolyte balance
- Evaluate for dysphagia/risk of aspiration
- Avoid indwelling urinary catheters if possible
- Deep venous thrombosis prophylaxis (low dose subcutaneously administered heparin or sequential compression stockings, →44)
- Rehabilitation

These measures are widely recommended and generally thought to reduce the frequency of complications and improve outcome.

10.6.2	Stroke Prevention		
	Antiplatelet drug (inhibition of platelet aggregation)	Aspirin - ASA (Ascriptin, Asprimox, Bayer Aspirin, Bufferin, Easprin, Ecotrin, Empirin, Genprin, Halfprin, Zorprin, Gens)	*50–1300mg PO qd*
		Clopidogrel (Plavix)	*75mg PO qd*
		Ticlopidine (Ticlid, Gens)	*250mg PO bid;* **Caution:** *need for monitoring WBC and risk for TTP*
		Aspirin + Dipyridamole-ER (Aggrenox)	*1 Cap (25+200mg ext.rel) PO bid*

For patients **with atrial fibrillation** and **CI to anticoagulation**, ASA 325 mg qd has shown to decrease the risk of stroke.

| or | Oral anticoagulant (inhibition of vitamin K-dependent coagulation factor synthesis) | Warfarin (Coumadin) | *Ini 2-5mg PO qd for 2-4d, maint 2-10mg/d PO; adj dose to maint INR 1.4 to 2.8; in AF adj dose to maint INR 2-3;* |

For patients **with prior stroke, without AF** and **without prosthetic heart valves** warfarin has shown to have approximately the same efficacy as ASA. In patients **with atrial fibrillation, without CI to anticoagulation** adjusted dose warfarin has shown to substantially reduce the risk of stroke.

For Patients with Coronary Artery Disease and Hypercholesterolemia

HMG Co-A reductase inhibitors (Statins)	Simvastatin (Zocor) Pravastatin (Pravachol)	*Ini 10-20mg qd, titrate based on cholesterol levels*

While specific evidence regarding efficacy of other agents in this class is not currently available, many practitioners use other statins in this setting.

For Patients with Carotid Artery Stenosis

Carotid Endarterectomy
- **Symptomatic carotid stenosis**: Patients with > 70% stenosis benefit from carotid endarterectomy compared to medical Tx alone when the surgery is done with low perioperative complication rates.
- **Asymptomatic carotid stenosis**: There is evidence that patients with > 60% asymptomatic carotid stenosis may benefit from endarterectomy when the surgery is done with low perioperative complication rates.

For All Patients

General Measures
- Hypertension control
- Smoking cessation
- Hyperlipidemia Tx (with statins)
- Avoiding heavy alcohol use
- Exercise
- Healthy dietary habits
- Control of diabetes

All of these measures have generally been shown to decr the risk of stroke. While tight control of diabetes has not been shown to decr stroke risk to date, tight control has been shown to decr many other complications and is appropriate.

Carter, 2003

10.7   Meningitis, Encephalitis

Before the initiation of the antibacterial Tx, consider consultation with an Infectious Disease specialist.

10.7.1   In General

Initial therapy (with no pathogen proven)

or	**Cephalosporin - 3rd gen. - nonpseudomonal** (broad spectrum antibiotic - cell wall mucopeptide synthesis ↓)	**Ceftriaxone** (Rocephin)	*1-2g IV q12h*
		Cefotaxime (Claforan, Gens)	*2g IV q6-8h (up to q4h)*

If significant local resistance to Pneumococcus exists

plus	**Glycopeptide**	**Vancomycin** (Vancocin, Vancoled, Gens)	*1g IV q12h*

If age > 50yr

plus	**Aminopenicillin**	**Ampicillin** (Omnipen, Principen, Totacillin, Gens)	*150-200 mg/kg/d IV (div q3-4h)*

10.7.2   In the Immunocompromised

	Aminopenicillin	**Ampicillin** (Omnipen, Principen, Totacillin, Gens)	*150-200 mg/kg/d IV (div q3-4h)*
plus	**Cephalosporin - 3rd gen** (broad spectrum antibiotic)	**Ceftazidime** (Ceptaz, Fortaz, Tazicef, Tazidime, Gens)	*2g IV q8h*

10.7.3   In Head Trauma, CSF Shunt, Neurosurgery

	Vancomycin (inhibition of cell wall and RNA synthesis)	**Vancomycin** (Vancocin, Vancoled, Gens)	*1g IV q12h*
plus	**Cephalosporin - 3rd gen** (broad spectrum antibiotic)	**Ceftazidime** (Ceptaz, Fortaz, Tazicef, Tazidime, Gens)	*2g IV q8h*

Tx must be modified according to the CSF culture, sensitivity results.

10.7.4 In Suspected Tuberculosis (3-Drug Therapy)

	Antimycobacterial (inhibition of lipid and nucleic acid synthesis)	Isoniazid (Laniazid, Nydrazid, Gens)	300mg PO qd (until ruled out)
plus/or	Antimycobacterial (inhibition of DNA-depend. RNA polymerase)	Rifampin (Rifadin, Rimactane, Gens)	600mg PO qd (until ruled out)
plus/or	Antimycobacterial (inhibition of metabolite synthesis)	Ethambutol (Myambutol, Gens)	10-20mg/kg/d (until ruled out)
plus/or	Antimycobacterial (MA unknown)	Pyrazinamide (Gens)	30mg/kg/d (until ruled out)

Any regimen must use multiple drugs to which M tuberculosis is susceptible. Therapy must be taken regularly and must continue for a period sufficient to resolve the illness.

Tyor, 2003

10.8 Seizures
10.8.1 Generalized Tonic-Clonic Status Epilepticus

	Antiepileptic, benzodiazepine (GABAergic effect↑)	Lorazepam (Ativan, Gens)	Adults: 4mg slowly IV (at 2mg/min), may rep after 10-15min, max 8mg
plus	Antiepileptic (ion permeability ↓, stabilizes Na⁺ channels ⇒ membrane stabilization)	Phenytoin (Dilantin, Gens)	Adults: 20mg/kg IV, max rate 50mg/min
		Fosphenytoin (Cerebryx)	Adults: 15-20mg PE/kg IV, max IV rate100-150mg PE/min

Preferable to use phosphenytoin, a pro-drug of phenytoin (PE = phenytoin equivalents); can be given more quickly IV without risk of local infiltration.

10.8.2 Prolonged Seizures, Seizure Clusters

Antiepileptic, benzodiazepine (GABAergic effect↑)	Diazepam (Diastat - Gel for rectal admin)	Adults: 10-20mg PR qd

10.8.3	Generalized Seizures: Myoclonic		
	Antiepileptic, benzodiazepine (GABAergic effect↑)	Clonazepam (Klonopin, Gens)	**Adults:** ini < 1.5mg/d (div tid), incr by 0.5-1.0mg/d until control achieved or AE encountered
or/plus	**Antiepileptic** (GABAergic effect↑)	Lamotrigine (Lamictal)	**>12yr:** ini 25mg/d, incr qwk, target 500mg/d: if pat. premedicated with valproate ini 25mg qod, incr qwk after first 2wk

Ini dose depends on whether patient already takes valproic acid (VPA), which increases risk of Stevens-Johnson syndrome and toxic epidermal necrolysis.

10.8.4	Generalized Seizures: Absence		
	Antiepileptic, T-calcium channel blocker (T-type Ca++ currents↓)	Ethosuximide (Zarontin, Gens)	**>6yr:** ini 500mg/d, incr by 250mg/d qwk, to 15-40mg/kg/d div qd-bid; **<6yr:** ini 10mg/kg/d, incr by 5-10mg/kg/d qwk to 15-40mg/kg/d
or/plus	**Antiepileptic** (blocks Na+ channels, GABAergic effects↑)	Valproic acid (Depacon, Depakene, Depakote, Myproic Acid, Gens)	**Ped** ini 10-15mg/kg/d (div bid), incr by 10-15mg/kg/d qwk to 30-60mg/kg/d, according to clinical response/serum levels

Caution: Cases of fatal hepatic necrosis have been reported in use of valproic acid, with peak incidence < age 2yr; analyze risk/benefit in younger patients!

10.8.5	Generalized Seizures: Primarily Generalized Tonic-Clonic Seizures		
adjunctive	**Antiepileptic, benzodiazepine** (GABAergic effect↑)	Clonazepam (Klonopin, Gens)	**Adults:** ini < 1.5mg/d (div tid), incr by 0.5-1.0mg/d until control achieved or AE encountered; **CH <10yr or <30kg:** ini 0.01-0.03mg/kg/d PO (div bid-tid), incr by 0.25-0.5mg q3d up to 0.1-0.2mg/kg/d (div tid)

last resort	Antiepileptic, glutamate modulator (inhibits NMDA subtype glutamate receptors)	Felbamate (Felbatol)	**Adults:** ini 400mg PO tid, incr by 600mg/d q2wk, max 3,600mg/d; **Ped:** ini 15mg/kg/d (div tid-qid), incr by 15mg/kg/d qwk, aim at 45mg/kg/d (div tid-qid)

Caution: Because of serious, potentially fatal complications of aplastic anemia and hepatotoxicity, use of Felbamate should be limited to patients with severe, uncontrolled seizures who have had an inadequate reponse to previous agents.

	Antiepileptic (GABAergic effect ↑)	Lamotrigine (Lamictal)	**>12yr:** ini 25mg/d, incr qwk, target 500mg/d: if pat. premedicated with valproate ini 25mg qod, incr qwk after first 2wk

Ini dose depends on whether patient already takes valproic acid (VPA), which increases risk of Stevens-Johnson syndrome and toxic epidermal necrolysis.

	Antiepileptic (Na^+ channel blocking, GABAergic effect ↑)	Topiramate (Topamax)	**>17yr:** ini 25-50mg/d, incr by 25-50mg/d qwk, target 400mg/d (div bid); smaller doses may be effective in some cases.

	Antiepileptic (blocks Na^+ channels, GABAergic effects ↑)	Valproic acid (Depacon, Depakene, Depakote, Myproic Acid, Gens)	**Ped** ini 10-15mg/kg/d (div bid), incr by 10-15mg/kg/d qwk to 30-60mg/kg/d, according to clinical response/serum levels; **Adults:** ini 250-500mg bid, incr to 1-3g/d, according to clinical response/serum levels

Caution: Cases of fatal hepatic necrosis have been reported in use of valproic acid, with peak incidence age < 2yr; analyze risk/benefit in younger patients!

10.8.6 Partial Seizures, Secondarily Generalized Tonic-Clonic Seizures

	Antiepileptic (stabilizes Na^+ channel)	Carbamazepine (Carbatrol, Epitol, Mazepine, Tegretol/-XR, Trileptal, Gens)	**Adults:** ini 200mg bid, incr by 200mg/d qwk, target 800-1200mg/d (div tid, ext.rel div bid)

Antiepileptic, glutamate modulator (inhibits NMDA subtype glutamate receptors)	**Felbamate** (Felbatol)	**Adults:** ini 400mg PO tid, incr by 600mg/d q2wk, max 3.6g/d; **Ped:** ini 15mg/kg/d (div tid-qid), incr by 15mg/kg/d qwk, up to 45mg/kg/d (div tid-qid)

Caution: Because of serious, potentially fatal complications of aplastic anemia and hepatotoxicity, use of Felbamate should be limited to patients with severe, uncontrolled seizures who have had an inadequate reponse to previous agents.

Antiepileptic (blockade of Na$^+$ channels, stabilization of hyperexcited neural membranes)	**Oxcarbazepine** (Trileptal)	**Adults:** ini 300mg bid, incr by 600mg/d qwk, maint 1.2g/d, max 2.4g/d. **Ped:** ini 8-10mg/kg/d (div bid), incr qwk by 10mg/kg/d to 20-45mg/kg/d (div bid). CH < 8yr may require higher dosage.
Antiepileptic (MA unknown)	**Levetiracetam** (Keppra)	**Adults:** ini 500mg bid, incr prn by 1000mg q2wk, max 3g/d (div bid)
Antiepileptic (brain GABA concentration↑)	**Gabapentin** (Neurontin)	**CH 3-12yr:** ini 10-15mg/kg/d (div tid), CH 3-4yr: incr q3d to 40mg/kg/d; CH 5yr or older: incr q3d to 25-35mg/kg/d **CH >12yr, adults:** ini 300mg tid, taper by 300-400mg/d q5d to max 1800mg; some patients may require higher doses
Antiepileptic (ion permeability↓, stabilizes Na$^+$ channels ⇒ membrane stabilization)	**Phenytoin** (Dilantin, Gens)	**Adults:** ini 300mg/d, maint usually 3-5mg/kg/d (div tid, ext.rel. qd), lower in the elderly, use serum levels; **Ped** typical maint dose 4-8mg/kg/d

Antiepileptic (GABAergic effects↑)	Primidone (Myidone, Mysoline, Gens)	**Adults:** *ini 50-100mg qhs. grad incr to 5-20mg/kg/d (div tid-qid)* **Ped** *ini 1-2 mg/kg/d, grad incr to 5-20mg/kg/d (div bid-qid)*
Antiepileptic (GABAergic effects↑)	Tiagabine (Gabitril)	*Ini 4mg/d, incr qwk by 4mg, usual maint dose 32-56mg/d (div bid-qid)*
Antiepileptic (Na+ channel blocking, GABAergic effect↑)	Topiramate (Topamax)	**Adults >17yr:** *ini 25-50mg/d, incr by 25-50mg qwk, target 20mg/d (div bid); smaller doses may be effective in some cases*
Antiepileptic (blocks Na+ channels, GABAergic effects↑)	Valproic acid (Depacon, Depakene, Depakote, Myproic Acid, Gens)	**Ped** *ini 10-15mg/kg/d (div bid), incr by 10-15mg/kg/d qwk to 30-60mg/kg/d, according to clinical response and serum levels;* **Adults:** *ini 250-500mg bid, incr to 1000-3000mg/d, according to clinical response + serum levels*

Caution: Cases of fatal hepatic necrosis have been reported in use of valproic acid, with peak incidence age < 2yr; analyze risk/benefit in younger patients!

Antiepileptic (modulates voltage dependent ion channels)	Zonisamide (Zonegram)	**Adults:** *ini 100mg/d, may incr q2wk by 100mg/d (qd or div bid), max 400mg/d*

10.8.7 Seizures in Suspected Herpes simplex Type I Infection

Antiepileptic (inhibits Na+ and Ca++ currents, GABAergic effects↑)	Topiramate (Topamax)	**Adults >17yr:** *Ini 25-50mg/d. incr by 25-50mg qwk, target 400mg/d (div bid); smaller doses may be effective in some cases*

Antiepileptic (blocks Na$^+$ channels, GABAergic effects ↑)	Valproic acid (Depacon, Depakene, Depakote, Myproic Acid, Gens)	*Ini 250-500mg tid, grad incr to 1-3g qd, according to clinical response + serum levels*

Pritchard, 2005

10.8.8   Surgical Interventions

Surgical interventions should be determined by an expert Epileptologist.

Vagus Nerve Stimulator

For medically intractable **partial seizures**: in selected patients reduces seizure frequency. Device must be programmed to meet individual needs + tolerance.

Ablative Surgery

For medically intractable **partial seizures**: Removal of the epileptogenic zone including local topectomy, temporal lobectomy, frontal lobectomy, and even hemispherectomy.

Pritchard, 2005

10.9   Parkinsonism

10.9.1   Parkinsonism in Patients < 50yr

	MAO-B inhibitor (irreversible inhibitor, dopaminergic activity ↑)	Selegiline (Eldepryl, Gens)	*5mg PO bid; Note: admin 2nd dose at noon to avoid insomnia.*
plus/or	Indir. dopamine agonist (glutamate receptor antagonism)	Amantadine (Symmetrel, Gens)	*100mg PO bid*
	Mainly if bradykinesia prominent.		
plus/or	Centrally acting anticholinergic (plus symptoms rigor, tremor ↓)	Trihexyphenidyl (Artane, Tremin, Trihexane, Gens)	*1mg PO bid, max 6-10mg/d*
		Benztropine (Cogentin, Gens)	*0.5mg PO bid, max 4-6mg/d*
	If tremor is prominent.		

Amantadine and the centrally acting Anticholinergics are not commonly used any more.

10.9.2	Parkinsonism in Patients 50 – 59yr		
1.	Dopamine agonist (mainly D2 dopamine receptor stimulation)	Bromocriptine (Parlodel)	*Ini 1.25mg PO qhs, usual effective dose 10-30mg/d (div tid), max 100mg/d*
		Pergolide (Permax)	*Ini 0.05mg PO qd, usual effective dose 2-3mg/d (div tid), max 5mg/d*
		Pramipexole (Mirapex)	*Ini 0.125mg PO tid, grad incr to 0.5-1.5mg PO tid*
		Ropinirole (Requip)	*Ini 0.25mg PO tid, grad incr to 1mg PO tid, max 24mg/d*
2.	MAO-B inhibitor (irreversible inhibitor, dopaminergic activity↑)	Selegiline (Eldepryl, Gens)	*5mg PO bid;* **Note:** *admin 2nd dose at noon to avoid insomnia.*
3.	Dopamine agonist (L-Dopa → dopamine in central dopaminerg. cells; Carbidopa inhibits periph. decarbox. of L-Dopa)	Levodopa + Carbidopa (Sinemet, Sinemet CR, Gens)	*Ini 25+100mg bid-tid, then incr q1-4d prn, max 200mg/d Carbidopa; ext.rel ini 25+100 - 50+200mg/d*
4. poss	Indirect dopamine agonist (glutamate receptor antagonism)	Amantadine (Symmetrel, Gens)	*100mg PO bid*
	May add for bradykinesia and rigidity.		
5. poss	Anticholinergic	Trihexyphenidyl (Artane, Tremin, Trihexane, Gens)	*1mg PO bid, max 6-10mg/d*
		Benztropine (Cogentin, Gens)	*0.5mg PO bid, max 4-6mg/d*
	May add for persisting tremor.		
6. poss	COMT Inhibitor (inhibition of catechol-O-methyltransferase COMT ⇒ levodopa ↑)	Entacapone (Comtan)	*200mg PO concomitantly with each Sinemet dose, max 1600mg/d (div 8x/d)*
	May also be added.		

10.9.3	Parkinsonism in Patients > 60yr		
	Dopamine agonist (L-Dopa → dopamine in central dopaminerg. cells; Carbidopa inhibits periph. decarbox. of L-Dopa)	**Levodopa + Carbidopa** (Sinemet, Sinemet CR, Gens)	*Ini 25+100mg bid-tid, then incr q1-4d prn, max 200mg/d Carbidopa; ext.rel ini 25+100 - 50+200mg PO bid*
plus/or	**Dopamine agonist** (mainly D2 dopamine receptor stimulation)	**Bromocriptine** (Parlodel)	*Ini 1.25mg PO qhs, usual effective dose 10-30mg/d (div tid), max 100mg/d*
		Pergolide (Permax)	*Ini 0.05mg PO qd, usual effective dose 2-3mg/d (div tid), max 5mg/d*
		Pramipexole (Mirapex)	*Ini 0.125mg PO tid, grad incr to 0.5-1.5mg PO tid*
		Ropinirole (Requip)	*Ini 0.25mg PO tid, grad incr to 1mg PO tid, max 24mg/d*

10.9.4	Surgical Interventions – Deep Brain Stimulation

Deep brain stimulation should be reserved for special cases, best identified by a Parkinson's disease expert:
- **Pallidum**: For tremor, stiffness, and rigidity
- **Subthalamic nucleas**: For tremor, stiffness, and rigidity
- **Thalamus**: For tremor

Kaliszky, 2003

10.10 Multiple Sclerosis
10.10.1 Acute Episode (Relapse) Treatment

1.	**Glucocorticoid** (anti-inflammatory, immuno-suppressive)	**Methylprednisolone** (Medrol, Depo-Medrol, Solu-Medrol, Gens)	*1000mg/d IV x 3-7d*
2.		**Prednisone** (Deltasone, Meticorten, Gens)	*Ini 60-80mg PO/d for 3-7d and taper over 8-12d; oral steroid taper with or without IV steroids*

10.10.2 Preventive Therapy for Relapsing-Remitting MS

1.	Beta-Interferon (many immuno-modulatory effects)	Interferon Beta-1A (Avonex)	30µg (6 M IU) IM qwk
		Interferon Beta-1A (Rebif)	44µg (12 M IU) SC tiw
		Interferon Beta-1B (Betaseron)	8 M IU (250µg) SC qod
2.	Immunomodulator (many immuno-modulatory effects)	Glatiramer acetate (Copaxone)	20mg SC qd

10.10.3 Preventive Therapy for Secondary Progressive MS

	Antineoplastic antibiotic (DNA-reactive, cytocidal)	Mitoxantrone (Novantrone)	$12mg/m^2$ IV q3mo, max total dose 140mg; Caution: needs cardiac, hematological and liver function monitoring.
or	Antimetabolite, immunosuppressant (inhibits dihydrofolate reductase, lymphocyte proliferation↓, cytokine synthesis↓)	Methotrexate sodium (Folex, Rheumatrex, Gens)	2.5mg PO/IM q12h for 3 doses once a week (=7.5mg/wk); based on limited trials
plus/or	Beta-Interferon (many immuno-modulatory effects)	Interferon Beta-1B (Betaseron)	8 M IU (250µg) SC qod
		Interferon Beta-1A (Avonex)	30µg (6 M IU) IM qwk

Conflicting results of trials but probably only effective for secondary progressive form of MS with continued relapses.

Tyor, 2003

10.11 Huntington's Chorea

Treatment for movement disorder component

1.	**Neuroleptic** (central dopamine D$_2$ receptor antagonism)	Haloperidol (Haldol)	0.5-5mg PO bid-tid; Caution: severe AE including Parkinsonism!
or	**Atypical antipsychotic** (Dopamine D$_2$ and serotonin 5-HT receptor antagonist)	Quetiapine (Seroquel)	Ini 25mg PO bid, max 150-750mg/d; eye exam q6mo for cataracts!
		Olanzapine (Zyprexa)	Ini 5-10mg PO qd, maint 10-15mg/d
plus/or	**Dopamine depleting agent** (depletes central biogenic monoamine stores)	Reserpine (Serpalan, Gens)	Ini 0.25mg PO bid, max 2-5mg/d; Caution: severe AE including orthostatic hypotension, depression
plus/or	**Benzodiazepine** (binds to benzodiazepine receptors; enhances GABA effects)	Clonazepam (Klonopin, Gens)	Ini 0.5mg PO bid, incr up to 3mg PO tid prn
poss	For akinetic/rigid form: - **L-dopa** (see Parkinsonism Tx, →222) - **Bromocriptine** (see Parkinsonism Tx, →222)		

Kaliszky, 2003

10.12 Myasthenia Gravis

	Cholinesterase inhibitor (⇒ acetylcholine ↑)	Pyridostigmine (Mestinon, Gens)	Titrate individually 30-120mg PO q3-6h; long acting, esp. effective qhs; Caution: monitor for cholinergic excess!
or	**Glucocorticoid** (anti-inflammatory, immunosuppressive)	Prednisone (Deltasone)	Ini low dose 10-20mg PO qd, monitor closely; incr slowly to 1mg/kg/d
		Methylprednisolone (Medrol, Depo-Medrol, Solu-Medrol)	Ini low dose 10-20mg PO qd, monitor closely; incr slowly to 1-1.5mg/kg/d
	Eventually reduce steroids to lowest possible dose, qod schedule		

or	**Immunosuppressive** (purine antangonist)	**Azathioprine** (Imuran)	*Ini 50mg PO qd, incr up to 2-3mg/kg PO qd*
or	**Immunosuppressive** (inhibition of interleukin-2 activation of T-lymphocytes)	**Cyclosporine** (Gengraf, Neoral, Sandimmune, SangCya, Gens)	*Ini 2.5 mg/kg bid, maint lowest effective dose*
or	**Sugical and intervenous Tx:** - **Elective thymectomy** (remove tumor thymoma) past the age of puberty; long-term clinical improvement - **Plasmapheresis** effective short-term Tx for acute exacerbations; removal of circulating antibodies including autoimmune antibodies responsible for MG; helpful to stabilize and used as prophylaxis qwk, qmo and/or bi-monthly; caution: need to evaluate for IgA deficiency		
or	**Immunotherapy** (MA unknown)	**IV Gamma globulin** (Sandoglobulin IV)	

Patients with myasthenic or cholinergic crisis require intensive care monitored setting/treatment, due to their unpredictable course.

Walker, 2005

11. Psychiatry

D. Cyril D'Souza, MD, Associate Professor
John H. Krystal, MD, Professor
Department of Psychiatry, School of Medicine
Yale University School of Medicine, New Haven, CT

11.1 Psychiatric Emergencies

11.1.1 Acute Agitation or Excitement

Acute Agitation or Excitement (e.g. in manic, schizophrenic disorder, schizoaffective psychosis). **Combine psychopharmacological approach** with **reducing environmental stimulation** e.g., seclusion room and in rare instances mechanical restraints until psychopharmacological treatment takes effect

prim. Tx	**Benzodiazepine** (facilitation of inhibitory GABA-A receptor transmission)	**Lorazepam** (Ativan, Gens)	*1-2mg IM or slowly IV*
		Diazepam (Diastat, Valium, Gens)	*5mg slowly IV*
		Midazolam (Versed, Gens)	*1-2mg slowly IV, rep after 30-45min sos*
	Caution: beware of respiratory depression!		
poss. augm. with	**High potency antipsychotic** (dopamine antagonism)	**Haloperidol** (Haldol, Gens)	*5mg PO or IM, rep after 30-45 min sos; synerg EF, less AE poss, if co-admin with benzodiazepine*
or	**Atypical antipsychotic** (D2-5HT2 antagonist)	**Olanzapine** (Zyprexa)	*5mg IM*
		Ziprasidone (Geodon)	*5-10mg IM (less extrapyram. side effects)*

11.1.2 Acute Suicidality

Secure patient in a **safe environment** e.g., in-patient unit, emergency room and assess for imminent risk and choose appropriate level of **monitoring**, including one-to-one observation. Treat underlying disorder e.g., psychosis or depression.

suppl Tx	**Benzodiazepine** (inhibitory transmitter GABA ↑)	**Lorazepam** (Ativan, Gens)	1-2mg PO tid-qid (non-specific relief of distress)
		Diazepam (Diastat, Valium, Gens)	5-10mg PO tid-qid
		Clonazepam (Klonopin)	0.5-1mg PO bid (long-acting!)

11.1.3 Catatonia

Secure patient in a **safe environment**.

prim. Tx	**Benzodiazepine** (inhibitory transmitter GABA ↑)	**Lorazepam** (Ativan, Gens)	2.5mg PO or 1-2mg slowly IV, rep sos
augm. with	**Atypical antipsychotic** (D_2-/5-HT_2-antagonist)	**Olanzapine** (Zyprexa)	10-20mg PO
		Risperidone (Risperdal)	1-4mg PO

11.1.4 Acute Alcohol Withdrawal (Delirium)

In general

Secure patient in a **safe environment** e.g., in-patient unit, emergency room and monitor for physiologic signs and symptoms of alcohol withdrawal.

Tx of choice	**Benzodiazepine** (facilitation of GABA receptor function)	**Lorazepam** (Ativan, Gens)	1-2mg PO q1-4h titrated according to autonomic signs of withdrawal
		Oxazepam (Serax)	15-30mg PO tid to qid
		Chlordiazepoxide (Chlordiazachel, Librium)	50-100mg PO rep q2-4h prn up to 300mg/d
	Adjust dose to the point at which withdrawal symptoms are subsiding and eventually taper slowly by 25-50% qd after symptoms have stabilized. Chlordiazepoxide (Librium) or other benzodiazepines may also be used.		
2nd line	**Anticonvulsant** (facilitation of GABA receptor function)	**Valproic acid** (Depakote)	500mg PO tid x 4d, then taper by 250-500mg/d

suppl. Tx	Vitamin B₁ (PRO of Wernicke's encephalopathy)	Thiamine (Gens)	5-10mg PO qd; 100mg PO/IM qd in suspected begin of Wernicke's encephalopathy
		Folate	1mg qd
suppl. Tx	Magnesium (PRO of hypomagnesemia and seizures)	Magnesium sulfate	1g/d IV or IM in sympt. hypomagnesemia or inablity to tolerate PO Tx

If psychotic symptoms

	Atypical antipsychotic (D₂-/5-HT₂-antagonist)	Olanzapine (Zyprexa)	10-20mg PO qd
		Risperidone (Risperdal)	0.5-2mg PO bid (less AE)
or	Typical antipsychotic	Haloperidol (Haldol, Gens)	5-15mg PO qd

If autonomic symptoms (BP > 180/120mmHg, tachycardia > 120/min) are not sufficiently treatable with benzodiazepines

poss. plus	Antihypertensive (central alpha₂-receptor agonist)	Clonidine (Catapres, Catapres-TTS, Gens)	Ini 0.1mg PO bid, incr slowly sos by 0.1-0.2mg/d, up to 0.3-0.6mg q6h; Caution: monitor vital signs cosely!

If seizures

plus	Anticonvulsant	Diphenylhydantoin (Dilantin, Gens)	Ini 10-15mg/kg IV, max rate 50mg/min, then 100mg IV/PO q6-8h

11.2   Dementia

11.2.1   In General

Investigate cause of dementia i.e., vascular, Alzheimers. For vascular dementia also treat hypertension, reduction of platelet aggregation, etc.

11.2.2   First Line

In Alzheimers dementia and possibly vascular dementia

1st	Reversible competitive-noncompetitive ACI	Donepezil (Aricept)	5mg PO qd over 1mo, then 10mg qd; discont if no change after 2mo

| 1st | Pseudoreversible ACI + butylcholine esterase inhibitor | Rivastigmine (Exelon) | *Ini 2mg PO qd, then titrate slowly over 12wk to 6-12mg* |
| | Reversible, competitive ACI + nicotinic agonist | Galantamine (Reminyl) | *Ini 4mg PO bid, incr by 8mg q4wk up to 16-32mg* |

EF/MA of ACI (= acetyl cholinesterase inhibitor): inhibition of centrally-active acetylcholinesterase ⇒ concentration of acetylcholine ↑ ⇒ synaptic transmission ↑ ⇒ cognitive function ↑. With all ACIs: the slower the titration the less GI side effects

11.2.3   Second Line

In mild to moderate dementia

| | Noncompetitive NMDA receptor antagonist | Memantine (Akatinol, Namenda) | *Wk1: 5mg PO qd, wk2: 10mg qd, then 15-20mg qd* |

In mild to moderate vascular dementias

| | Ca++ channel blocker (brain vessel dilation + modulation of neuronal Ca++ homeostasis) | Nimodipine (Nimotop) | *30mg PO tid* |

11.2.4   Psychosis associated with Dementias

	Atypical antipsychotic, low dose (D_2-/5-HT_2-partial - antagonist)	Aripiprazole (Abilify)	*2-10mg PO qd*
	Atypical antipsychotic, low dose (D_2-/5-HT_2-antagonist)	Olanzapine (Zyprexa, Zyprexa Zydis)	*1.25-2.5mg PO qd; Zydis, if Pat unable to swallow*
		Quetiapine (Seroquel)	*25mg PO bid up to max 200mg bid;* **Caution:** *monitor BP and pulse!*
		Risperidone (Risperdal)	*0.5-1.0mg PO qd*

Caution: possible risk of CVA in the elderly with atypical antipsychotics

or	**Typical antipsychotic, low dose, high potency** (dopamine antagonism)	**Haloperidol** (Haldol, Gens)	*0.5-2mg PO qd*
	Caution: since the elderly are more vulnerable to develop tardive dyskinesia, chronic Tx with typical antipsychotics should be avoided		
poss.	**Benzodiazepine**	**Lorazepam** (Ativan, Gens)	*Low doses;* **Caution:** *paradoxical effects poss*

11.3   Alcoholism
11.3.1   Acute Alcohol Withdrawal

See Acute Alcohol Withdrawal (Delirium) →229

11.3.2   Chronic Alcoholism

	Deterrent (deterrant acetaldehyde formed during normal catabolism of alcohol ⇒ unpleasant symptoms)	**Disulfiram** (Antabuse)	*250–500mg qd PO after discussion of interactions with alcohol and alcohol containing preparations*
	Glutamate modulating (craving ↓ ⇒ period of abstinence ↑)	**Acamprosate** (Campral)	*BW <60kg: 1.3g/d PO; >60kg: 2g/d PO div bid; available as 333mg enteric-coated Tab*
	Opioid antagonism (craving ↓)	**Naltrexone** (Revia)	*50mg PO qd*

11.4   Depressive Disorders
11.4.1   Acute Treatment

With all antidepressants assessment of success at the earliest after 2-3 wk of Tx with target/Tx dose! After depressive symptoms cease, cont drug Tx for at least 6 mo.

	SSRI (selective serotonin reuptake inhibition)	**Citalopram** (Celexa)	*Incr slowly to 20-60mg PO qd*
		Fluoxetine (Prozac)	
		Paroxetine (Paxil, Paxil CR)	

	SSRI (selective serotonin reuptake inhibition)	**Sertraline** (Zoloft)	*Incr slowly to 50-150mg PO qd*
		Fluvoxamine (Luvox, Gens)	
		Escitalopram (Lexapro)	*Incr slowly to 10-20mg PO qd*
or	**NASA** (norepinephrine and serotonin antagonism)	**Mirtazapine** (Remeron, Remeron Soltab)	*Incr slowly to 15-45mg PO qd*
or	**Non-Tricyclic SNRI** (serotonin-norepinephrine reuptake inhibition)	**Venlafaxine** (Effexor, Effexor XR)	*Incr slowly to 75-225mg PO qd*
		Duloxetine (Cymbalta)	*20-30mg PO bid*
or	**Tricyclic SNRI** (serotonin-norepinephrine reuptake inhibition plus additional (side)effects due to cholinergic and histaminergic actions)	**Amitriptyline** (Clavil, Elavil, Endep, Gens)	*Incr slowly to 150-200mg/d PO in div doses prn*
		Clomipramine (Anafranil, Gens)	
		Desipramine (Norpramin, Gens)	*Incr slowly to 50-200mg PO in div doses prn*
		Doxepin (Sinequan, Gens)	*Incr slowly to 150-200mg PO in div doses prn*
		Nortriptyline (Aventyl, Pamelor, Gens)	
		Protryptilline (Vivacty)	*Incr slowly to 15-40mg PO in div doses prn*
		Trimipramine (Surmontil)	*Incr slowly to 150-200mg PO in div doses prn*
		Amoxapine (Asendin)	
		Maprotiline (Ludiomil)	*Incr slowly to 100-150mg PO in div doses prn*
or	**DRI** (dopamine reuptake inhibition)	**Bupropion** (Wellbutrin)	*Incr slowly to 150-450mg PO qd (div tid); seizures at higher doses*

or	**SARI** (serotonin 5-HT$_2$-antagonism and reuptake inhibition)	**Trazodone** (Desyrel, Gens)	*Incr slowly to 200-600mg PO qd in div doses*
		Nefazodone (Serzone)	*Incr slowly to 200-500mg PO qd in div doses*
or	**Irreversible MAO inhibitor** (norepinephrine and serotonine breakdown ↓)	**Tranylcypromine** (Parnate)	*Incr slowly to 20-50mg PO qd in div doses prn*
		Phenelzine (Nardil)	*45-60 mg PO qd; low tyramine diet req!*

11.4.2   If No Response or Partial Response

	Change to an antidepressant from a different substance class (s.a.)		
or	Augment with: **SSRI, tricyclic SNRI** or **previously described antidepressant. Caution**: do not combine with MAOIs!		
or	**Lithium augmentation** (complex mechanism of action)	**Lithium** (Eskalith, Eskalith CR, Lithane, Lithobid, Gens)	*Ini 300mg PO bid, titrate to serum level of 0.4-0.8meq/l*
or	**Stimulant** (DA release)	**Dextroamphetamine**	*5-30mg/d PO in div doses*
or	**Electroconvulsive Tx** (induction of a grand mal seizure in anesthesia)		*e.g. three times a week*

11.4.3   Psychotic Depression

plus	**Atypical antipsychotic** (D$_2$-/5-HT$_2$-antagonist)	**Olanzapine** (Zyprexa)	*Incr slowly to 5-20mg/d PO*
		Risperidone (Risperdal)	*Incr slowly to 2-6mg/d PO*
		Quetiapine (Seroquel)	*Incr slowly to 200-400mg PO bid*
		Ziprasidone (Geodon)	*Incr slowly to 40-80mg PO bid*
	Atypical antipsychotic (D$_2$-/5-HT$_2$-partial-antagonist)	**Aripiprazole** (Abilify)	*15-45mg PO qd*

11.5 Manic Disorders

11.5.1 Acute Mania

First line

either	**Lithium** (complex mechanism of action)	**Lithium** (Eskalith, Eskalith CR, Lithane, Lithobid, Gens)	*Ini 300mg PO bid, then titrate to serum level of 0.8–1.2meq/l;* **Caution:** *overdose!*
or	**Anticonvulsant** (facilitation of GABA receptor function)	**Valproic acid** (Depakene, Depakote, Myproic Acid, Gens)	*Titrate to serum level of 75-100mg/l ; „IV-loading" also poss: 20mg/kg/d*

Second line

	Atypical antipsychotic (D$_2$-/5-HT$_2$-antagonist)	**Olanzapine** (Zyprexa)	*Incr slowly to 5-20mg/d PO*
		Risperidone (Risperdal)	*Incr slowly to 2-6mg/d PO*
		Quetiapine (Seroquel)	*Incr slowly to 200-400mg/d PO (div bid-tid)*
		Ziprasidone (Geodon)	*Incr slowly to 40-120mg/d PO bid*
	Atypical antipsychotic (D$_2$-/5-HT$_2$-partial-antagonist)	**Aripiprazole** (Abilify)	*15-45mg PO qd*

May be used as standalone Tx (without mood stabilizer) regardless of whether the patient has psychotic symptoms

Supplementary Tx for agitation, excitement, insomnia

Benzodiazepine (increase in inhibitory transmitter GABA)	**Lorazepam** (Ativan, Gens)	*1-2mg IM or slowly IV*
	Diazepam (Diastat, Valium, Gens)	*5-10mg slowly IV, rep prn*

11.5.2 Prophylaxis, Maintenance

Continue mood stabilizer, but lower dose

either	**Lithium** (established antimanic effects, complex MA)	**Lithium** (Eskalith, Eskalith CR, Lithane, Lithobid, Gens)	*Titrate dose for serum level of 4-8meq/l*
or	**Anticonvulsant** (facilitation of GABA function)	**Valproic acid** (Depakene, Depakote, Myproic acid, Gens)	*Titrate dose for serum level of 50-100mg/l*

11.6 Psychotic Disorders (Schizophrenia, Delusional Disorder,
11.6.1 Acute or Subacute Psychosis

First line

Atypical antipsychotic (Balanced D$_2$- : 5-HT$_2$- receptor antagonism)	**Risperidone** (Risperdal)	*Incr slowly to 4-8mg PO qd; in higher dose more frequently extrapyram. symptoms*
	Olanzapine (Zyprexa, Zyprexa Zydis)	*Incr slowly to 5-20mg PO qd*
	Quetiapine (Seroquel)	*Incr slowly to 200-400mg PO bid*
	Ziprasidone (Geodon)	*Incr slowly to 40-120mg PO bid*
	Zotepine (Zoleptil)	*Ini 75-150mg PO (div tid), incr to 300mg/d sos*
	Amisulpride (Solian)	*400-800mg PO qd*
Atypical antipsychotic (D$_2$-/5-HT$_2$-partial-antagonist)	**Aripiprazole** (Abilify)	*15-45mg qd*

Second line (in order of decreasing potency)			
Typical antipsychotic (central dopamine receptor antagonism)	**Haloperidol** (Haldol, Gens)	*5-20mg PO qd*
	Fluphenazine (Prolixin)	*5-20mg PO qd*
	Pimozide (Orap)	*1-8mg PO qd*
	Perphenazine (Trilafon, Gens)	*16-64mg PO qd*

In drug-induced dose-related extrapyramidal disorder (dystonia, parkinsonism)

Anticholinergic Parkinsonian drug (inhibition of central cholinergic neurons)	**Biperiden** (Akineton)	*2mg PO or 5mg slowly IV*
	Benztropine mesylate (Cogentin)	*1-2mg PO or IM/IV*

In dose-related akathisia

Betablocker (central sympathic act. ↓)	**Propranolol** (Inderal, Inderal LA, Gens)	*10-30mg PO tid*

11.6.2   Treatment-resistant Psychosis or Intolerable Side-effects (e.g. Treatment Failure with at least 2 Other Antipsychotics)

	SDA (serotonin dopamine receptor antagonist)	**Clozapine** (Clozaril, Gens)	*Ini 12.5-25mg qd, then titrate up to 300-600mg qd;* **Caution:** *monitor granulocyte (neutrophil) count (agranulocytosis!)*
or	**Electroconvulsive Tx** (Induction of a grand mal seizure in anesthesia)		*e.g. 3 x per wk*
or	Combination of antipsychotics		

11.6.3   Acute Catatonia

	Benzodiazepine (inhib. transmit. GABA ↑)	**Lorazepam** (Ativan, Gens)	*1-2.5mg PO or IM, rep sos*
plus	Treat as for acute psychosis with **atypical** or **typical antipsychotics**: - If negative symptoms predominant, lower doses and atypical antipsychotics preferred - Comorbid substance abuse disorders: atypical antipsychotics preferred - Relapse prophylaxis, maintenance of remission: consider reducing dose to minimum effective dose		

11.6.4	In Noncompliant Patients		
	Depot Neuroleptic (delayed release after IM-injection through bond to oily medium)	**Haloperidol Decanoate** (Haldol Decanoate)	*50-200mg IM q3-4wk*
		Fluphenazine Decanoate (Prolixin Decanoate)	*12.5-50mg IM q2wk*
		Flupentixol (Fluanxol)	*20-40mg IM q2wk*
		Risperidone (Consta)	*25-75mg IM q2wk*

For first time recipients, test dose with oral equivalent, followed by continued oral supplementation till 3rd injection

11.7 Anxiety Disorders

11.7.1 Acute Fear or Acute Panic Attack

	Benzodiazepine (inhibitory transmitter GABA ↑)	**Lorazepam** (Ativan, Gens)	*1-2mg PO*
		Diazepam (Diastat, Valium, Gens)	*5-10mg PO*

11.7.2 Generalized Anxiety Disorder (GAD)

either	**SSRI antidepressant** (selective serotonin reuptake inhibition)	**Citalopram** (Celexa)	*Incr slowly to 20-60mg PO qd*
		Fluoxetine (Prozac)	*Incr slowly to 20-60mg PO qd*
		Paroxetine (Paxil, Paxil CR)	*Incr slowly to 20-60mg PO qd*
		Sertraline (Zoloft)	*Incr slowly to 50-150mg PO qd*
		Fluvoxamine (Luvox, Gens)	*Incr slowly to 50-150mg PO qd*
		Escitalopram (Lexapro)	*Incr slowly to 10-20mg PO qd*

Effects often seen only after several weeks of treatment.

or	**Non-Tricyclic SNRI** (serotonin-norepineph-rine reuptake inhibition)	**Venlafaxine** (Effexor, Effexor XR)	*Incr slowly to 225-375mg PO qd*
	Effects often seen only after several weeks of treatment.		
and/ or	**Benzodiazepine** (inhibitory transmitter GABA ↑)	**Clonazepam** (Klonopin)	*1-4 mg PO qd*
		Lorazepam (Ativan, Gens)	*up to 1-2mg tid PO*
		Diazepam (Diastat, Valium, Gens)	*5-10mg PO tid*
		Alprazolam (Xanax)	*0.5-1 mg PO tid-qid*
	Tolerance and dependence may emerge over time.		
and/ or	**Anxiolytic** (partial serotonin 5-HT1a receptor agonism)	**Buspirone** (Buspar, Gens)	*Ini 5mg tid, incr up to 20mg tid*

1.7.3 Panic Disorder and Agoraphobia

	SSRI antidepressant (selective serotonin reuptake inhibitor)	**Paroxetine** (Paxil, Paxil CR)	*40-80mg PO qd; effects often only after several wks' Ts*
or	**Tricyclic SNRI antidepressant** (especially serotonin reuptake inhibition)	**Imipramine** (Tofranil, Gens)	*100-300mg PO qd*
		Clomipramine (Anafranil, Gens)	*150-225mg PO qd*
	Effects often only after several weeks' treatment. Tricyclics may lead to cardiac toxicity.		
and/ or	**Benzodiazepine** (inhibitory transmitter GABA ↑)	**Clonazepam** (Klonopin)	*1-4 mg PO qd*
		Lorazepam (Ativan, Gens)	*up to 1-2mg PO tid*
		Diazepam (Diastat, Valium, Gens)	*5-10mg PO tid*
		Alprazolam (Xanax)	*0.5-1 mg PO qid*
	Tolerance and dependence may emerge over time.		

1.7.4 Social Phobia

	SSRI antidepressant (selective serotonin reuptake inhibitor)	**Paroxetine** (Paxil, Paxil CR)	*40-60mg PO qd; effects often only after several weeks' treatment*

or	**Reversible MAO inhibitor** (inhibition of MAO ⇒ norepinephrine and serotonine breakdown↓)	Moclobemide (Manerix)	*Ini 300mg PO qd, incr to 300mg bid; effects often only after several weeks Tx*

11.8   Obsessive-Compulsive Disorders

either	**SSRI** (selective serotonin reuptake inhibition)	**Fluvoxamine** (Luvox, Gens)	*Incr slowly to 100-300mg PO qd*
		Fluoxetine (Prozac)	*Incr slowly to 20-80mg PO qd*
		Sertraline (Zoloft)	*Incr slowly to 75-225mg PO qd*
		Paroxetine (Paxil, Paxil CR)	*Incr slowly to 40-80mg PO qd*
or	**Tricyclic Antidepressant** (reuptake inhibition of serotonin and norepinephrine)	**Clomipramine** (Anafranil, Gens)	*Incr slowly to 150-300mg PO qd*

Improvement takes 5-10 weeks of treatment.

11.8.1   Treatment resistant patients

Augm Tx	**Atypical antipsychotic** (Balanced D_2- : 5-HT_2-receptor antagonism)	**Risperidone** (Risperdal)	*Incr slowly to 4-8mg PO qd; in higher dose more frequently extrapyram. symptoms*
		Olanzapine (Zyprexa, Zyprexa Zydis)	*Incr slowly to 5-20mg PO qd*
		Quetiapine (Seroquel)	*Incr slowly to 200-400mg PO bid*
		Ziprasidone (Geodon)	*Incr slowly to 40-120mg PO bid*
		Zotepine (Zoleptil)	*Ini 75-150mg PO (div tid), incr to 300mg/d so*
		Amisulpride (Solian)	*400-800mg PO qd*

12. Ophthalmology

Daniel S. Casper, MD, Assistant Clinical Professor
Director of Ophthalmology, Naomi Berrie Diabetes Center,
Columbia University Medical Center, New York, NY
Pamela Cheung, MD, Assistant Professor
Department of Ophthalmaology, College of Physicians & Surgeons of
Columbia University, New York, NY

12.1 Hordeolum, Chalazion

	- **Warm compresses** - **Massage** - **Lid hygiene**		
plus or	**Topical Antibiotic** (broad-spectrum)	**Bacitracin oint** (Gens)	*apply ½ inch ribbon tid-qid for 7-10d*
		Erythromycin oint 0.5% (Ilotycin)	
con- sider	**Intralesional corticosteroid**	**Triamcinolone 40mg/ml** (Kenalog, Aristocort)	*0.2-1.0ml Inj directly into lesion*

Intralesional corticosteroid may be associated with localized permanent skin depigmentation. If these measures do not eliminate the lesion, then **incision with drainage and curettage** may be considered.

12.2 Blepharitis

12.2.1 Anterior Blepharitis

	Lid hygiene with eyelid scrubs + warm compresses		
Plus	**Artificial tears, lubricant** (lubricate ocular surface, maintain ocular tonicity)	**Methyl, ethyl, and propyl cellulose preparations; Glycerin** (Celluvisc, GenTeal, Hypo Tears, Refresh Tears, Tears Naturale II, Gens)	*1 Gtt qid-qh* *(short or long-term)*
or		**Preservative-free Tears** (Bion Tears, GenTeal, Hypo Tears PF, OcuCoat PF, Refresh Plus, Tears Naturale Free, Thera Tears)	*1 Gtt qid-qh (long-term)*

or		Petrolatum/lanolin/ mineral oil oint comb. (Lacri-lube, Duolube, Duratears Naturale, Refresh PM, Gens)	½ inch qhs-qid
Plus	Topical antibiotic (gram-positive coverage)	Bacitracin oint (Gens)	apply ½ inch ribbon qhs-tid
or	Topical macrolide	Erythromycin oint 0.5% (Ilotycin)	
Or	Topical antibiotic + corticosteroid (antiinflammatory)	Tobramycin + Dexamethasone 0.1% (Tobradex aq or oint)	1 Gtt qd-qid or ½ inch oint qhs
		Tobramycin 0.3% + Loteprednol etabonate 0.5% (Zylet)	1-2 Gtt q4-6h adjusted accordingly

12.2.2 Posterior Blepharitis, Meibomianitis

	Topical antibiotic (gram-positive coverage)	Bacitracin oint (Gens)	apply ½ inch ribbon qhs-tid
or	Topical macrolide	Erythromycin oint 0.5% (Ilotycin)	
Plus	Oral tetracycline	Doxycycline (Doryx, Periostat, Vibramycin, Gens)	100mg PO bid for 2wk, then decr slowly
or		Minocycline (Dynacin, Minocin, Vectrin, Gens)	
or		Tetracycline (Achromycin, Sumycin, Gens)	250mg PO qid for 2wk, then decr slowly
or	Oral macrolide	Erythromycin (E-Base, E-mycin, Eryc, Gens)	

Note: Doxycycline, minocycline and tetracycline are contraindicated in children, pregnant women and nursing women.

153. Lederman C, Miller M: Hordeola and chalazia. Pediatr Rev 1999; 20(8): 283-284.
154. Cohen EJ: Cornea and external disease in the new millennium. Arch Ophthalmol 2000; 118(7): 979-981.
155. Fraunfelder FT, Roy FH, Steinemann TL: Current Ocular Therapy. 5th ed. 2000: 72, 374, 378, 450.

12.3 Abscess, Furuncle of the Eyelids

12.3.1 In General

	- Warm compresses - Debridement (prn) - Incision and drainage (prn)		
plus	Topical antibiotic	Bacitracin + Polymyxin B oint (Polysporin, Gens)	½ inch tid-qid
or		Tobramycin oint 0.3% (Tobrex)	
plus	Systemic cephalosporin	Cefaclor (Ceclor, Gens)	250-500mg PO q8h, Ped 20-40mg/kg PO qd (div tid), for 7-10d
or	Systemic broad- spectrum penicillin + beta-lactamase Inhibit.	Amoxicillin + Clavulanate (Augmentin)	250-500mg PO q8h, Ped 20-40mg/kg qd (div tid) for 7-10d

12.3.2 In Severe Cases in Adults

Systemic cephalosporin	Cefuroxime (Kefurox, Zinacef, Gens)	750-1500mg IM/IV q8h

12.3.3 In Severe Cases in Children

Systemic broad- spectrum penicillin	Ampicillin (Omnipen, Principen, Totacillin, Gens)	Ped 50-100mg/kg PO qd (div q6h), or 100- 200mg/kg IM/IV qd (div q6h)

156. Barza M, Baum J: Ocular infections. Med Clin North Am 1983;67(1):131-152.
157. Schwartz G: Etiology, Diagnosis, and Treatment of Orbital Infections. Curr Infect Dis Rep 2002;4(3):201-205.
158. Weiss A, Friendly D, Eglin K, et al: Bacterial periorbital and orbital cellulitis in childhood. Ophthalmology 1983; 90(3): 195-203.

12.4 Viral Infections of the Eyelids
12.4.1 Herpes Simplex

	Warm compresses to lesions tid		
Plus	Topical antiviral	Trifluridine 1% (Viroptic)	*1 Gtt 5x/d for 7-14d*
or		Vidarabine oint 3% (Vira-A)	*½ inch 5x/d*
+/-	Oral antiviral	Acyclovir (Zovirax, Gens)	*400mg PO 5x/d for 7-14d; systemic in primary herpetic infection*

12.4.2 Herpes Zoster

	Warm compresses to lesions tid		
Plus	Topical antibiotic	Bacitracin oint (Gens)	*½ inch bid-tid;*
or		Erythromycin oint 0.5% (Ilotycin)	*Note: trifluridine not effective in HZV*
Plus	Oral antiviral	Acyclovir (Zovirax, Gens)	*800mg PO 5x/d for 7d*
or		Famciclovir (Famvir)	*500mg PO tid for 7d*
or		Valacyclovir (Valtrex)	*1g PO tid for 7d*

159. Chern KC, Margolis TP: Varicella zoster virus ocular disease. Int Ophthalmol Clin 1998; 38(4): 149-160.
160. Pavan-Langston D: Viral diseases of the cornea and external eye. In: Albert DM, Jakobiec FA, eds.
161. Principles and Practices of Ophthalmology. Vol. 1. 1994: 117-161.

12.5 Dacryoadenitis
12.5.1 Acute Bacterial Dacryoadenitis

	In general		
	Systemic broad-spectrum penicillin + beta-lactamase Inhibit.	Amoxicillin + Clavulanate (Augmentin)	*250-500mg PO q8h, **Ped** 20-40mg/kg PO qd (div tid) for ca. 7-14d*
or	Systemic cephalosporin	Cephalexin (Keflex, Keftab, Gens)	*250-500mg PO q6h, **Ped** 20-50mg/kg PO qd (div qid) for ca. 7-14d*

In severe cases IV Tx			
	Systemic cephalosporin	Cefazolin (Ancef, Kefzol, Gens)	1g IV tid-qid for 7-14d, Ped 50-100mg/kg qd (div tid-qid) for 7-14d
In Gonococci			
	Systemic cephalosporin	Ceftriaxone (Rocephin)	125mg IM once
In Staphylococci			
	Systemic penicillin	Oxacillin (Bactocill)	1g IM/IV q6h, Ped 50-100mg/kg qd (div qid) for 7-14d
In Streptococci			
	Systemic broad-spectrum penicillin	Ampicillin (Omnipen, Principen, Totacillin, Gens)	500mg q6h, Ped 50-100mg/kg PO qd (div q6h), or 100-200mg/kg IM/IV (div q6h)

12.5.2 Acute Viral Dacryoadenitis

- Mumps, Mononucleosis, EBV, HZV, CMV
- Supportive measures: cool compresses, analgesics prn

12.5.3 Chronic Dacryoadenitis in Tuberculosis

	Tuberculostatic	Isoniazid (Gens)	300mg PO qd for 2mo; PRO of isoniazid neuropathy: Pyridoxine (Gens) 25-50mg PO qd suppl
or		Rifampin (Rifadin, Rimactane, Gens)	600mg PO qd for 2mo
or		Pyrazinamide (Gens)	2g PO qd for 2mo
or		Ethambutol (Myambutol, Gens)	15mg/kg PO qd, max 2500mg qd

162. Boruchoff SA, Boruchoff SE: Infections of the lacrimal system. Infect Dis Clin North Am 1992; 6(4): 925-932.
163. Fitzsimmons TD, Wilson SE, Kennedy RH: Infectious dacryoadenitis. In: Ocular Infection and Immunity. St. Louis: CV Mosby; 1996:1341-1345.
164. Massaro BM, Tabbara KF: Infections of lacrimal apparatus. In: Infections of the Eye. Boston: Little Brown & Co; 1996:551-558.

12.6 Dacryocystitis

12.6.1 In General

- Warm compresses
- Massage
- Poss incision/drainage if abscess

12.6.2 Acute Dacryocystitis in Adults (modify depending on etiology)

	Systemic cephalosporin	Cephalexin (Keflex, Keftab, Gens)	*500mg PO q6h for 10-14d*
or	Systemic penicillin + beta-lactamase Inhibit.	Amoxicillin + Clavulanate (Augmentin)	*500mg PO q8h for 10-14d*
severe	Systemic cephalosporin	Cefazolin (Ancef, Kefzol, Gens)	*1g IV q8h*
or	Systemic penicillin + beta-lactamase Inhibit.	Ampicillin + Sulbactam (Unasyn)	*1.5g IV q6h*

12.6.3 Acute Dacryocystitis in Children

	Systemic penicillin + beta-lactamase Inhibit.	Amoxicillin + Clavulanate (Augmentin)	*20-40mg/kg qd (div tid) for 10-14d*
severe	Systemic cephalosporin	Cefuroxime (Kefurox, Zinacef, Gens)	*50-100mg/kg IV qd (div tid) for 10-14d*

165. Dryden RM, Wulc AE: Lacrimal inflammations and infections. In: Oculoplastic, Orbital and Reconstructive Surgery. Vol. 2. 1417-1423.
166. Hurwitz JJ, Rodgers KJ: Management of acquired dacryocystitis. Can J Ophthalmol 1983; 18(5): 213-216.

12.7 Conjunctivitis

12.7.1 Keratoconjunctivitis Sicca

Artificial tears, lubricant (lubricate ocular surface, maintain ocular tonicity)	Methyl, ethyl, and propyl cellulose preparations; Glycerin (Celluvisc, GenTeal, Hypo Tears, Refresh Tears, Tears Naturale II, Gens)	*1 Gtt qid-qh (long-term)*

or	Artificial tears, lubricant (lubricate ocular surface, maintain ocular tonicity)	Preservative-free Tears (Bion Tears, GenTeal, Hypo Tears PF, OcuCoat PF, Refresh Plus, Tears Naturale Free, Thera Tears)	1 Gtt qid-qh (long-term)
or		Petrolatum/lanolin/ mineral oil oint comb. (Lacri-lube, Duolube, Duratears Naturale, Refresh PM, Gens)	½ inch qhs-qid

Consider placement of punctal plugs in puncta of nasolacrimal ducts to decrease tear egress and prolong tear presence in conjunctival sac

12.7.2 Allergic Conjunctivitis

	Vasoconstrictor + antihistamine	Naphazoline + Pheniramine (Naphcon-A, Opcon-A, Visine-A)	1 Gtt qid prn
or	Topical mast cell stabilizer	Cromolyn sodium (Crolom, Opticrom, Gens)	1 Gtt qid *may take wk for effect
or		Nedocromil (Alocril)	1 Gtt bid prn
or		Pemirolast (Alamast)	1 Gtt qid prn
or		Lodoxamide (Alomide)	1 Gtt bid-qid prn
+/ or	Topical antihistamine (H1 receptor antagonist)	Azelastine (Optivar)	1 Gtt bid prn
or	Antihistamine (selective H1 receptor antagonist with affinity for H2 receptor)	Epinastine HCl 0.05% (Elestat)	1 Gtt bid
or	Antihistamine/ mast cell stabilizer	Olopatadine (Patanol)	1 Gtt bid prn
		Ketotifen (Zaditor)	1 Gtt bid prn
or	Topical corticosteroid (low-medium potency)	Loteprednol (Alrex, Lotemax)	1 Gtt bid-qid
+/-	Oral antihistamine	Diphenhydramine (Benadryl, Gens)	25-50mg q4-6h

12.7.3   Bacterial Conjunctivitis

In general

	Topical antibiotic (broad-spectrum)	**Polymyxin B + Trimethoprim** (Polytrim, Gens)	*1 Gtt qid for 5-7d*
or		**Bacitracin oint** (Gens)	*½ inch qid for 5-7d*
or		**Erythromycin oint 0.5%** (Ilotycin)	
or	Topical fluoroquinolone	**Ciprofloxacin** (Ciloxan)	*1 Gtt (0.3%) qid for 5-7d*
		Ofloxacin (Ocuflox)	

In Gonococci

	– Irrigate with saline QID – Treat concurrent Chlamydia		
	Topical antibiotic (broad-spectrum)	**Bacitracin oint** (Gens)	*½ inch q2-4h*
	Systemic cephalosporin	**Ceftriaxone** (Rocephin)	*1g IM once;* **Neonatal:** *125mg IM once*

Chlamydia conjunctivitis

	Topical antibiotic	**Erythromycin oint 0.5%** (Ilotycin)	*½ inch qid*
or		**Sulfacetamide oint** (Bleph-10, Gens)	
Plus	Systemic antibiotic	**Tetracycline** (Achromycin, Sumycin, Gens)	*250-500mg qid for 3-6wk*
or		**Doxycycline** (Doryx, Periostat, Vibramycin, Gens)	*100mg bid for 3-6wk*
	Note: Doxycycline and tetracycline are contraindicated in children, pregnant women and nursing women		
or	Systemic macrolide	**Erythromycin** (E-Base, E-mycin, Eryc, Gens)	*250-500mg qid,* **Neonate:** *50mg/kg qd (div qid) for 3-6wk*

12.7.4 Viral Conjunctivitis

	- Cool compresses - Spread precautions		
	Artificial tear preparations and lubricants	**Methyl, ethyl, and propyl cellulose preparations; Glycerin** (Celluvisc, GenTeal, Hypo Tears, Refresh Tears, Tears Naturale II, Gens)	*1 Gtt qid-qh*
+/-	**Vasoconstrictor + antihistamine**	**Naphazoline + Pheniramine** (Naphcon-A, Opcon-A, Visine-A)	*1 Gtt qid prn*
+/-	**Topical NSAID** (anti-inflammatory)	**Diclofenac** (Voltaren)	*1 Gtt qid prn*

167. Allansmith MR, Ross RN: Ocular allergy and mast cell stabilizers. Surv Ophthalmol 1986; 30(4): 229-244.
168. Friedlaender MH: A review of the causes and treatment of bacterial and allergic conjunctivitis. Clin Ther 1995;17(5):800-810.
169. Hingorani M, Lightman S: Therapeutic options in ocular allergic disease. Drugs 1995;50(2):208-221.
170. Nelson JD: Diagnosis of keratoconjunctivitis sicca. Int Ophthalmol Clin 1994; 34(1): 37-56.
171. Pavan-Langston D: Viral diseases of the cornea and external eye. In: Albert DM, Jakobiec FA, eds.
172. Principles and Practices of Ophthalmology. Vol. 1. 1994:117-161.

12.7.5 Keratitis Sicca (Dry Eye Syndrome)

	Artificial tears, lubricant (lubricate ocular surface, maintain ocular tonicity)	**Methyl, ethyl, and porpyl, cellulose preparations; Glycerin** (Celluvisc, GenTeal, Hypo Tears, Refresh Tears, Systane, Tears Naturale II, Gens)	*1 Gtt qid-qh (short or long-term)* **Caution:** *avoid any drops containing vasoconstrictive components*
or		**Preservative-free Tears** (Bion Tears, GenTeal, Hypo Tears PF, OcuCoat PF, Refresh Plus, Tears Naturale Free, Thera Tears)	*1 Gtt qid-qh (long-term)*

| and/or | **Artificial tears, lubricant** (lubricate ocular surface, maintain ocular tonicity) | **Petroleum/lanolin/ mineral oil oint comb.** (Lacri-lube, Duolube, Duratears Naturale, Refresh PM, Gens) | *1/2 inch qhs-qid* |
| Consider | **Topical immunomodulator with anti-inflammatory effects** | **Cyclosporine ophthalmic emulsion 0.05% (Restasis)** | *1 Gtt bid (long-term) (some practitioners use a mild topical steroid either before or during cyclosporine initiation due burning)* |

Note: Used to treat dry eye irritation. Many types of artificial tears are available over the counter. In mild cases, preserved tears can be used. In severe cases only nonpreserved tears should be used.

173. Strong B, Farley W, Stern ME, Pflugfelder SC. Topical cyclosporine inhibits conjunctival epithelial apoptosis in experimental murine keratoconjunctivitis sicca. Cornea 2005;24:80-5
174. Stevenson D, Tauber J, Reis BL. Efficacy and safety of cyclosporin A ophthalmic emulsion in the treatment of moderate-to-severe dry eye disease: a dose-ranging, randomized trial. The cyclosporin A phase 2 study group. Ophthalmology 2000;107:967-74
175. Gunduz K, Ozdemir O. Topical cyclosporin treatment of keratoconjunctivitis sicca in secondary Sjogren's syndrome. Acta Ophthalmol (Copenh.) 1994;72:438-42

12.8 Keratitis
12.8.1 Bacterial Ulcers

Note: Any ulcer at or near the visual axis, and > 1mm in diameter, or any lesion > 2-3mm in diameter requires culturing.

Topical therapy

	Topical broad-spectrum antibiotic	**Ciprofloxacin** (Ciloxan)	*1 Gtt (0.3%) qid-qh (may use loading dose as directed)*
or		**Ofloxacin** (Ocuflox)	
or		**Moxifloxacin HCL 0.5%** (Vigamox)	*1 Gtt tid x 7d*
or		**Gatifloxacin 0.3%** (Zymar)	*1 Gtt q2h WA x 2d, then qid WA x 5d*
or		**Tobramycin** (Tobrex)	*1 Gtt (0.3%) qid-qh (may use loading dose as directed)*

+/–	Topical broad-spectrum antibiotic	Ciprofloxacin oint (Ciloxan)	½ inch (0.3%) qhs
or		Tobramycin oint (Tobrex)	
or if severe	Fortified topical antibiotics (-gram-positive coverage)	Fortified Cefazolin (50mg/ml)	1 Gtt q1-2h
or		Fortified Vancomycin (25-50mg/ml)	1 Gtt q1-2h
or	Fortified topical antibiotics (-gram-neg. coverage)	Fortified Tobramycin (15mg/ml)	1 Gtt q1-2h alternating
plus	Cycloplegic (ciliary spasm ↓)	Cyclopentolate 1-2% (AK-Pentolate, Cyclogyl, Gens)	1 Gtt bid-tid
or		Homatropine 2%, 5% (Isopto Homatropine)	
or		Atropine 1.0% (Atropine care, Atropisol, Isopto Atropine, Gens)	
+/–	Topical corticosteroid (anti-inflammatory)	Prednisolone 1% (Predforte, Econopred Plus)	1 Gtt qd-qid; recommend referral to ophthalmologist

Systemic therapy in Gonococci, Haemophilus, +/– Pseudomonas

	Systemic cephalosporin	Cefazolin (Ancef, Kefzol, Gens)	1-2g IV bid
or		Ceftriaxone (Rocephin)	1g IV qd
H. Flu	Systemic broad-spectrum penicillin + beta-lactamase Inhibit.	Amoxicillin + Clavulanate (Augmentin)	500mg PO q8h for 10-14d, **Ped** 20-40mg/kg qd (div tid) for 10-14d

12.8.2 Fungal Keratitis

	Topical antifungal (molds: ex/Fusarium)	Natamycin 5% (Natacyn)	*1 Gtt q1-2h;* **Note:** *only topical antifungal commercially available*
or	Topical antifungal (-yeasts: ex/Candida)	Amphotericin B 0.15% (Fungizone)	*1 Gtt q1-2h*
or	Topical antifungal	Clotrimazole 0.1-1% (Mycelex)	*1 Gtt q1-2h*
or		Miconazole 0.1-1% (Monistat)	
+/-	Oral antifungal	Ketoconazole (Nizoral, Gens)	*200-400mg PO qd*
or		Fluconazole (Diflucan)	*100-400mg PO qd*
or		Itraconazole (Sporanox)	*200mg PO qd-bid*
plus	Cycloplegic (ciliary spasm↓; see bacterial ulcer, →250)	Cyclopentolate 1-2% (AK-Pentolate, Cyclogyl, Gens)	*1 Gtt bid-tid*
or		Homatropine 2%, 5% (Isopto Homatropine)	

12.8.3 Herpes Simplex Keratitis

Epithelial HSV keratitis

	Topical antiviral	Trifluridine 1% (Viroptic)	*1 Gtt 9x/d*
or		Vidarabine oint 3% (Vira-A)	*½ inch 5x/d*
+/-	Cycloplegic (ciliary spasm↓; see bacterial ulcer, →250)	Cyclopentolate 1-2% (AK-Pentolate, Cyclogyl, Gens)	*1 Gtt bid-tid*
or		Homatropine 2%, 5% (Isopto Homatropine)	

Stromal HSV keratitis

	Antiviral prophylaxis	Trifluridine 1% (Viroptic)	*1 Gtt tid-qid*

plus	**Topical corticosteroid** (anti-inflammatory)	**Prednisolone 1%** (Predforte, Econopred Plus)	*1 Gtt qid*
+/-	**Cycloplegic** (ciliary spasm ↓; see bacterial ulcer, →250)	**Cyclopentolate 0.5-2%** (AK-Pentolate, Cyclogyl, Gens)	*1 Gtt bid-tid*
or		**Homatropine 2%, 5%** (Isopto Homatropine)	

HSV keratouveitis, in addition to above:

+/-	**Systemic Antiviral**	**Acyclovir** (Zovirax, Gens)	*400mg PO 5x/d*

Neurotrophic/Metaherpetic keratopathy

	Artificial tears, lubricant (lubricate ocular surface, maintain ocular tonicity; see Keratoconjunctivitis →246)	**Preservative-free Tears** (Bion Tears, GenTeal, Hypo Tears PF, OcuCoat PF, Refresh Plus, Tears Naturale Free, Thera Tears)	*1 Gtt q1-2h*
+/-	**Topical antibiotic** (broad-spectrum)	**Bacitracin oint** (Gens)	*½ inch tid-qid*
or		**Erythromycin oint 0.5%** (Ilotycin)	

12.8.4 Herpes Zoster Keratitis

or	**Topical antibiotic** (broad-spectrum)	**Bacitracin oint** (Gens)	*½ inch tid-qid*
		Erythromycin oint 0.5% (Ilotycin)	
plus	**Artificial tears, lubricant** (lubricate ocular surface, maintain ocular tonicity; see Keratoconjunctivitis sicca →246)	**Preservative-free Tears** (Bion Tears, GenTeal, Hypo Tears PF, OcuCoat PF, Refresh Plus, Tears Naturale Free, Thera Tears)	*1 Gtt q1-2h*
plus	**Systemic virostatic** (purine antagonist, DNA polymerase inhibit.)	**Acyclovir** (Zovirax, Gens)	*800mg PO 5x/d for 7d*

In HZV disciform keratitis

+/-	**Topical corticosteroid** (anti-inflammatory)	**Prednisolone 1%** (Predforte, Econopred Plus)	*1 Gtt q1-4h*

Note: A biomicroscopic exam must precede any **use of topical corticosteroids**, which should be used only with extreme caution in the presence of a corneal epithelial defect, or evidence of ocular viral, fungal, or bacterial infection. Some clinicians feel that topical steroids are absolutely contraindicated for many corneal infections, particularly active HSV, viral epithelial keratitis, and fungal keratitis. Long-term effects of topical steroids can include cataract formation, and glaucoma.

176. Baum J, Barza M: The evolution of antibiotic therapy for bacterial conjunctivitis and keratitis: 1970-2000. Cornea 2000;19(5): 659-672.
177. Chern KC, Margolis TP: Varicella zoster virus ocular disease. Int Ophthalmol Clin 1998 Fall; 38(4):149-160.
178. Herpetic Eye Disease Study Group: Oral acyclovir for herpes simplex virus eye disease: effect on prevention of epithelial keratitis and stromal keratitis. Arch Ophthalmol 2000;118(8): 1030-1036.
179. Mabon M: Fungal keratitis. Int Ophthalmol Clin 1998; 38(4): 115-23.
180. Stern GA, Buttross M: Use of corticosteroids in combination with antimicrobial drugs in the treatment of infectious corneal disease. Ophthalmology 1991 Jun; 98(6): 847-853.
181. Wilhelmus KR et al:Herpetic Eye Disease Study. A controlled trial of topical corticosteroids for herpes simplex stromal keratitis. Ophthalmology 1994;101(12):1883-95; discussion 1895-96

12.9 Chemical Burns of the Conjunctiva and Cornea

12.9.1 Immediate Treatment

Topical anesthetic	**Proparacaine** (Alcaine, Ophthaine, Ophthetic, Gens)	*1 Gtt; apply topical anesthetic prior to irrigation*

Caution: do not prescribe topical anesthetic for patient use, due to potential for corneal infections or toxicity

Irrigation (dilutes substance, flushes it away)	**Saline 0.9%, Ringer's lactate**	*Irrigate conjunctival sac and fornices for >½h until neutral pH=7.0; may use IV tubing*

12.9.2 Further Treatment

Depending on severity of burns

	Artificial tears, lubricant (lubricate ocular surface)	**Preservative-free Tears** (Bion Tears, GenTeal, Hypo Tears PF, OcuCoat PF, Refresh Plus, Tears Naturale Free, TheraTears)	*1 Gtt qh*
plus or	**Topical antibiotic** (broad-spectrum)	**Bacitracin oint** (Gens)	*½ inch qid*
		Erythromycin oint 0.5% (Ilotycin)	
plus or	**Topical corticosteroid** (anti-inflammatory)	**Prednisolone 1%** (Pred Forte, Econopred Plus)	*1 Gtt qid-q2h for 7d*
	Topical antibiotic + corticosteroid	**Tobramycin + Dexamethasone 0.1%** (Tobradex)	*1 Gtt qid-q2h*
		Tobramycin 0.3% + Loteprednol etabonate 0.5% (Zylet)	*1-2 Gtt q4-6h adjusted accordingly*
plus or	**Cycloplegic** (ciliary spasm↓; see bacterial ulcer, →250)	**Cyclopentolate 1-2%** (AK-Pentolate, Cyclogyl, Gens)	*1 Gtt bid-tid*
		Homatropine 2%, 5% (Isopto Homatropine)	
+/- severe	**Oral anti-collagenase** (inhibits breakdown of collagen fibers)	**Doxycycline** (Doryx, Periostat, Vibramycin, Gens)	*100mg PO bid*
+/- severe	**Oral vitamin C**	**Ascorbic acid** (Gens)	*1g PO bid*
Plus or	**Oral analgesic**	**Indomethacin** (Indocin, Indocin SR, Gens)	*25-50mg PO tid prn*
		Acetaminophen 300mg + Codeine 30mg (Tylenol, Gens)	*1-2 tabs PO q4h prn*

Avoid phenylephrine, lyse symblepharon, and treat glaucoma

182. Pfister RR, Pfister DA: Alkali injuries of the eye. In: Fundamentals of Cornea and External Disease. Cornea. Vol 1. 1997: 1443-1451.
183. Wagoner MD: Chemical injuries of the eye: current concepts in pathophysiology and therapy. Surv Ophthalmol 1997; 41(4): 275-313.

12.10 Corneal Edema

Hypertonic solution + preservative (used most commonly with recurrent erosion syndrome)	Sodium chloride 2% and 5% + Thimerosol (Adsorbonac)	Solution: 1 Gtt bid or prn Ointment: Apply 1/4" to conjunctival sac qhs or 3-4h prn
Hypertonic solution perservative free	Sodium chloride 2% and 5% (solution and ointment) (Muro 128)	

12.11 Episcleritis

mild	Artificial tears, lubricant (lubricate ocular surface)	Methyl, ethyl, and propyl cellulose preparations; Glycerin (Celluvisc, GenTeal, Hypo Tears, Refresh Tears, Tears Naturale II, Gens)	Gtt qid-6x/d (chilling of tear preparations may provide relief)
or	Topical corticosteroid (anti-inflammatory)	Fluorometholone 0.1% (Flarex, Fluor-Op, FML)	1 Gtt bid-qid
or	Topical NSAID (anti-inflammatory)	Diclofenac 0.1% (Voltaren)	1 Gtt qid
or		Ketorolac 0.5% (Acular, Acular preservative free)	
+/-	Oral NSAID (anti-inflammatory)	Ibuprofen (Advil, Children's advil, Motrin, Gens)	200-600mg PO tid-qid
or		Indomethacin (Indocin, Indocin SR, Gens)	25mg PO tid

12.12 Scleritis

	Oral NSAID (inhibits cyclooxygenase ⇒ prostaglandins ↓ ⇒ anti-inflammatory, analgesic)	**Ibuprofen** (Advil, Children's advil, Motrin, Gens)	400-600mg PO qid
or		**Naproxen** (Anaprox, Naprelan, Naprosyn, Gens)	250-500mg PO bid
or		**Indomethacin** (Indocin, Indocin SR, Gens)	25mg PO tid, 75mg SR PO qd-bid
or		**Diclofenac** (Voltaren, Voltaren-XR, Gens)	75mg PO bid-tid
plus	**Plus** antacid or H_2-blocker, →142		
+/-	**Oral corticosteroid** (anti-inflammatory)	**Prednisone** (Deltasone, Meticorten, Gens)	1-1.5mg/kg PO qd for 1wk, then taper slowly
+/-	**Systemic immunosuppressant** (Antimetabolite, cytokine synthesis ↓)	**Methotrexate** (Rheumatrex)	7.5-15mg PO qwk, or 15mg IM qwk; **Plus:** folate suppl.
or		**Azathioprine** (Imuran, Gens)	1-2mg/kg PO/IV qd for 6-8wk
or	(Cytotoxic agent)	**Cyclophosphamide** (Cytoxan, Neosar)	1-3mg/kg PO qd
or	(T-Cell Suppressor)	**Cyclosporine** (Neoral, Sandimmune, Gens)	2.5mg/kg PO qd (div bid)
	Note: systemic immunosuppressant in consultation with internist		

Note: Subconjunctival/tenon's corticosteroid injection is contraindicated. If scleritis progresses or worsens despite Tx, an underlying cause, such as Lupus, or Wegener's Granulomatosis must be suspected, and would require aggressive systemic Tx.

184. Jabs DA et al: Episcleritis and scleritis: clinical features and treatment results. Am J Ophthalmol 2000;130(4):469-476.
185. Sainz de la Maza M, Jabbur NS, Foster CS: An analysis of therapeutic decision for scleritis. Ophthalmology 1993;100(9):1372-1376.
186. Watson PG: Episcleritis. Current Ocular Therapy. 5th ed. 809.

12.13 Anterior Uveitis (All Etiologies, Including Post-surgical)
12.13.1 Mild to Moderate Anterior Uveitis

con-sider	**Topical corticosteroid, medium potency** (anti-inflammatory)	Fluorometholone (Flarex, Fluor-Op, FML)	*1 Gtt bid-qid*
or		Loteprednol (0.2%, Alrex; 0.5%. Lotemax)	
or		Prednisolone 0.12% (Econopred, Pred Mild)	
or	**Topical corticosteroid, high potency** (anti-inflammatory)	Dexamethasone 0.1% (Decadron, Maxidex, Gens)	*1 Gtt qid-6x/d*
or		Prednisolone 1% (Pred Forte, Inflamase Forte, Econopred Plus)	
or	**Non-steroidal anti-inflammatory**	Brofemac 0.09% (Xibrom)	*1 Gtt bid*
Plus con-sider	**Cycloplegic** (pain of ciliary muscle spasm↓, posterior synechiae formation↓)	Tropicamide 0.5-1.0% (Mydriacyl, Tropicacyl, Gens)	*1 Gtt qd-tid*
or		Cyclopentolate 0.5-2% (AK-Pentolate, Cyclogyl, Gens)	
or		Homatropine 2%, 5% (Isopto Homatropine)	

12.13.2 Moderate to Severe Anterior Uveitis

	Topical corticosteroid, high potency (anti-inflammatory)	Prednisolone 1% (Pred Forte, Inflamase Forte, Econopred Plus)	*1 Gtt 6-10x/d*
Plus	**Cycloplegic** (ciliary spasm↓; see bacterial ulcer, →250)	Tropicamide 0.5-1.0% (Mydriacyl, Tropicacyl, Gens)	*1 Gtt qd-qid*
or		Cyclopentolate 0.5-2% (AK-Pentolate, Cyclogyl, Gens)	

or	Cycloplegic (ciliary spasm ↓; see bacterial ulcer, →250)	Homatropine 2%, 5% (Isopto Homatropine)	1 Gtt qd-qid
or		Atropine 1.0% (Atropine care, Atropisol, Isopto Atropine, Gens)	1 Gtt qd-bid

12.13.3 Severe Anterior Uveitis

	Topical corticosteroid (anti-inflammatory)	Prednisolone 1% (Pred Forte, Inflamase Forte, Econopred Plus)	qh when awake; consider adding corticosteroid oint hs
Consider	Local corticosteroid, subconjunctival or sub-tenon injection (anti-inflammatory)	Triamcinolone (Kenalog, Aristocort)	20-40mg Inj (0.5-1ml) q2-4wk
or		Methylprednisolone 80mg/ml (Depo-Medrol, Solu-Medrol)	40mg Inj (0.5ml) q2-4wk
Plus	Cycloplegic (ciliary spasm ↓; see bacterial ulcer, →250)	Tropicamide 0.5-1.0% (Mydriacyl, Tropicacyl, Gens)	1 Gtt bid-qid
or		Cyclopentolate 0.5-2% (AK-Pentolate, Cyclogyl, Gens)	
or		Homatropine 2%, 5% (Isopto Homatropine)	
or		Atropine + Phenylephrine 2.5% (Neo-Synephrine)	
consider	Systemic corticosteroid (anti-inflammatory)	Prednisone (Deltasone, Meticorten, Gens)	1-1.5mg/kg PO qam, taper over 2-4wk
and/ or	Oral NSAID (inhibits cyclooxygenase ⇒ prostaglandins ↓⇒ anti-inflammatory, analgesic)	Diclofenac (Voltaren, Voltaren-XR, Gens)	75mg bid-tid
		Indomethacin (Indocin, Indocin SR, Gens)	25-50mg PO tid prn

12.13.4 Very Severe Anterior Uveitis

Systemic immunosuppressive Tx (in addition to above)

Consider in consultation with internist (!)

	Systemic immunosuppressant (cytokine synthesis ↓, T-Cell Suppressors)	**Cyclosporine** (Neoral, Sandimmune, Gens)	*Ini 5mg/kg PO qd (div bid), taper according to disease activity*
or	(alkylating agent, cytotoxic agent)	**Cyclophosphamide** (Cytoxan, Neosar)	*1-3mg/kg PO qd*
or	(antimetabolite, cytokine synthesis ↓)	**Azathioprine** (Imuran, Gens)	*1-2 mg/kg PO qd, max 2.5 mg/kg qd; keep dose as low as possible*
or		**Methotrexate** (Rheumatrex, Gens)	*7.5mg PO qwk, incr grad to 17.5-20 mg/wk prn;* **Plus** *folate suppl.*
or		**Mycophenolate** (CellCept)	*Ini 500mg PO bid, max 1.5g bid*

In addition, if herpetic kerato-uveitis

consider	**Topical antiviral**	**Trifluridine 1%** (Viroptic)	*1Gtt tid-5x/d*
	Systemic antiviral	**Acyclovir** (Zovirax, Gens)	*400mg PO 5x/d*

If secondary glaucoma (see glaucoma for more details, →268)

sos	**Topical carbonic anhydrase inhibitor** (aqueous humor prod.↓ ⇒ IOP↓)	**Dorzolamide** (Trusopt)	*Gtt bid-tid*
plus	**Topical betablocker** (aqueous humor production ↓ or inflow ↓)	**Timolol 0.25-0.5%** (Betimol, Timoptic, Timoptic-XE, Gens)	*1 Gtt bid (avoid metipranolol and prostaglandin analogues with intraocular inflam.)*

Note: In all cases of recurrent or bilateral uveitis, a determination of etiology must be attempted. If a treatable cause is determined, such as an infection (e.g. syphilis, tuberculosis), this must be treated initially, sometimes prior to institution of uveitis medications.

187. American Academy of Ophthalmology: Intraocular inflammation and uveitis. In: Basic and Clinical Science Course, Section 9. San Francisco: American Academy of Ophthalmology; 1999-2000.
188. Bloch-Michel E, Nussenblatt RB: International Uveitis Study Group recommendations for the evaluation of intraocular inflammatory disease. Am J Ophthalmol 1987; 103(2): 234-235.
189. Herndon LW:Glaucoma associated with anterior uveitis. Current Ocular Therapy 2000;5:470-1
190. Nussenblatt RB, Whitcup SM, Palestine AG: Uveitis: Fundamentals and Clinical Practice. 2nd ed. St. Louis: CV Mosby, 1996.

12.14 Intermediate and Posterior Uveitis

12.14.1 Mild Intermediate/Posterior Uveitis

- No significant visual impairment (20/40 or worse)
- No macular edema
- No significant vasculitis
- No peripheral retinal neovascularization
- ⇒ No therapy required

12.14.2 Moderate Intermediate/Posterior Uveitis, if Associated Iritis

consider	Topical corticosteroid	Prednisolone 1% (Pred Forte, Inflamase Forte, Econopred Plus)	1 Gtt tid-qh

12.14.3 Severe Intermediate/Posterior Uveitis, or if Cystoid Macular Edema

	Depot corticosteroid or sub-tenon injection (anti-inflammatory)	Triamcinolone (Kenalog, Aristocort)	20-40mg Inj (0.5-1ml) q2-4wk
		Methylprednisolone 80mg/ml (Depo-Medrol, Solu-Medrol)	40mg Inj (0.5ml) q2-4wk

If insufficient response, consider

	Systemic corticosteroid (anti-inflammatory)	Prednisone (Deltasone, Meticorten, Gens)	1mg/kg PO qd
sos	Systemic immunosuppressive	Cyclosporine, Methotrexate, or Azathioprine (→260; in consultation with internist)	
sos	Surgical therapy (cryotherapy, vitrectomy) Specific therapy (e.g., antibiotics, chemotherapy) to treat underlying diseases		
sos	Topical Betablocker and Carbonic Anhydrase inhibitor, as above (may be required in future if secondary glaucoma develops; see glaucoma section for further medications and guidelines, →268)		

sos	**Topical carbonic anhydrase inhibitor** (aqueous humor prod.↓ ⇒ IOP↓)	**Dorzolamide** (Trusopt)	*1 Gtt bid-tid*
plus	**Topical betablocker** (aqueous humor production↓ or inflow↓)	**Timolol 0.25-0.5%** (Betimol, Timoptic, Timoptic-XE, Gens)	*1 Gtt bid (avoid metipranolol and prostaglandin analogues with intraocular inflam.)*

Note: In the setting of persistent severe uveitis and systemic inflammatory disease (including Behcet's , Reiters, rheumatoid arthritis, ankylosing spindylitis, inflammatory bowel disease and others), many clinicians are adding some of the newer medication being introduced (such as anti-Tumor Necrosis Factor, Interleukin inhib., T-lymphocyte inhibitors, and others) in addition to those already listed above. Some of those which have begun clinical testing include Infliximab (Remicade), Etanercept (Enbrel) Daclizumab (Zenaprax), Sirolimus (Rapamune) and others.

191. American Academy of Ophthalmology: Intraocular inflammation and uveitis. In: Basic and Clinical Science Course, Section 9. San Francisco: American Academy of Ophthalmology; 1999-2000.
192. Bloch-Michel E, Nussenblatt RB: International Uveitis Study Group recommendations for the evaluation of intraocular inflammatory disease. Am J Ophthalmol 1987; 103(2): 234-235.
193. Henderly DE, Genstler AJ, Smith RE, Rao NA: Changing patterns of uveitis. Am J Ophthalmol 1987; 103(2): 131-136.
194. Jabs DA et al: Guidelines for the use of immunosuppressive in patients with ocular inflammatory disorders: recommendations of an expert panel. Am J Ophthalmol 2000;130(4): 492-513.
195. Joseph A, Raj D, Dua HS, Powell PT, Lanyon PC, Powell RJ. Infliximab in the treatment of refractory posterior uveitis. Ophthalmology 2003;110(7):1449-53Kaplan HJ: Intermediate Uveitis- A four step approach to treatment. In: Saari KM, ed. Uveitis Update. Amsterdam: Excerpta Medica; 1984: 169-172.
196. Kulkarni P. Review: Uveitis and immunosuppressive drugs. J Ocul Pharmacol Ther 2001;17(2):181-7
197. Moorthy RS et al: Glaucoma associated with uveitis. Surv Ophthalmol 1997;41(5):361-394.
198. Opremcek EM: Uveitis: A Clinical Manual for Ocular Inflammation. New York: Springer-Verlag; 1995.
199. Smith JA, Thompson DJ, Whitcup SM, Suhler E, Clarke G, Smith S, Robinson M, Kim J, Barron KS. A randomized, placebo-controlled, double-masked clinical trial of etanercept for the treatment of uveitis associated with juvenile idiopathic arthritis. Arthritis Rheum 2005;53(1):18-23
200. Smith JR, Levinson RD, Holland GN, Jabs DA, Robinson MR, Whitcup SM, Rosenbaum JT. Differential efficacy of tumor necrosis factor in inhibition in the management of inflammatory eye disease and associated rheumatic disease. Arthritis Rheum 2001;45:252-7
201. Smith RE, Nozik RA: Uveitis: A Clinical Approach to Diagnosis and Management. 2nd ed. Baltimore: Williams & Wilkins; 1988.

12.15 Optic Neuritis
12.15.1 With Acute Visual Loss

Note: Corticosteroid treatment is controversial, and although there is evidence that high doses of IV methylprednisolone given for an isolated acute attack of optic neuritis reduces the rate at which multiple sclerosis develops over a 2-year period, there is no evidence that long-term outcome is enhanced. IV steroid is instituted to decrease the likelihood of developing clinical multiple sclerosis if brain lesions are already noted on MRI. Oral steroid use alone, however, has been shown to be associated with increased rate of recurrence

Con-	Systemic corticosteroid (anti-inflammatory)	Methylprednisolone (Solu-Medrol, Gens)	*Pulse Tx: 250mg IV q6h for 3d (if brain lesions are also noted on MRI), followed by Prednisone*
then		Prednisone (Deltasone, Meticorten, Gens)	*1mg/kg qd PO for taper for 12d*

202. Beck R et al: A randomized controlled trial of corticosteroids in the treatment of acute optic neuritis. N Engl J Med 1992;326:581-588.
203. Beck R et al: The effect of corticosteroids for acute optic neuritis on the subsequent development of multiple sclerosis.The Optic Neuritis Study Group. N Engl J Med 1993;329(4):1764-1769.
204. Optic Neuritis Study Group: The clinical profile of optic neuritis. Experience of the Optic Neuritis Treatment Trial. Arch Ophthalmol 1991; 109(12): 1673-1678.
205. Trobe JD, et al: The impact of the optic neuritis treatment trial on the practices of ophthalmologists and neurologists. Ophthalmology 1999;106(11):2047-2053.

12.16 Ischemic Optic Neuropathy
12.16.1 Non-arteritic

	Antiplatelet drug (phosphodiesterase/platelet aggregation-adhesion inhibition)	Aspirin – ASA (Ascriptin, Asprimox, Bayer Aspirin, Bufferin, Easprin, Ecotrin, Empirin, Genprin, Halfprin, St. Joseph Pain Reliever, ZORprin, Gens)	*80-325mg PO qd;* **Note**: *use controversial*
plus	Oral corticosteroid (anti-inflammatory) (controversial; usually not recommended)	Prednisone (Deltasone, Meticorten, Gens)	*100mg PO qd*

12.16.2 Arteritic (Giant Cell Arteritis, Temporal Arteritis)

Consider initial pulse	**Systemic corticosteroid** (anti-inflammatory)	**Methylprednisolone** (Solu-Medrol, Gens)	*0.5-1g IV bid for 3-5d (followed by Prednisone)*
then		**Prednisone** (Deltasone, Meticorten, Gens)	*80-100mg PO qd; taper slowly (over months) based on symptoms and lab results*

206. Ghanchi FD, Dutton GN: Current concepts in giant cell (temporal) arteritis. Surv Ophthalmol 1997; 42(2): 99-123.
207. Hoffman GS et al: A multicenter, randomized, double-blind, placebo-controlled trial of adjuvant methotrexate treatment for giant cell arteritis. Arthritis Rheum 2002;46(5):1309-1318.
208. Neff AG, Greifenstein EM: Giant cell arteritis update. Semin Ophthalmol 1999 ;14(2): 109-12.
209. Weyand CM, Bartley GB: Giant cell arteritis: new concepts in pathogenesis and implications for management. Am J Ophthalmol 1997; 123(3):392-395.

12.17 Central Retinal Artery Occlusion

12.17.1 Acute Measures

Reduction of intraocular pressure (see section on glaucoma, →268)

	Topical carbonic anhydrase inhibitor (aqueous humor prod.↓)	**Dorzolamide 2%** (Trusopt)	*1 Gtt bid-tid*
plus/ or		**Acetazolamide** (Diamox, Gens)	*500mg PO/IV qd, max 1g/d*
plus	**Topical betablocker** (aqueous humor production↓ or inflow↓, IOP↓)	**Timolol 0.25-0.5%** (Betimol, Timoptic, Timoptic-XE, Gens)	*1 Gtt qd or bid*
or		**Levobunolol** (Akbeta, Betagan, Gens)	

- Immediate digital ocular massage
- Consider anterior chamber paracentesis

12.17.2 Additional Measures

Inhalation of carbogen (5% CO2, 95% O2) or hyperbaric oxygen

plus	**Antiplatelet drug** (phosphodiesterase/ platelet aggregation- adhesion inhibition)	**Aspirin – ASA** (Ascriptin, Asprimox, Bayer Aspirin, Bufferin, Easprin, Ecotrin, Empirin, Genprin, Halfprin, St. Joseph Pain Reliever, Zorprin, Gens)	*80-325mg PO qd*

In suspected giant cell arteritis (→264) additionally

	Systemic corticosteroid (anti-inflammatory)	**Methylprednisolone** (Solu-Medrol, Gens)	*1000mg IV (once, followed by Prednisone)*
then		**Prednisone** (Deltasone, Meticorten, Gens)	*60-100mg PO qd*
plus	- Obtain CBC with platelets + - Sedimentation Rate (ESR) + - C-Reactive protein + - Consider temporal artery biopsy.		

210. Atebara NH, Brown GC, Cater J: Efficacy of anterior chamber paracentesis and Carbogen in treating acute nonarteritic central retinal artery occlusion. Ophthalmology 1995; 102(12): 2029-2034.
211. Augsburger JJ, Magargal LE: Visual prognosis following treatment of acute central retinal artery obstruction. Br J Ophthalmol 1980 ; 64(12): 913-917.
212. Brown G: Retinal arterial occlusive disease. In: Guyer DR, ed. Retina-Vitreous-Macula. Vol. 1. WB Saunders; 1999: 271-285.
213. Mangat HS: Retinal artery occlusion. Surv Ophthalmol 1995;40(2): 145-156.

12.18 Central Retinal Vein Occlusion

Most practitioners do not treat CRVO with any medications except aspirin.
Close follow-up is required to monitor for secondary glaucoma.

Possible treatments (controversial)

con- sider	**Antiplatelet drug** (phosphodiesterase/ platelet aggregation- adhesion inhibition)	**Aspirin – ASA** (Ascriptin, Asprimox, Bayer Aspirin, Bufferin, Easprin, Ecotrin, Empirin, Genprin, Halfprin, St. Joseph Pain Reliever, Zorprin, Gens)	*80-325mg PO qd*

or	**IV anticoagulant** (unfractionated Heparin → coagulation factor inhibition↑, embolism prophylaxis)	**Heparin** (Gens)	*With primary care MD*
then	**Oral anticoagulant** (vit. K antagonism ⇒ clotting factors II, VII, IX, X↓ ⇒ longterm anticoag.)	**Warfarin** (Coumadin, Gens)	*With primary care MD*
consider or	**Oral NSAID** (inhibits cyclooxygenase ⇒ prostaglandins ↓ ⇒ anti-inflammatory, analgesic)	**Ibuprofen** (Advil, Children's advil, Motrin, Gens)	*400-600mg PO qid*
or		**Naproxen** (Anaprox, Naprelan, Naprosyn, Gens)	*250-500mg PO bid*
or		**Indomethacin** (Indocin, Indocin SR, Gens)	*25mg PO tid, 75mg SR PO qd-bid*
or		**Diclofenac** (Voltaren, Voltaren-XR, Gens)	*75mg PO bid-tid*
or	**Plus** antacid or H$_2$-blocker, →142		
or	**Systemic corticosteroid** (anti-inflammatory)	**Prednisone** (Deltasone, Meticorten, Gens)	*Recommended dose not established (e.g. 5-60 mg PO qd (div qd-qid), max 80 mg/d, taper over 2wk as symptoms resolve)*
or	**Intravitreal corticosteroid** (PRO of macular edema after CRVO, recently reported, controversial)	**Triamcinolone** (Kenalog, Aristocort)	*4mg intravitreal Inj*
sos	**Topical betablocker** (aqueous humor production ↓, IOP↓)	**Timolol 0.25- 0.5%** (Betimol, Timoptic, Timoptic-XE, Gens)	*1 Gtt bid*
plus/or	**Topical carbonic anhydrase inhibitor** (aqueous humor prod.↓)	**Dorzolamide 2%** (Trusopt)	*1 Gtt bid-tid*
	Note: may be required in future if secondary neovascularization glaucoma develops; see glaucoma section for further medications and guidelines, →268		

214. Central Vein Occlusion Study: Baseline and early natural history report. Arch Ophthalmol 1993; 111(8): 1087-1095.
215. Central Vein Occlusion Study Group: Natural history and clinical management of central retinal vein occlusion. Arch Ophthalmol 1997; 115(4): 486-491.
216. Hayreh SS: Classification of central retinal vein occlusion. Ophthalmology 1983; 90: 458-47.
217. Ip MS: Intravitreal triamcinolone acetonide as treatment for macular edema from central retinal vein occlusion. Arch Ophthalmol.2002;120:1217-1219.

12.19 Neovascular ("Wet") Age-Related Macular Degeneration (ARMD)

Anti-angiogenesis treatment

Photodynamic therapy (PDT)	Verteporfin (Visudyne)	*Intravenous infusion, 15mg (7.5ml solution comtaining 2.5mg/ml) subsequently activated by nonthermal red light (at 689nm)application, administered over 83 seconds, q3mo*
Selective vascular endothelial growth factor (VEGF) antagonist	Pegatanib (Macugen)	*Intravitreal injection 0.3mg q3wk*

Note: A large number of new medications and treatments are currently in development for the treatment of neovascular growth from various causes, including ARMD, diabetic retinopathy, trauma, myopia and others. These include Anecortave (Retaane), rhuFabV2 (Lucentis), Sqalamine (Evizon), Bevacizumab (Avastin), Fluocinolone (Retisert), SnET2 (PhotoPoint), and others

218. Comer GM, Ciulla TA, Criswell MH, Tolentino M. Current and further treatment options for nonexsudative and exsudative age-related macular degeneration. Drugs Aging 2004;21:967-92
219. Gragoudas ES, Adamis AP Cunningham ET Jr, Feinsod M, Guyer DR. VEGF inhibition study in ocular neovascularization clinical trial group. Pegaptanib for neovascular age-related macular degeneration. Engl J Med 2004;351:2805-16
220. Liu M, Regillo CD. A review of treatment for macular degeneration: a synopsis of currently approved treatments and ongoing clinical trials. Curr Opin Ophthalmol 2004;15:221-6
221. Schachat AP. New treatment for age-related macular degeneration. Ophthalmology 2005;112:531-2
222. van Wijngaarden P, Coster DJ, Williams KA. Inhibitors of ocular neovascularization: promises and potential problems. JAMA 2005;293:1509-13
223. Woodburn KW, Engelman CJ, Blumenkranz MS. Photodynamic therapy for choroidal neovascularization: a review. Retina 2002;22:391-405; quiz:527-8

12.20 Non-Exsudative ("Dry") Age-Related Macular Degeneration (ARMD)

Vitamin and antioxidant therapy	"Over-the-counter preparations" (Ocuvite, PreserVision soft gels, Viteyes, Icaps, Gens)	*Daily recommended dosages are: Vitamin C 500mg, Vitamin E 400IU, Beta carotene 15mg, Zinc (as zinc oxide) 80mg, copper (as cupric oxide) 2mg*

Note: No accepted medical or surgical therapy exists for treatment of non-exsudative ARMD. Vitamin and anti-oxidant therapy, along with control of hypertension and smoking cessation, are recommended for prevention of possible progression of ARMD.

Note: Beta carotene use is not recommended for smokers or ex-smokers, as a possible link with lung carcinomas has been reported.

224. Age-related eye disease study research group. A randomized, placebo-controlled, clinical trial of high-dose supplementation with vitamins C and E, beta carotene, and zinc for age-related macular degeneration and vision loss:AREDS report no.8. Arch Ophthalmol 2001;119:1417-36
225. Comer GM, Ciulla TA, Criswell MH. Current and future treatment options for nonexsudative age-related macular degeneration. Drugs Aging 2004;21:967-92

12.21 Glaucoma

12.21.1 Primary Open-Angle Glaucoma

Stage 1: Monotherapy

	Topical betablocker, non-selective (aqueous humor prod. ↓)	Timolol 0.25% or 0.5% (Betimol, Istalol, Timoptic, Timoptic-XE, Gens)	*1 Gtt qd or bid*
or		Levobunolol (Betagan, Gens)	
or		Carteolol 1% (Ocupress, Gens)	
or		Metipranolol 0.3% (Optipranolol)	*1 Gtt bid*

or	Topical betablocker, β-1 selective (aqueous humor prod.↓)	Betaxolol 0.25% (Betoptic S, Gens)	1 Gtt bid

If intolerance, insufficient pressure reduction, contraindication or unstable visual field situation, → Stage 2

	Stage 2: Alternative Monotherapy		
	Topical carbonic anhydrase inhibitor (aqueous humor prod.↓ ⇒ IOP↓)	Dorzolamide 2% (Trusopt)	1 Gtt bid-tid
or		Brinzolamide 1% (Azopt)	1 Gtt (1%) bid-tid
or	Topical prostaglandin analogue (uveoscleral outflow/ drainage of aqueous↑)	Latanoprost 0.005% (Xalatan)	1 Gtt qhs
or		Unoprostone 0.15% (Rescula)	1 Gtt bid
or		Travoprost 0.004% (Travatan)	1 Gtt qhs
or		Bimatoprost 0.03% (Lumigan)	1 Gtt qhs
or	Topical alpha-2 selective adrenergic agonist (aqueous production↓)	Apraclonidine 1% (Iopidine)	1 Gtt bid-tid
or		Brimonidine 0.15% (Alphagan P)	1 Gtt bid-tid
or	Topical miotic, cholinergic (ciliary muscle contraction ⇒ outflow of aqueous↑)	Pilocarpine 0.5, 1, 2, 3, 4, 6% (Isopto Carpine, Ocusert Pilo-40, Ocusert Pilo-20, Gens)	1 Gtt tid-qid
or		Carbachol 0.75, 1.5, 2.25, 3% (Carbastat, Miostat)	1 Gtt up to tid
or	Topical adrenergic agonist (outflow of aqueous↑, aqueous production↓)	Dipivefrin 0.1% (Akpro, Propine, Gens)	1 Gtt bid
or		Epinephrine 0.5, 1, 2% (Epinal, Epifrin, Glaucon)	1Gtt qd-bid

or	**Topical cholinesterase inhibitor** (aqueous humor drainage↑)	**Echothiophate Iodide** (Phospholine Iodide)	*Gtt qd-bid; absolutely contraindicated prior to general anesthesia with succinylcholine*
or		**Physostigmine** (Eserine)	*1 Gtt or ½ inch oint qhs-tid*
or		**Demecarium** (Humorsol)	*Up to 1 Gtt bid*

Note: Anticholinesterase inhibitors are no longer commonly used!

If insufficient pressure reduction, progression of visual field defects, optic nerve deterioration, → Stage 3

Stage 3: Fixed Combination Therapy (2 Drugs)

	Topical betablocker + carb. anhydr. inhibitor (aqueous humor prod.↓)	**Timolol + Dorzolamide** (Cosopt 0.5/2%)	*1 Gtt bid*

If insufficient pressure reduction, progression of visual field defects, optic nerve deterioration, → Stage 4

Stage 4: Combination Therapy (3 drugs)

	Topical betablocker + carb. anhydr. inhib. + Alpha-2-agonist	**Timolol/Metipranolol + Dorzolamide/Brinzolamide + Brimonidine**	
or	**Topical prostaglandin + betablocker + sympathomimetic**	**Latanoprost + Timolol + Brimonidine**	
or	**Topical prostaglandin + carb. anhydr. inhib. + Alpha-2 Agonist**	**Latanoprost + Dorzolamide + Brimonidine**	
or	**Topical betablocker + cholinergic + carb. anhydr. inhib.**	**Timolol/Metipranolol + Pilocarpine + Dorzolamide/Brinzolamide**	

If persistent high pressure, progressive visual field and/or optic nerve deterioration, on maximal topical therapy, or if intolerant of topical therapy:

	Systemic carbonic anhydrase inhibitor (aqueous humor prod.↓)	Acetazolamide 125, 250, 500mg (Diamox, Diamox Sequels, Gens)	250-1000mg, PO qd, split dosage bid or qid
or		Methazolamide 25, 50, 100mg (Neptazane)	25-100mg PO, bid to tid

Note: **topical** carbonic anhydrase inhibitors should be stopped.

If persistent high pressure, progressive visual field and/or optic nerve deterioration, on maximal medical therapy, → Stage 5

Stage 5: Non-Medical Treatments

SOS **Laser procedures**
 - e.g., trabeculoplasty
 Surgical procedures
 - e.g., trabeculectomy, shunt/valve placement

226. American Academy of Ophthalmology Preferred Practice Pattern: Primary Open-Angle Glaucoma. 2000.
227. Foundation of the American Academy of Ophthalmology: Medical management of glaucoma. In: Basic and Clinical Science Course, Section 10. San Francisco: American Academy of Ophthalmology;2000-2001; 130-146.
228. David, R: Changing therapeutic paradigms in glaucoma management. Exp Opin Invest Drugs. 1998;7(7):1063-1066.
229. Hugues FC, Jeunne CL, Munera Y: Systemic effects of topical antiglaucomatous drugs. Glaucoma. 1992;14:100-104.
230. Hutzelmann J et al, and International Clinical Equivalence Study Group:Comparison of the safety and efficacy of the fixed combination of dorzolamide/timolol and the concomitant administration of dorzolamide and timolol: A clinical equivalence study. Br J Ophthalmol. 1998;82:1249-1253.
231. The Advanced Glaucoma Intervention Study (AGIS): The relationship between control of intraocular pressure and visual field deterioration. The AGIS Investigators. Am J Ophthalmol. 2000; 130:429-440.

12.21.2 Angle-Closure Glaucoma

In General

	Miotic, cholinergic (ciliary muscle contraction ⇒ miosis, outflow of aqueous↑)	**Pilocarpine 0.5-1%** (Isopto Carpine, Pilo, Gens)	*1 Gtt q15min for 1h (during attack); also 1 Gtt 0.5 or 1% once in contralateral eye*
	Systemic carbonic anhydrase inhibitor (aqueous humor prod.↓)	**Acetazolamide** (Diamox, Gens)	*500 mg PO, then 125-250mg q4h; in nausea IV (during attack)*
consider	**Topical betablocker, non-selective** (aqueous humor prod.↓)	**Timolol 0.25% or 0.5%** (Betimol, Istalol, Timoptic, Timoptic-XE, Gens)	*1 Gtt qd or bid (caution with obstructive pulmonary disease)*
or		**Levobunolol** (Betagan, Gens)	
or		**Carteolol 1%** (Ocupress, Gens)	
or		**Metipranolol 0.3%** (Optipranolol)	*1 Gtt bid*
consider	**Topical alpha-2-agonist** (alpha-2 sympathomimetic)	**Apraclonidine 1%** (Iopidine)	*1 Gtt once*
or		**Brimonidine 0.15%** (Alphagan)	
consider	**Systemic analgesic**	**Meperidine** (Demerol, Gens)	*50-150mg PO/SC/IM q3-h prn*
consider	**Systemic antiemetic**	**Trimethobenzamide** (Tigan)	*200mg PR/IM tid prn*
poss.	**Systemic hyperosmotic** (osmotic gradient blood-ocular fluids↑ ⇒ H₂O loss from vitreous ⇒ IOP↓)	**Mannitol 20%** (Osmitrol, Gens)	*1-2g/kg IV Inf (during attack); extreme caution with diabetics*
or		**Glycerin 50% solution** (Osmoglyn)	*1-1.5g/kg PO*
or		**Isosorbide 45% solution** (Ismotic)	*1.5g/kg PO*
consider	**Topical corticosteroid**	**Prednisolone acetate** (Pred Forte)	*1% q15min for 1h, then qh*

Note: If medical Tx of angle-closure glaucoma does not sufficiently lower intraocular pressure, an emergency laser iridotomy or surgical iridotomy may be necessary.

Malignant Glaucoma (Aqueous Misdirection Syndrome)

	Topical anticholinergic (mydriasis and cycloplegia)	**Atropine + Phenylephrine 2.5%** (Neo-Synephrine)	*1 Gtt tid-qid (during attack), then qd* *1 Gtt qid*
plus	**Systemic carbonic anhydrase inhibitor** (aqueous humor prod. ↓)	**Acetazolamide** (Diamox, Gens)	*250-500 mg PO, then 250mg qid; in nausea IV (during attack)*
plus	**Systemic hyperosmotic agent** (osmotic gradient blood-ocular fluids↑ ⇒ H$_2$O loss from vitreous ⇒ IOP↓)	**Mannitol 20%** (Osmitrol, Gens)	*0.5-2g/kg IV Inf*
or		**Glycerin 50% solution** (Osmoglyn)	*1-1.5g/kg PO*
or		**Isosorbide 45% solution** (Ismotic)	*1.5g/kg PO*
Plus	**Topical betablocker, non-selective** (aqueous humor prod. ↓)	**Timolol 0.25% or 0.5%** (Betimol, Istalol, Timoptic, Timoptic-XE, Gens)	*1 Gtt qd or bid (caution with obstructive pulmonary disease)*
or		**Levobunolol** (Betagan, Gens)	
or		**Carteolol 1%** (Ocupress, Gens)	
or		**Metipranolol 0.3%** (Optipranolol)	*1 Gtt bid*
or	**Topical alpha-2-agonist** (alpha-2 selective sympathomimetic)	**Apraclonidine** (Iopidine)	*1 Gtt once*
		Brimonidine (Alphagan)	

232. American Academy of Ophthalmology:Laser peripheral iridotomy for pupillary-block glaucoma. Ophthalmology.1994;101(10):1749-1758.
233. Fourman S: Malignant glaucoma. Surv Ophthalmol. 1987;32(2):73-93.
234. Foundation of the American Academy of Ophthalmology: Angle-Closure Glaucoma In: Basic and Clinical Science Course, Section 10. San Francisco: American Academy of Ophthalmology;2000-2001; 100-121.
235. Foundation of the American Academy of Ophthalmology: Medical management of glaucoma. In: Basic and Clinical Science Course, Section 10. San Francisco: American Academy of Ophthalmology;2000-2001; 130-146.
236. Ching-Costa A, Chen TC: Malignant glaucoma. Int Ophthalmol Clin. 2000; 40(1):117-125.

12.22 Thyroid-Related Exophthalmos

Treatment of thyroid dysfunction (Graves' thyroid ophthalmopathy)

See Endocrinology, →126

Lid retraction, exposure keratopathy, keratoconjunctivitis sicca

See Keratitis sicca, →246

Exophthalmos; acute diplopia; optic neuropathy w/visual loss

	Systemic corticosteroid (anti-inflammatory)	Prednisone (Deltasone, Meticorten, Gens)	*80-100mg PO qd; Note: in consultation with internist, use is controversial!*
plus	Systemic immunosuppressive (reduction of dosage of corticosteroid possible)	Azathioprine (Imuran, Gens) Cyclosporine (Neoral, Sandimmune, Gens) *Dosage in consultation with internist or rheumatologist. Note: use is controversial!*	
poss. plus	Megavolt Radiotherapy: *2000 cGy in fractionated doses over 10d*		
sos	Acute thyroid ophthalmopathy with severe exposure or visual loss from optic neuropathy may require emergent orbital decompression surgery.		

237. Brennan MW, Leone C, Janaki L: Radiation therapy for Graves' disease. Am J Ophthalmol 1983;96:195-199.
238. Day RM, Carroll RD: Corticosteroids in the treatment of optic nerve involvement associated with thyroid dysfunction. Arch Ophthalmol 1968;79:279-282.
239. Feldon SE, Weiner JM: Clinical significance of extraocular muscle volume in Graves' ophthalmolopathy. Arch Ophthalmol 1982;100:1266-1269.
240. Kazim M, Trokel, SL, Moore, S: Treatment of acute Graves orbitopathy. Ophthalmology 1991;98:1443-1448.
241. Sergott RC et al: Graves' ophthalmopathy. Immunologic parameters related to corticosteroid therapy. Invest Ophthalmol Vis Sci 1981; 20:173-182.

13. ENT

Gayle Ellen Woodson, MD, FACS, FRCS (C)
Professor, Division of Otolaryngology
Southern Illinois University, Springfield, IL

13.1 Rhinosinusiitis

13.1.1 Acute Viral Rhinosinusiitis

	Topical alpha-sympathomimetic (mucosal detumescence, nasal decongestant)	Oxymetazoline (Afrin)	2-3 sprays/nostril bid; **Caution:** *do not use > 5d, may cause rebound!*
and/or	Systemic sympathomimetic (nasal decongestant)	Pseudoephedrine (Pediacare, Sudafed, Triaminic, Gens)	30-60mg PO q4-6h prn
plus/ or	Anticholinergic (antisecretory)	Ipratropium bromide (Atrovent)	1-2 sprays tid

13.1.2 Acute Bacterial Rhinosinusiitis

For patients with mild symptoms, with no antibiotics for past 4-6 weeks

	Aminopenicillin + beta-lactamase inhibitor	Amoxicillin + Clavulanate (Augmentin)	250mg PO q8h or 500mg PO q12h for 10-14d
or	Oral cephalosporin	Cefuroxime-Axetil (Ceftin, Veftin)	250-500mg PO bid for 10-14d
		Cefpodoxime proxetil (Vantin)	200mg PO q12h
		Cefdinir (Omnicef)	300mg PO q12h or 600mg PO q24h for 10d

For patients with mild symptoms and antibiotics in past 4-6 weeks or moderate disease

	Fluorquinolone	Moxifloxacin (Avelox)	400mg PO/IV q24h for 10d
		Gatifloxacin (Tequin)	400mg PO q24h for 10d
		Levofloxacin (Levaquin)	500mg PO q24h for 10-14d **or** 750mg PO q24h for 5d

or	Aminopenicillin + beta-lactamase inhibitor	Amoxicillin + Clavulanate (Augmentin)	*500mg PO q8h or 875 mg PO q12h*

Or combination therapy

	Aminopenicillin	Amoxicillin (Amoxil)	*250-500mg PO tid*
or	Lincosamide	Clindamycin (Cleocin, Gens)	*300-450mg q6h*
plus		Cefixime (Suprax)	*400mg/d PO*
or		Rifampin (Rifadin, Rimactane)	*600mg/d PO*

242. Sinus and Allergy Health Partnership. Otolaryngology - Head & Neck Surgery. 2004:130:1-44

13.1.3   Chronic Sinusitis

	Aminopenicillin + beta-lactamase inhibitor	Amoxicillin + Clavulanate (Augmentin)	*500-875mg PO bid for 3-6wk*
or	Fluoroquinolone	Moxifloxacin (Avelox)	*400mg PO od for 3-6wk*
or	Lincosamide	Clindamycin (Cleocin, Gens)	*300mg PO qid for 3-6wk*
or	Nitroimidazole	Metronidazole (Flagyl)	*500mg PO q6-8h for 3-6wk*
Plus	Topical glucocorticoid	Beclomethasone (Beconase AQ, Vancenase AQ)	*1 spray each nostril bid-qid*
		Flunisolide (Nasalide, Nasarel)	*2 sprays in each nostril bid-tid*
		Fluticasone (Flonase)	*2 sprays each nostril qd or 1 spray each nostr. bid*
		Mometason (Nasonex)	*2 sprays each nostril qd*
		Triamcinolone (Nasacort/AQ, Tri-nasal)	*2 sprays each nostril bid, prn decr to 2 sprays/nostril qd*

243. Benninger MS, Anon, J, Mabry RL: The medical management of rhinosinusitis. Otolaryngology-Head & Neck Surgery 1997;117:41-49.

13.1.4	Allergic Rhinitis		
	Topical antihistamine (histamine release in allergic response ↓)	**Azelastine** (Astelin)	*2 sprays each nostril bid*
and/or	**Mast cell stabilizer** (degranulation of mast cells after Ag exposure ↓)	**Cromolyn** (NasalCrom, Gens)	*1 spray each nostril tid-qid*
plus	**Topical glucocorticoid** (anti-inflammatory)	**Beclomethasone** (Beconase AQ, Vancenase AQ)	*1 spray each nostril bid-qid*
		Flunisolide (Nasalide, Nasarel)	*2 sprays in each nostril bid-tid*
		Fluticasone (Flonase)	*2 sprays each nostril qd or 1 spray each nostr. bid*
		Mometason (Nasonex)	*2 sprays each nostril qd*
		Triamcinolone (Nasacort/AQ, Tri-nasal)	*2 sprays each nostril bid, prn decr to 2 sprays/nostril qd*
plus/or	**Systemic antihistamine** (histamine release in allergic response ↓)	**Cetirizine** (Zyrtec)	*5-10mg PO qd*
		Fexofenadine (Allegra)	*60-80mg PO bid*
or	**Leukotriene inhibitor**	**Montelukast** (Singulair)	*10mg/d*

13.2 Furuncles of the Nose

Initially			
	Tetracycline	**Doxycycline** (Doryx, Monodox, Periostat, Vibramycin, Gens)	*d1: 200mg PO, d2-8(10): 100mg PO qd for 8-10d*
or	**Penicillin – penicillinase resistant**	**Dicloxacillin** (Dycill, Dynapen, Pathocil, Gens)	*125-250mg q6h PO for 8-10d*
In betalactam allergy			
	Macrolide	**Clarithromycin** (Biaxin)	*250mg PO bid for 10-14d*

244. Recommendations of the Paul-Ehrlich Society, Chemother J, 1999, 8, 2-49

13.3 Tonsillitis
13.3.1 Acute Tonsillitis

Initially

	Benzylpenicillin	Penicillin V (Pen-vee K, Veetids, Gens)	*250-500mg PO q6-8h for 10d*
or	Oral cephalosporin	Cefuroxime-Axetil (Ceftin, Veftin)	*250-500mg PO bid for 10d*
or	Macrolide	Azithromycin (Zithromax)	*500mg PO for 1d, then 250mg PO qd for 4d*
		Clarithromycin (Biaxin)	*500mg PO for 10d; Ped 12mg/kg PO qd*
or	IM penicillin	Benzathine Penicillin (Bicillin L-A, Permapen)	*<27.3kg: 600,000 U IM, >27.3kg:1,200,000 U IM, as single dose*
poss.	Analgesic – aniline derivative (inhibits cyclooxygenase ⇒ prostaglandins ↓, analgesic, antipyretic)	Acetaminophen (Acephen, Infants' feverall, Neopap, Tylenol, Gens)	*In pain or fever: 500-1000mg PO/PR tid-qid; Ped 500mg/d; infants max 125mg/d, toddler 250mg/d*

In resistance to therapy

	Aminopenicillin + beta-lactamase inhibitor	Amoxicillin + Clavulanate (Augmentin)	*500-875mg PO bid for 10d*
or	Lincosamide	Clindamycin (Cleocin, Gens)	*300mg PO qid for 10d*

13.4 Pharyngitis
13.4.1 Viral Pharyngitis, Symptomatic

Salicylate (analgesic, anti-inflammatory, antipyretic)	Aspirin – ASA (Ascriptin, Asprimox, Bayer Aspirin, Bufferin, Easprin, Ecotrin, Empirin, Genprin, Halfprin, St. Joseph Pain Reliever, Zorprin, Gens)	*0.5-1g PO bid-tid*

13.4.2 Bacterial Pharyngitis, Superinfection			
1sr Choice			
	Benzylpenicillin	**Penicillin V** (Pen-vee K, Veetids, Gens)	*250-500mg PO q6-8h for 10d*
In penicillin allergy			
or	Macrolide	**Azithromycin** (Zithromax)	*500mg PO on d1, then 250mg PO qd for 4d*
		Clarithromycin (Biaxin)	*250mg PO bid for 10-14d*

13.5 Laryngitis
13.5.1 Symptomatic

poss.	**Expectorant** (sputum viscosity ↓)	**Guafenesin** (Humibid, Robitussin, Gens)	*200-400mg PO q4h, max 2400mg/d*
or		**Guaifenesin – sustained release** (Humibid, Gens)	*SR: 600-1200mg PO q12h, plenty of water, max 2400mg/d*
poss.	**Antitussive** (acts on cough center in medulla oblongata)	**Dextromethorphan** (Benylin, Delsym, Hold, Pertussin, Robitussin DM, Sucrets, Vicks, Gens)	*10-20mg PO q4h prn, or 30-60mg SR q12h*
poss.	**Glucocorticoid** (anti-inflammatory, immunosuppressive)	**Methylprednisolone** (Medrol, Depo-Medrol, Solu-Medrol, Gens)	*2-60mg PO qd*
		Prednisone (Deltasone, Meticorten, Prednisone Intensol, Gens)	*5-60mg PO qd*

13.5.2 Bacterial Superinfection, Epiglottitis			
Initially			
	Cephalosporin 2nd gen.	**Cefuroxime-Axetil** (Ceftin, Veftin)	*0.75-1.5g IV tid for 7d*
or	Cephalosporin 3rd gen.	**Ceftriaxone** (Rocephin)	*1-2g IV qd for 7d, **Ped** 75mg/kg IV qd for 7d*

For tuberculous laryngitis			
poss.	Tuberculostatic	**Rifampin** (Rifadin, Rimactane, Gens)	*10mg/kg PO qd (div bid) for 4d*
For diphtheria			
	Antitoxin (from horse serum, passive immunization)	**Diphtheria antitoxin**	*30,000-50,000 IU IV inf over 1h, max 120,000 IU*
Plus	Benzylpenicillin	**Penicillin G** (Penicillin, Penicillin G Potassium, Pfizerpen, Gens)	*0.5-10 M IU IV qid-6x/d for 14d*
or	Macrolide	**Clarithromycin** (Biaxin)	*250mg PO bid for 10d*

13.6 Perichondritis

	Fluoroquinolone	**Ciprofloxacin** (Cipro)	*500mg PO bid for 14d*

13.7 External Otitis
13.7.1 Acute Otitis Externa

	Fluoroquinolone	**Ciprofloxacin** (Cipro)	*3 Gtt qd for 14d*
		Ofloxacin (Floxin)	*1 Gtt tid for 14d*
Plus	Glucocorticoid (anti-inflammatory, immunosuppressive)	**Triamcinolone acetonide** (Aristocort, Kenalog, Oracort, Oralone)	*Apply qd-bid with finger*
or	Antibiotic + glucocorticoid	**Polymyxin B + Hydrocortisone** (Otobiotic)	*5 Gtt tid-qid*
or	Anti-bacterial	**Acetic acid Sol 2%** (Acetasol, Domeboro, VoSol)	*4-6 Gtt q2-3h in canal or on ear wick*
Plus poss	NSAID - proprionic acid derivate (inhibits cyclooxygenase ⇒ prostaglandins ↓⇒ anti-inflamm., analgesic)	**Ibuprofen** (Advil, Children's advil, Ibu, Ibu-Tab, Motrin, Gens)	*400mg PO tid*

13.7.2	Otitis Externa Circumscripta (Acoustic Duct Furuncle)		
	Oral cephalosporin	**Cephalexin** (Keflet, Keflex, Keftab, Gens)	*1g PO tid for 7d*
	NSAID – proprionic acid derivate (inhibits cyclooxygenase ⇒ prostaglandins ↓ ⇒ anti-inflammatory, analgesic)	**Ibuprofen** (Advil, Children's advil, Ibu, Ibu-Tab, Motrin, Gens)	*400mg PO tid*
13.7.3	**Chronic Otitis Externa**		
	Anti-bacterial + glucocorticoid	**Acetic acid 2% + Hydrocortisone 1%** (VoSol HC)	*5 Gtt tid-qid*
13.7.4	**Fungal Otitis Externa**		
	Antifungal	**Clotrimazole Sol 1%** (Lotrimin, Mycelex, Gens)	*3 Gtt tid*
or		**Nystatin cream** (Mycostatin, Gens)	*Fill canal, leave 5-7d*
or	**Anti-bacterial + glucocorticoid**	**Acetic acid 2% + Hydrocortisone 1%** (VoSol HC)	*5 Gtt tid-qid*
13.7.5	**Otitis Externa Maligna**		
	Fluoroquinolone	**Ciprofloxacin** (Cipro)	*1000-1500mg PO qd*
poss plus	**Fluoroquinolone + glucocorticoid**	**Ciprofloxacin + Hydrocortisone** (Cipro HC Otic)	*Instill Gtt tid-5x/d*
poss plus	**NSAID – proprionic acid derivate** (inhibits cyclooxygenase ⇒ prostaglandins ↓ ⇒ anti-inflammatory, analgesic)	**Ibuprofen** (Advil, Children's advil, Ibu, Ibu-Tab, Motrin, Gens)	*400mg PO tid*

245. Louie TJ: Ciprofloxacin: and oral quinolone for the treatment of infections with gram-negative pathogens. Committee on Antimicrobial Agents. Canadian Infectious Disease Society. CMAJ 1994; 150:669-76.

13.8 Herpes Zoster Oticus

poss. plus	Virostatic (purine antagonist, DNA polymerase inhibitor)	Acyclovir (Zovirax, Gens)	Moderately severe: 800mg PO 5x/d; severe: 10mg/kg IV qd (div tid-5x/d)

13.9 Otitis Media

Symptomatic

	Analgesic – aniline derivative (inhibits cyclooxygenase ⇒ prostaglandins ↓, analgesic, antipyretic)	Acetaminophen (Acephen, Infants' feverall, Neopap, Tylenol, Gens)	500-1000mg PO/PR tid-qid prn; Ped 500mg/d PR; Infants: 125mg/d; toddler: 250mg/d; Max dose 4g in adults and 90 mg/kg in CH

Initially

	Aminopenicillin	Amoxicillin (Amoxil, Larotid, Trimox, Wymox, Gens)	250-500mg PO tid for 7-10d; Ped 80-90mg/kg PO qd (div q8h) for 7-10d
or	Oral cephalosporin	Cefixime (Suprax)	400mg PO qd for 7-10d; Ped 8mg/ky PO qd for 7-10d
		Cefuroxime-Axetil (Ceftin, Veftin)	250-500mg PO bid for 7-10d
or	Aminopenicillin + beta-lactamase inhibitor	Amoxicillin + Clavulanate (Augmentin)	500+250mg tid for 10d; Ped 50-100mg/kg PO qd for 10d
or	Cephalosporin 3rd gen.	Ceftriaxone (Rocephin)	Ped 60mg/kg IV/IM qd (single dose)
or	Folate antagonist + p-aminobenzoic acid antagonist	Sulfamethoxazole + Trimethoprim (Cotrimoxazole) (Bactrim, Cotrim, Septra, Sulfamethoprim, Sulfatrim, Gens)	800+160mg PO bid for 10d

In resistance to therapy, complications			
	Fluoroquinolone	**Ciprofloxacin** (Cipro)	*500mg PO bid for 14d*
plus	Lincosamide	**Clindamycin** (Cleocin, Gens)	*150-450mg PO tid-qid, 200-600mg IV tid-qid, for 14d*

13.10 Mastoiditis

Acute empiric treatment, pending culture			
	Aminopenicillin + beta-lactamase inhibitor	**Ampicillin + Sulbactam** (Unasyn)	*1-3g IV q6h; Ped 100-200mg/kg qd (div q6h)*
or	Cephalosporin 3rd gen.	**Cefotaxime** (Claforan, Gens)	*6g IV qd, Ped 50mg/kg IV q12h*

Treatment should be adjusted based on culture & sensitivity

13.11 Ménière Disease
13.11.1 During Acute Attack

	Antiemetic, antihistamine (inhibition of histamine receptors ⇒ antiemetic)	**Dimenhydrinate** (Dramamine, Marmine, Gens)	*50-100mg PO/IM/IV q4-6h*
or	Benzodiazepine (sedation)	**Diazepam** (Diastat, Diazepam Intensol, Valium, Gens)	*2-10mg PO/IM q4h*
poss.	Loop diuretic (volume relief)	**Furosemide** (Lasix, Gens)	*40mg IV*

13.11.2 Prevention

	Diuretic (excretion of Na^+, H_2O, K^+, H^+ ↑, volume relief)	**Hydrochlorothiazide** (Esidrix, Hydrodiuril, Microzide, Oretic, Gens)	*50mg PO qd*
poss.	Vestibulosuppressant (excitability of middle ear labyrinth ↓)	**Meclizine** (Antivert, Gens)	*25-50mg PO bid-tid*

or	**Anticholinergic** (suppressing conduction in vestibular cerebellar pathways)	**Scopolamine** (Transderm Scop)	*Transdermal patch: apply 2.5cm^2 patch to hairless area behind the ear q3d*
plus	- Reduce salt intake - Stop smoking - Avoid significant noise exposure - Reduce stress		

13.12 Sudden Deafness

	Glucocorticoid (anti-inflammatory immunosuppressive)	**Prednisolone** (Onapred, Pediapred, Prelone, Gens)	*IV inf in 500ml Ringer's solution over >4-6h on d1-8, then PO on d9-14, d1: 250mg, d2: 200mg, d3-4: 150mg, d5-6: 100mg, d7: 75mg, d8: 50mg, d9: 40mg, d10: 20mg, d11: 16mg, d12: 12mg, d13: 8mg, d14: 4mg (14d)*

13.13 Inflammation of the Salivary Glands (Sialadenitis)

poss.	**Oral cephalosporin**	**Cefuroxime-Axetil** (Ceftin, Veftin)	*250-500mg PO bid for 7-14d*

14. Dermatology

Norman Levine, MD
Professor of Medicine (Dermatology),
Arizona Health Sciences Center, University of Arizona, Tucson, AZ

14.1 Abscess

	Penicillin – penicillinase resistant	Oxacillin (Bactocill)	*Adults, Ped > 40kg: 500mg PO q6h for 10d; Ped < 40kg: 25mg/kg PO qid for 10d*
or		Dicloxacillin (Dycill, Dynapen, Pathocil, Gens)	*Adults, Ped > 40kg: 250mg PO qid for 10d; Ped < 40kg: 6.25mg/kg PO q6h for 10d*
or	Oral cephalosporin	Cephalexin (Biocef, DisperDose, Keflex, Keftab, Panixine, Gens)	*250-500mg PO tid for 10d; Ped: 12.5-25mg/kg PO tid for 10d*

14.2 Acne Vulgaris
14.2.1 Comedonal Acne

	Retinoid (sebaceous gland size↓, sebum production↓)	Tretinoin (Avita, Renova, Retin-A, Retin A Micro, Gens)	*Apply gel/crm/sol qpm until clear*
or		Adapalene (Differin)	*Apply gel/crm qpm until clear*
or		Tazarotene (Avage, Tazorac)	

14.2.2 Papulopustular Acne

Topical agents

	Retinoid (sebaceous gland size↓, sebum production↓)	Tretinoin (Avita, Renova, Retin-A, Retin A Micro, Gens)	*Apply gel/crm/sol qhs until clear*
or		Adapalene (Differin)	*Apply gel/crm qhs until clear*
or		Tazarotene (Avage, Tazorac)	

Plus	**Antibiotic** (oxidization of bacterial proteins, keratolytic, comedolytic)	**Benzoyl peroxide** (Benzac, Buf-Oxal, Desquam)	*Apply sol/gel bid until clear*
or	**Dicarboxylic acid** (antimicrobial, normalization of keratinization)	**Azelaic acid** (Azelex, Finevin)	*Apply crm bid until clear*
Plus	**Macrolide**	**Erythromycin 2%** (Akne-mycin, Eryderm, EryMax, Emgel, Erygel, Gens)	*Apply crm/gel bid until clear*
or	**Lincosamide**	**Clindamycin 1%** (Cleocin T, Clinda-Derm, Clindets, Gens)	*Apply sol/gel bid until clear*
Or	**Antibiotic + Macrolide**	**Benzoyl peroxide + Erythromycin** (Benzamycin)	*Apply gel bid until clear*
or	**Antibiotic + Lincosamide**	**Benzoyl peroxide + Clindamycin** (Benzaclin, Duac)	*Apply gel bid until clear*
Systemic agents			
1.	**Tetracycline**	**Tetracycline** (Achromycin, Bristacycline, Panmycin, Robitet, Sumycin, Gens)	*500mg PO bid until improvement, maint Tx 250-500mg PO qd indef.*
or		**Minocycline** (Dynacin, Minocin, Vectrin, Gens)	*50-100mg PO bid until improvement, maint Tx 50-100mg PO qd indef.*
or		**Doxycycline** (Adoxa, Doryx, Monodox, Vibramycin, Gens)	*100mg PO bid until improvement, maint Tx 50-100mg PO qd indef.*
2.	**Oral contraceptive**	**Desogestrel + Ethinyl Estradiol** (Desogen, Ortho-Cept, Gens)	*1 Tab PO qd for 21d indef. (monophasic)*
or		**Ethinyl Estradiol + Norgestimate** (Ortho Tri-Cyclen)	*1 Tab PO qd for 21d indef. (triphasic)*

14.2.3	Nodulocystic Acne		
	Retinoid (sebaceous gland size↓, sebum production↓)	**Isotretinoin** (Accutane, Amnesteem, Sotret, Claravis, Gens)	*1mg/kg PO qd for 5mo*
	Caution: in women of childbearing potential mandatory oral contraception during Tx and until 4wk after Tx!		

14.3 Alopecia

14.3.1 Androgenetic in Men

	Topical hair growth stimulator (vasodilation ⇒ hair growth↑)	**Minoxidil 5%** (Rogaine)	*Apply sol bid indef.*
and/or	**Systemic 5-α-reductase inhibitor** (conversion of testosterone to dihydrotestosterone ↓)	**Finasteride** (Propecia)	*1mg PO qd indefintely*

14.3.2 Androgenetic in Women

	Topical hair growth stimulator (vasodilation ⇒ hair growth↑)	**Minoxidil 2%** (Rogaine)	*Apply sol bid indef.*

14.3.3 Alopecia Areata

	Intralesional corticosteroid (locally immunosuppressive)	**Triamcinolone** (Kenalog)	*3-4mg/ml intralesional Inj q6wk until hair regrowth*
or	**Systemic corticosteroid** (anti-inflammatory, immunosuppressive)	**Prednisone** (Deltasone, Meticorten, Prednisone Intensol, Gens)	*20-60mg PO qd until full regrowth;* **Caution:** *AE of chronic Tx!*

14.4   Bullous Pemphigoid

Topical therapy

	Topical corticosteroid, very high potency (anti-inflammatory)	Clobetasol 0.05% (Cormax, Temovate, Gens)	*Apply crm/oint bid for max 2wk, then 1wk rest, rep cycle until clear*
or		Diflorasone 0.05% (Psorcon)	*Apply crm/oint bid for max 2wk, then 1wk rest, rep cycle until clear*
or		Halobetasol 0.05% (Ultravate)	*Apply crm/oint bid for max 2wk, then 1wk rest, rep cycle until clear*

Systemic therapy

	Systemic corticosteroid (anti-inflammatory, immunosuppressive)	Prednisone (Deltasone, Meticorten, Prednisone Intensol, Gens)	*0.5-1.5mg/kg PO qd until clear;* **Caution:** *AE of chronic corticosteroid Tx!*
OR	Tetracycline (anti-inflammatory)	Tetracycline (Achromycin, Bristacycline, Panmycin, Robitet, Sumycin, Gens)	*500mg PO bid-tid until clear*
or		Minocycline (Dynacin, Minocin, Vectrin, Gens)	*50-100mg PO bid until clear*
or		Doxycycline (Adoxa, Doryx, Monodox, Vibramycin, Gens)	*100mg PO bid until clear*
Poss plus	Vitamin B3	Niacinamide (Nicotinamide)	*500mg PO bid-tid until clear*
OR	Anti-inflammatory	Dapsone (Gens)	*25-200mg PO qd until clear*

14.5 Condyloma Acuminata

	Antiviral (antimitotic)	**Podofilox 0.5%** (=Podophyllotoxin) (Condylox, Gens)	*Apply sol/gel bid for 3d, hold for 4d, then rep for 4 cycles*
or	**Antiviral, immune response modifier** (secretion of cytokines/ interferon alpha ↑)	**Imiquimod 5%** (Aldara)	*Apply crm tiw for max 6wk*

14.6 Dermatophytosis (Superficial Fungal Infection)
14.6.1 Tinea Capitis

Topical therapy

	Antifungal, azole (change in membrane fluidity, fungistatic)	**Clotrimazole 1%** (Lotrimin, Mycelex, Gens)	*Apply crm/sol bid for 6-8wk*
or		**Miconazole 2%** (Monistat-Derm, Micatin, Gens)	*Apply crm/sol bid for 6-8wk*
or		**Ketoconazole 2%** (Ketozole, Nizoral, Gens)	*Apply crm bid for 6-8wk*
or		**Oxiconazole 1%** (Oxistat)	*Apply crm/lot bid for 6-8wk*
or	**Antifungal, allylamine** (keratophilic, chitin synthesis ↓, fungicidal)	**Terbinafine 1%** (Lamisil AT)	*Apply crm/sol bid for 1-4wk*
or		**Naftifine 1%** (Naftin)	*Apply crm/gel bid for 6-8wk*

Plus systemic therapy

	Antifungal (keratophilic, inhibition of cell wall synthesis)	**Griseofulvin** (Fulvicin, Grifulvin-V, Grisactin, Gris-Peg, Ultragris, Gens)	*500mg PO bid for 6-8wk,* **Ped** *20mg/kg qd for 6-8wk*
or	**Antifungal, allylamine** (keratophilic, chitin synthesis ↓, fungicidal)	**Terbinafine** (Lamisil)	*250mg PO qd for 4wk,* **Ped** *125mg PO qd for 4wk*
or	**Antifungal, azole** (change in membrane fluidity, fungistatic)	**Itraconazole** (Sporanox)	*200mg PO qd for 4wk,* **Ped** *200mg PO qd for 4wk*

14.6.2 Tinea Cruris, Tinea Pedis, Tinea Corporis

Topical therapy

	Antifungal, azole (change in membrane fluidity, fungistatic)	**Clotrimazole 1%** (Lotrimin, Mycelex, Gens)	*Apply crm/sol bid for 3-4wk*
or		**Miconazole 2%** (Monistat-Derm, Micatin, Gens)	*Apply crm/sol bid for 3-4wk*
or		**Ketoconazole 2%** (Ketozole, Nizoral, Gens)	*Apply crm bid for 3-4wk*
or		**Oxiconazole 1%** (Oxistat)	*Apply crm/lot bid for 3-4wk*
or	**Antifungal, allylamine** (keratophilic, chitin synthesis↓, fungicidal)	**Terbinafine 1%** (Lamisil AT)	*Apply crm/sol bid for 1wk*
or		**Naftifine 1%** (Naftin)	*Apply crm/gel bid for 3-4wk*

Or systemic therapy in severe or recurrent disease

	Antifungal (keratophilic, inhibition of cell wall synthesis)	**Griseofulvin** (Fulvicin, Grifulvin-V, Grisactin, Gris-Peg,, Ultragris, Gens)	*500mg PO bid for 4-6wk,* **Ped** *20mg/kg PO qd for 6-8wk*
or	**Antifungal, allylamine** (keratophilic, chitin synthesis↓, fungicidal)	**Terbinafine** (Lamisil)	*250mg PO qd for 4wk,* **Ped** *125mg PO qd for 4wk*
or	**Antifungal, azole** (change in membrane fluidity, fungistatic)	**Itraconazole** (Sporanox)	*200mg PO qd for 4wk,* **Ped** *200mg PO qd for 4wk*

14.6.3 Onychomycosis (Tinea Unguium)

Topical therapy

	Antifungal, pyridone (Inhibit synthesis of DNA, RNA, protein)	**Ciclopirox 12%** (Loprox, Penlac)	*Apply qd for 48wk*

Plus systemic therapy

	Antifungal (keratophilic, inhibition of cell wall synthesis)	Griseofulvin (Fulvicin, Grifulvin-V, Grisactin, Gris-Peg, Ultragris, Gens)	*1000mg PO qd for 6-12mo, Ped 20mg/kg PO qd for 6-12mo*
or	**Antifungal, allylamine** (keratophilic, chitin synthesis↓, fungicidal)	Terbinafine (Lamisil)	*250mg PO qd for 3mo, Ped 125mg PO qd for 3mo*
or	**Antifungal, azole** (change in membrane fluidity, fungistatic)	Itraconazole (Sporanox)	*400mg PO qd for 7d, hold for 21d, then rep for 2 cycles, Ped 200mg PO qd for 7d, hold for 21d, then rep for 2 cycles*

14.6.4 Candidiasis, Including Candida Vulvovaginitis

Topical therapy

or	**Antifungal, azole** (change in membrane fluidity, fungistatic)	Clotrimazole 1% (Lotrimin, Mycelex, Gens)	*Apply crm/sol bid for 3-4wk*
or		Miconazole 2% (Monistat-Derm, Micatin, Gens)	*Apply crm/sol bid for 3-4wk*
or		Ketoconazole 2% (Ketozole, Nizoral, Gens)	*Apply crm bid for 3-4wk*
or		Oxiconazole 1% (Oxistat)	*Apply crm/sol bid for 3-4wk*
or	**Antifungal, allylamine** (keratophilic, chitin synthesis↓, fungicidal)	Terbinafine 1% (Lamisil AT)	*Apply crm/sol for 1wk*
or		Naftifine 1% (Naftin)	*Apply crm/gel bid for 3-4wk*

Systemic therapy in severe or extensive disease

or	**Antifungal, azole** (change in membrane fluidity, fungistatic)	Fluconazole (Diflucan)	*150mg PO once*
or		Itraconazole (Sporanox)	*200mg PO qd for 1-2wk*

14.7 Eczema
14.7.1 Contact, Stasis, Atopic, Xerotic, Nummular, Dyshidrotic Eczema

Topical Agents

	Topical corticosteroid, medium potency (anti-inflammatory)	**Hydrocortisone 1%** (Alphaderm, Anusol-HC, Cetacort, Cortaid, Texacort, Locoid, Nutracort)	*In mild disease or facial involvement: apply crm/oint bid until clear*
or	**Topical corticosteroid, high potency** (anti-inflammatory)	**Triamcinolone 0.1%** (Aristocort, Kenalog)	*In moderate disease: apply crm/oint bid until clear*
or		**Fluocinonide 0.05%** (Lidex)	*In severe disease: apply crm/oint bid until clear*
OR	**Topical immunomodulator** (humoral immunity/ T-lymphocyte activity↓)	**Tacrolimus 0.03% or 0.1%** (Protopic)	*Apply oint bid until clear*
or		**Pimecrolimus** (Elidel)	*Apply crm bid until clear*

Systemic Agents in severe, recalcitrant, extensive disease

	Antipruritic, oral antihistamine (relief of pruritus)	**Diphenhydramine** (AllerMax, Benadryl, Diphen, Sominex, Gens)	*25–50mg PO qhs prn*
or		**Hydroxyzine** (Atarax, Vistaril, Gens)	*10–25mg PO tid prn*
or		**Doxepin** (Sinequan, Gens)	*10–25mg PO qhs prn*
	Systemic corticosteroid (anti-inflammatory, immunosuppressive)	**Prednisone** (Deltasone, Meticorten, Prednisone Intensol, Gens)	*1mg/kg PO qd for max 3wk;* **Caution:** *AE of chronic corticosteroid Tx!*
or		**Triamcinolone** (Kenalog, Gens)	*40–80mg IM, not > q6–8wk*
or	**Immunosuppressant**	**Cyclosporine** (Neoral, Sandimmune, Gens)	*3–5mg/kg PO qd for max 6mo;* **Caution:** *potent drug to be used only in severe cases!*

14.7.2 Seborrheic Eczema

	Shampoo	**Zinc pyrithione** (Head and Shoulders, Zincon, ZNP, Neutrogena T Gel Daily Control)	*Use shampoo qd indef.*
or	**Shampoo, antifungal**	**Ketoconazole** (Nizoral)	*Use shampoo biw indef.*
or	**Shampoo, keratolytic**	**Coal Tar** (Polytar, T Gel, Zetar, Gens)	*Use shampoo qd indef.*
poss	**Topical corticosteroid, medium potency** (anti-inflammatory)	**Hydrocortisone 1%** (Alphaderm, Anusol-HC, Cetacort, Cortaid, Texacort, Locoid, Nutracort)	*In mild disease or facial involvement: apply crm/ oint qd-bid prn*
or	**Topical corticosteroid, high potency** (anti-inflammatory)	**Triamcinolone 0.1%** (Aristocort, Kenalog)	*In moderate disease: apply crm/oint/lotion qd-bid prn*
or	**Topical corticosteroid, medium potency** (anti-inflammatory)	**Betamethasone** (Betatrex, Betaval, Luxiq)	*In scalp involvement: apply lot (0.1%) qd-bid prn; apply aerosol (0.12%, Luxiq) qd-bid prn*

14.8 Erysipelas

Oral antibiotic therapy

	Oral penicillin – penicillinase resistant	**Dicloxacillin** (Dycill, Dynapen, Pathocil, Gens)	**Adults, Ped > 40kg:** *500mg PO qid for 10d,* **Ped < 40kg:** *6.25mg/kg PO q6h for 10d*
or	**Oral cephalosporin**	**Cephalexin** (Biocef, DisperDose, Keflex, Keftab, Panixine, Gens)	*500mg PO qid for 10d,* **Ped** *12.5-25mg/kg PO qid for 10d*
or	**Oral macrolide**	**Azithromycin** (Zithromax)	*500mg PO on d1; 250mg qd on d2-5,* **Ped** *10mg/kg PO on d1; 5mg/kg PO on d2-5*
or		**Clarithromycin** (Biaxin)	*250mg PO q12h for 5-7d*

Intravenous antibiotic therapy, when systemically ill			
	IV penicillin, penicillinase resistant	Nafcillin (Nallpen, Unipen, Gens)	*0.5-1.5g IV q4h for 3-7d, Ped 10-20mg/kg IV q4h for 3-7d*
or	IV cephalosporin	Cefotaxime (Claforan, Gens)	*1-2g IV q8h for 3-7d, Ped 12.5-45mg/kg IV q6h for 3-7d*

14.9 Erythrasma

	Topical antifungal, azole (change in membrane fluidity, fungistatic)	Miconazole 2% (Monistat-Derm, Micatin, Gens)	*Apply crm/sol bid for 14d*
or	Topical macrolide	Erythromycin 2% (Akne-mycin, Emgel, Erygel, Gens)	*Apply crm/gel bid for 7-10d*
or	Systemic macrolide	Erythromycin base (E-base, E-Mycin, Eryc, Ery-Tab, Gens)	*250mg PO qid for 7-10d*
or		Clarithromycin (Biaxin)	*1g PO once*

14.10 Folliculitis
14.10.1 Bacterial Folliculitis

Topical therapy			
	Topical antiseptic	Povidone-iodine (Betadine)	*Cleanse (sol) qd-bid until clear*
or		Chlorhexidine (Hibiclens)	*Cleanse (sol) qd-bid until clear*

Systemic antibiotic therapy in extensive disease			
	Penicillin - penicillinase resistant	Dicloxacillin (Dycill, Dynapen, Pathocil, Gens)	**Adults, Ped > 40kg:** *500mg PO qid for 10d;* **Ped < 40kg:** *6.25mg/kg PO q6h for 10d*

or	Oral cephalosporin	Cephalexin (Biocef, DisperDose, Keflex, Keftab, Panixine, Gens)	*500mg PO qid for 10d;* **Ped** *12.5-25mg/kg PO qid for 10d*

14.10.2 Inflammatory Folliculitis

Topical therapy

	Topical antiseptic	Povidone-iodine (Betadine)	*Cleanse (sol) qd-bid until clear*
or		Chlorhexidine (Hibiclens)	*Cleanse (sol) qd-bid until clear*

Systemic therapy in extensive or chronic disease

	Systemic tetracycline	Tetracycline (Achromycin, Bristacycline, Panmycin, Robitet, Sumycin, Gens)	*500mg PO bid until improvement, maint Tx 250-500mg PO qd indef.*
or		Minocycline (Dynacin, Minocin, Vectrin, Gens)	*50-100mg PO bid until improvement, maint Tx 50-100mg PO qd indef.*
or		Doxycycline (Adoxa, Doryx, Monodox, Vibramycin, Gens)	*100mg PO bid until improvement, maint Tx 50-100mg PO qd indef.*

14.11 Herpes Simplex Virus Infection (Including Herpes Vulvovaginitis)

Topical therapy

	Virostatic (purine antagonist, inhibits DNA polymerase)	Acyclovir 0.5% (Zovirax)	*Apply oint q4h for 5-7d (only useful in primary infection)*
or		Penciclovir 1% (Denavir)	*Apply crm q2h for 4d, while awake*

Plus systemic therapy

	Virostatic (purine antagonist, inhibits DNA polymerase)	Acyclovir (Zovirax, Gens)	*200mg PO 5x/d for 7d*
or		Valacyclovir (Valtrex)	*500mg PO q12h for 7d*
or		Famciclovir (Famvir)	*500mg PO tid for 7d*

Systemic prophylaxis			
	Virostatic (purine antagonist, inhibits DNA polymerase)	**Acyclovir** (Zovirax, Gens)	*200mg PO bid-tid indef.*
or		**Valacyclovir** (Valtrex)	*500mg PO qd-bid indef.*
or		**Famciclovir** (Famvir)	*250mg PO bid indef.*

14.12 Ichthyosis

Topical therapy			
	Emollients	Lotion, cream	*Apply at least bid indef.*
	Desquamating agent (epidermal keratinization↓)	**Ammonium lactate** (AmLactin, Lac-Hydrin)	*Apply crm/lot bid indef.*

Systemic therapy in severe disease, lamellar ichthyosis or epidermolytic hyperkeratosis			
	Retinoid (normalizes skin/ mucosa cell differentiation)	**Acitretin** (Soriatane)	*25-75mg PO qd indef.*
	Caution: in women of childbearing potential mandatory oral contraception!		

14.13 Impetigo

Topical therapy			
	Topical antibiotic	**Mupirocin** (Bactroban)	*Apply oint tid for 7-10d*
	Antibacterial soap	(Lever 2000, Dial, Hibiclens)	*Use at least bid for 7-10d*

Systemic antibiotic therapy, if multiple lesions			
	Penicillin - penicillinase resistant	**Oxacillin** (Bactocill)	**Adults, Ped > 40kg:** *500mg PO q6h for 10d,* **Ped < 40kg:** *25mg/kg PO qid for 10d*
or		**Dicloxacillin** (Dycill, Pathocil, Dynapen, Gens)	**Adults, Ped > 40kg:** *250mg PO qid for 10d,* **Ped < 40kg:** *6.25mg/kg PO q6h for 10d*

or	**Oral cephalosporin**	**Cephalexin** (Biocef, DisperDose, Panixine, Keflex, Keftab, Gens)	*250-500mg PO qid for 10d, Ped 12.5-25mg/kg PO qid for 10d*

14.14 Lichen Planus

Topical therapy

	Topical corticosteroid, high potency (anti-inflammatory)	**Triamcinolone 0.1%** (Kenalog, Aristocort)	*In moderate disease: apply crm/oint bid until clear*
or		**Fluocinonide 0.05%** (Lidex)	*In severe disease: apply crm/oint bid until clear*
or	**Topical corticosteroid, very high potency** (anti-inflammatory)	**Clobetasol 0.05%** (Cormax, Temovate, Gens)	*In severe disease: apply crm/oint bid for max 2wk, then 1wk rest, then rep cycle*
or		**Diflorasone 0.05%** (Psorcon)	*In severe disease: apply crm/oint bid for max 2wk, then 1wk rest, then rep cycle*
or		**Halobetasol 0.05%** (Ultravate)	*In severe disease: apply crm/oint bid for max 2wk, then 1wk rest, then rep cycle*

Systemic therapy in severe, widespread disease

	Systemic corticosteroid (anti-inflammatory, immunosuppressive)	**Prednisone** (Deltasone, Meticorten, Prednisone Intensol, Gens)	*20-60mg PO qd for max 3wk per course; Caution: AE of chronic Tx!*
or		**Triamcinolone** (Kenalog, Gens)	*40-60mg IM, not > q8wk*
	Retinoid (normalizes skin/ mucosa cell differentiation)	**Acitretin** (Soriatane)	*25-75mg PO qd until clear*
	Caution: in women of childbearing potential mandatory oral contraception!		

14.15 Lyme Disease (Lyme Borreliosis)

	Tetracycline	Doxycycline (Adoxa, Doryx, Monodox, Vibramycin, Gens)	*100mg PO bid for 3wk*
or	Aminopenicillin	Amoxicillin (Amoxil, Polymox, Trimox)	*250-500mg PO tid for 3wk, Ped 20-50mg/kg PO tid for 3wk*
or	Oral cephalosporin, 2nd gen.	Cefuroxime-Axetil (Ceftin, Veftin)	*500mg PO bid for 3wk, Ped 250mg PO bid for 3wk*
or	Macrolide	Erythromycin base (E-base, E-Mycin, Eryc, Ery-Tab, Gens)	*250mg PO qid for 3wk, Ped 30-50mg/kg qd PO (div tid) for 3wk*

14.16 Melasma

	Depigmenting agent (melanocyte metabolic processes ↓ ⇒ reversible depigmentation)	Hydroquinone 4% (Eldopaque Forte, Eldoquin Forte, Lustra AF, Solaquin Forte)	*Apply crm/gel to affected areas bid until clear*
and/or	Dicarboxylic acid (antimicrobial)	Azelaic acid (Azelex, Finevin)	*Apply crm bid until clear*
and/or	Retinoid (regulate cell growth/ proliferation, formation of microcomedos ↓)	Tretinoin (Avita, Renova, Retin-A, Gens)	*Apply gel/crm/sol qpm until clear*
		Adapalene (Differin)	*Apply gel/crm qpm until clear*
		Tazarotene (Avage, Tazorac)	*Apply crm/gel qpm until clear*

14.17 Parasitic Infestation
14.17.1 Scabies

	Topical anti-parasitic	Permethrin (Elimite)	*Apply overnight; rep in 7d*
Or	Systemic anti-parasitic	Ivermectin (Stromectol)	*200µg/kg PO once, rep in 7d*

14.17.2 Pediculosis

	Topical Anti-parasitic	**Lindane** (Kwell, Scabene, Kwildane, Thionex)	*Apply to wet hair, rinse in 30min; rep in 7d sos*
or		**Malathion** (Ovide)	*Apply to dry hair; wash out in 8–12h*
or		**Permethrin 1%** (Nix)	*Apply crm to dry hair; rinse in 10–15min*
or		**Pyrethrin 4% shampoo/ foam** (A-200, Rid)	*Apply to dry hair; rinse in 10–15min*

14.18 Pemphigus Vulgaris

Topical therapy

	Topical corticosteroid, high potency (anti-inflammatory)	**Triamcinolone 0.1%** (Aristocort, Kenalog)	*In moderate disease: apply crm/oint bid until clear*
or		**Fluocinonide 0.05%** (Lidex)	*In severe disease: apply crm/oint bid until clear*
or	**Topical corticosteroid, very high potency** (anti-inflammatory)	**Clobetasol 0.05%** (Cormax, Temovate, Gens)	*In severe disease: apply crm/oint bid for max 2wk per course, hold for 1wk, then rep until clear*
or		**Diflorasone 0.05%** (Psorcon)	
or		**Halobetasol 0.05%** (Ultravate)	

Systemic therapy

	Systemic corticosteroid (anti-inflammatory, immunosuppressive)	**Prednisone** (Deltasone, Meticorten, Prednisone Intensol, Gens)	*1–2mg/kg PO qd until clear;* **Caution:** *AE of chronic Tx!*
Plus	**Immunosuppressant** (synthesis of DNA, RNA, proteins ↓, proliferation of immune cells ↓)	**Azathioprine** (Imuran, Gens)	*2–3mg/kg PO qd until clear*
or	(cytokine synthesis ↓)	**Methotrexate** (Folex, Rheumatrex, Gens)	*10–25mg PO per wk until clear*
or	(alkylating agent)	**Cyclophosphamide** (Cytoxan, Neosar)	*75–200mg PO qd until clear*

or	**Immunosuppressant**	**Aurothioglucose** (Solganal)	*25-50mg IM qwk until clear*
or	(proliferation of immune cells↓)	**Mycophenolate Mofetil** (CellCept)	*2-3g PO qd until clear*
or	(cytokine synthesis ↓)	**Cyclosporine** (Neoral, Sandimmune, Gens)	*3-5mg/kg PO qd until clear*

14.19 Pityriasis Rosea

	Macrolide	**Erythromycin base** (E-base, E-Mycin, Eryc, Ery-Tab, Gens)	*250mg PO qid for 2wk,* **Ped** *30-50mg/kg PO qd (div tid) for 2wk*

14.20 Psoriasis

Topical therapy

	Topical corticosteroid, high potency (anti-inflammatory)	**Triamcinolone 0.1%** (Aristocort, Kenalog)	*In mild disease: apply crm/oint bid until clear*
or		**Fluocinonide 0.05%** (Lidex)	*In moderate disease: apply crm/oint bid until clear*
or	**Topical corticosteroid, very high potency** (anti-inflammatory)	**Clobetasol 0.05%** (Cormax, Temovate, Gens)	*In severe disease: apply crm/oint bid for max 2wk per course, hold for 1wk, then rep until clear*
or		**Diflorasone 0.05%** (Psorcon)	
or		**Halobetasol 0.05%** (Ultravate)	
and/or	**Antiproliferative** (cell proliferation↓, keratolytic)	**Anthralin** (Anthra-Derm, Drithocreme, Lasan)	*Apply for 10-30min qd until clear*
and/or	(vitamin D3 analog, regulate skin cell production)	**Calcipotriene 0.005%** (Dovonex)	*Apply crm/sol/oint qd-bid until clear*
and/or	**Retinoid** (regulate cell growth/proliferation)	**Tazarotene** (Avage, Tazorac)	*Apply crm/gel qd-bid until clear*

and/or or	**Tar** (antimitotic)	**Coal Tar** (Estar)	*Apply gel qd until clear*
		LCD (Liquor carbonis detergens) 5%	*Apply qd until clear*

Systemic Therapy

	Retinoid (normalizes skin/ mucosa cell differentiation)	**Acitretin** (Soriatane)	*25-75mg PO qd until clear*
	Caution: in women of childbearing potential mandatory oral contraception!		
or	**Immunosuppressant** (cytokine synthesis ↓)	**Methotrexate** (Folex, Rheumatrex, Gens)	*5-25mg PO qwk indef.*
or		**Thioguanine**	*120-160mg PO biw-tiw indef.*
or	(cytokine synthesis ↓)	**Cyclosporine** (Neoral, Sandimmune, Gens)	*3-5mg/kg PO qd for max 6mo*
or	(proliferation of immune cells ↓)	**Mycophenolate Mofetil** (CellCept)	*2-3g PO qd indef.*

14.21 Rosacea

Topical therapy

	Antiinfective	**Metronidazole** (Noritate, MetroCream, MetroGel, MetroLotion)	*Apply crm/lot/gel qd indef.*
or		**Sulfur + Sodium Sulfacetamide** (Plexion, Sulfacet-R)	*Apply lot bid indef.*
or or	**Retinoid** (regulate cell growth/ proliferation)	**Tretinoin** (Avita, Renova, Retin-A, Gens)	*Apply gel/crm/sol qpm indef.*
		Adapalene (Differin)	*Apply gel/crm qpm indef.*

Systemic Therapy

	Tetracycline	**Tetracycline** (Achromycin, Bristacycline, Panmycin, Robitet, Sumycin, Gens)	*500mg PO bid until improvement, then maint Tx 250-500mg PO qd indef*

or	Tetracycline	**Minocycline** (Dynacin, Minocin, Vectrin, Gens)	*50-100mg PO bid until improvement, then maint Tx 50-100mg PO qd indef*
or		**Doxycycline** (Adoxa, Doryx, Monodox, Vibramycin, Gens)	*100mg PO bid until improvement, then maint Tx 50-100mg PO qd indef*

14.22 Sexually Transmitted Diseases

14.22.1 Syphilis (Treponema pallidum)

	Depot Benzylpenicillin	**Benzathine Penicillin** (Bicillin L-A, Permapen)	*<1y of infection: 2.4 M U IM; >1y of infection: 2.4 M U IM qwk for 3 wk*
or	Tetracycline	**Tetracycline** (Achromycin, Bristacycline, Panmycin, Robitet, Sumycin, Gens)	*Prim./sec. or early latent disease: 500mg PO tid for 14d; late latent or tertiary disease: 500mg PO qid for 28d*

14.22.2 Chancroid (Haemophilus ducreyi)

	Macrolide	**Azithromycin** (Zithromax)	*1g PO once*
or	Cephalosporin 3rd Gen.	**Ceftriaxone** (Rocephin)	*250mg IM once*
or	Fluoroquinolone	**Ciprofloxacin** (Cipro)	*500mg PO bid for 3d*

14.22.3 Granuloma Inguinale (Calymmatobacterium granulomatis)

	Folate antagonist + p-Aminobenzoic acid antagonist	**Sulfamethoxazole + Trimethoprim** (Bactrim, Cotrim, Septra, Sulfamethoprim, Sulfatrim, Gens)	*800+160mg PO bid for 14d*
or	Tetracycline	**Doxycycline** (Adoxa, Doryx, Monodox, Vibramycin, Gens)	*100mg PO bid for 14d*
or	Fluoroquinolone	**Ciprofloxacin** (Cipro)	*500mg PO bid for 3d*

14.22.4 Lymphogranuloma Venereum (Chlamydia trachomatis)			
	Tetracycline	Doxycycline (Adoxa, Doryx, Monodox, Vibramycin, Gens)	100mg PO bid for 21d
or	Macrolide	Erythromycin base (E-base, E-Mycin, Eryc, Ery-Tab, Gens)	500mg PO qid for 21d

14.22.5 Chlamydia Urethritis (Chlamydia trachomatis)			
	Tetracycline	Tetracycline (Achromycin, Bristacycline, Panmycin, Robitet, Sumycin, Gens)	500mg PO bid until improvement, then 250-500mg qd indef.
or		Minocycline (Dynacin, Minocin, Vectrin, Gens)	50-100mg PO bid until improvement, then 50-100mg qd indef.
or		Doxycycline (Adoxa, Doryx, Monodox, Vibramycin, Gens)	100mg PO bid until improvement, then 50-100mg qd indef.

14.23 Tinea Versicolor (Malassezia furfur)

Topical therapy

or	Antifungal, azole (change in membrane fluidity, fungistatic)	Clotrimazole 1% (Lotrimin, Mycelex, Gens)	Apply crm/sol bid for 3-4wk
or		Miconazole 2% (Monistat-Derm, Micatin, Gens)	Apply crm/sol bid for 3-4wk
or		Ketoconazole 2% (Ketozole, Nizoral, Gens)	Apply crm bid for 3-4wk
or		Oxiconazole 1% (Oxistat)	Apply crm/lot bid for 3-4wk
or	Antifungal, allylamine (keratophilic, chitin synthesis ↓, fungicidal)	Terbinafine 1% (Lamisil AT)	Apply crm bid for 1wk
or		Naftifine 1% (Naftin)	Apply crm/gel bid for 3-4wk

or	**Selenium sulfide**	**Selenium sulfide** (Selsun Blue, Exsel, Head and Shoulders)	*Apply shampoo qod for 2wk; apply lot qd for 2wk*
or	**Zinc pyrithione**	**Zinc pyrithione shampoo** (Zincon, ZNP, T-Gel Complete)	*Apply shampoo qod for 2wk*

Systemic therapy in extensive disease

	Antifungal, azole (fungistatic)	**Ketoconazole** (Nizoral, Gens)	*400mg PO once; rep in 7d*
or		**Itraconazole** (Sporanox)	*200mg PO qd for 7-10d*

14.24 Urticaria
14.24.1 Acute Urticaria

	Antihistamine (suppress histamine activity)	**Diphenhydramine** (AllerMax, Benadryl, Diphen, Sominex, Gens)	*25-50mg PO qid 7-21d*
or		**Hydroxyzine** (Atarax, Vistaril, Gens)	*10-25mg PO tid 7-21d*
or		**Doxepin** (Sinequan, Gens)	*10-25mg PO qhs 7-21d*
or		**Cetirizine** (Zyrtec)	*10mg PO qd for 7-21d*
or	(nosedating)	**Loratadine** (Claritin, Clarinex)	*10mg PO qd 7-21d*

14.24.2 Chronic Urticaria

	Antihistamine (suppress histamine activity)	**Diphenhydramine** (AllerMax, Benadryl, Diphen, Sominex, Gens)	*25-50mg PO qhs indef.*
or		**Hydroxyzine** (Atarax, Vistaril, Gens)	*10-25mg PO tid indef.*
or		**Doxepin** (Sinequan, Gens)	*10-25mg PO qhs indef.*
or		**Cetirizine** (Zyrtec)	*10mg PO qd indef.*
or	(nosedating)	**Loratadine** (Claritin, Clarinex)	*10mg PO qd indef.*

poss plus	Ca⁺⁺ channel blocker (stabilize mast cells and inhibit degranulation)	Nifedipine (Adalat, Procardia, Gens)	20-40mg PO qid indef.
poss plus	Systemic corticosteroid (anti-inflammatory, immunosuppressive)	Prednisone (Deltasone, Meticorten, Prednisone Intensol, Gens)	0.5-1.0mg/kg PO qd indef.; Caution: AE of chronic Tx!

14.25 Varicella Zoster Virus Infection
14.25.1 Varicella

	Virostatic (purine antagonist, inhibits DNA polymerase)	Valacyclovir (Valtrex)	1000mg PO tid for 7d
or		Famciclovir (Famvir)	500mg PO tid for 7d

14.25.2 Herpes Zoster

	Virostatic (purine antagonist, inhibits DNA polymerase)	Valacyclovir (Valtrex)	1000mg PO tid for 7d
or		Famciclovir (Famvir)	500mg PO tid for 7d

14.26 Warts (Verruca; Human Papilloma Virus, HPV)

	Keratolytic (dissolving intercellular cement, desquamating horny layer of skin)	Salicylic acid +/- Lactic acid (Duofilm, Occlusal-HP, Wart-Off, Medi-Plast)	Apply qd until clear
or	Retinoid (regulate cell growth/ proliferation, formation of microcomedos ↓)	Tretinoin (Avita, Renova, Retin-A, Retin A Micro, Gens)	Apply gel/crm/sol qpm (flat warts only) until clear
or		Adapalene (Differin)	Apply gel/crm qpm (flat warts only) until clear
or		Tazarotene (Avage, Tazorac)	Apply crm/gel qpm (flat warts only) until clear
or	Vesicating agent (epidermal necrosis and blistering)	Cantharidin (Cantharone, Canthacur)	Apply 0.7% sol once; rep in 4-6wk prn
or	Cytotoxic agent (inhibit cell growth and proliferation)	Bleomycin (Blenoxane, Gens)	0.5-1U/ml sol intralesional Inj, not to exceed 1.5 U/Tx; rep prn

15. Oncology

Abdul-Rahman Jazieh, MD, M.P.H.
Professor, Acting Division Director, Hematology/Medical Oncology,
Department of Internal Medicine, University of Cincinnati, Cincinnati, OH

15.1 Supportive Treatment

15.1.1 Depending on Symptom

	Antiemetic (inhibits dopamine receptors)	**Prochlorperazine** (Compazine, Compro, Gens)	*5-10mg IM/PO q6h prn*
or	**Antiemetic** (serotonine receptor antagonist = 5-HT3-receptor antagonist)	**Dolasetron** (Anzemet)	*100mg PO/IV qd*
		Granisetron (Kytril)	*1mg IV qd before chemo-Tx or 2mg PO*
		Ondansetron (Zofran)	*8mg PO/IV qd, max 8mg tid*
		Palonosetron (Aloxi)	*0,25mg IV*
Plus	**Glucocorticoid** (anti-inflammatory, immunosuppressive)	**Dexamethasone** (Decadron, Hexadrol, Mymethasone, Gens)	*10-20mg PO/IV (premed of chemo-Tx)*
Plus	**Antiemetic** (Neurokinin-1 receptor inhibitor)	**Aprepitant** (Emend)	*125mg PO day 1, then 85mg PO day 2 and 3*
Additional Options			
	Antiemetic (dopamine rec. antag.)	**Metoclopramide** (Reglan, Gens)	*10-20mg PO q4h prn, 10mg IV (max 2mg/kg)*
or	**Antiemetic** (inhibits histamine rec.)	**Promethazine** (Phenergan)	*25mg IV/PO q6h*
or	**Benzodiazepine** (anxiolytic)	**Lorazepam** (Ativan, Gens)	*0.5-1mg PO/IV q6h*

15.2   Anal Cancer

Primary Chemotherapy + Radiation

	Cytostatic antibiotic (bifunctional alkylating)	**Mitomycin C** (Mutamycin, Mytozytrex, Gens)	$10mg/m^2$ IV as bolus on d1, rep cyc in 6-8wk
plus	**Pyrimidine antagonist** (inhibition of thymidine nucleotide synthesis)	**Fluorouracil** (Adrucil, Gens)	$1000mg/m^2$ IV on d1-4, rep cyc in 6-8wk

246. Flam 1996

Salvage Chemotherapy

	Pyrimidine antagonist (inhibition of thymidine nucleotide synthesis)	**Fluorouracil** (Adrucil, Gens)	$1000mg/m^2$ IV on d1-4, rep cyc from d22-29
plus	**Alkylating agent** (intrastrand cross-linking of DNA)	**Cisplatin** (Platinol, Platinol AQ, Gens)	$100mg/m^2$ IV on d1, rep cyc from d22-29

247. Mahjoubi et al. 1990

15.3   Bladder Cancer
15.3.1   Monotherapy

	Antimetabolite (cytidine analog, inhibits ribonucleotide reductase)	**Gemcitabine** (Gemzar)	$1200mg/m^2$ IV over 30min on d1, d8, d15; rep cyc from d29
or	**Spindle poison** (microtubule inhibitor, tubulin polymerization, mitosis inhibition)	**Paclitaxel** (Taxol, Gens)	$175-225mg/m^2$ IV inf over 3h rep q3wk
Plus	**Alkylating agent** (intrastrand cross-linking of DNA)	**Carboplatin** (Paraplatin)	AUC 6 IV over 30min on d1

To calculate the dosage of carboplatin with the AUC-method (AUC=area under the curve of plasma concentration), use formula by A. Calvert:
Dosage of carboplatin (mg) = AUC 6 (mg/ml x min) x [GFR (ml/min) + 25]

15.3.2   Polychemotherapy

M–VAC Methotrexate + Vinblastine + Adriamycin + Cisplatin)

	Antimetabolite (folate antagonist)	**Methotrexate** (Folex, Mexate, Trexall, Gens)	*30mg/m² IV bolus on d1, d15, d22, rep cyc from d29*
plus	**Spindle poison** (inhibits microtubule formation, mitosis ↓)	**Vinblastine** (Velban, Gens)	*3mg/m² IV bolus on d2, d15, d22, rep cyc from d29*
plus	**Cytostatic antibiotic** (binds to DNA, impairs nucleic acid synthesis)	**Doxorubicin** (Adriamycin, Rubex, Gens)	*30mg/m² IV on d2, rep cyc from d29*
plus	**Alkylating agent** (intrastrand cross-linking of DNA)	**Cisplatin** (Platinol, Platinol AQ, Gens)	*70mg/m² IV on d2, rep cyc from d29*

248. Droz et al. 1998
249. Pollera et al. 1994

CISCA (Cisplatin + Cyclophosphamide + Adriamycin)

	Alkylating agent (intrastrand cross-linking of DNA)	**Cisplatin** (Platinol, Platinol AQ, Gens)	*100mg/m² IV on d1 rep cyc from d22*
plus	**Alkylating agent** (cross-linking of DNA)	**Cyclophosphamide** (Cytoxan, Neosar, Gens)	*650mg/m² IV on d1, rep cyc from d22*
plus	**Cytostatic antibiotic** (binds to DNA, impairs nucleic acid synthesis)	**Doxorubicin** (Adriamycin, Rubex, Gens)	*50mg/m² IV on d29*

Carboplatin and Taxol

	Spindle poison (microtubule inhibitor, tubulin polymerization, mitosis inhibition)	**Paclitaxel** (Taxol, Gens)	*80mg/m² IV inf over 1h qwk*
Plus	**Alkylating agent** (intrastrand cross-linking of DNA)	**Carboplatin** (Paraplatin)	*AUC 6 IV over 30min on d1*

To calculate the dosage of carboplatin with the AUC-method (AUC=area under the curve of plasma concentration), use formula by A. Calvert:
Dosage of carboplatin (mg) = AUC 6 (mg/ml x min) x [GFR (ml/min) + 25]

15.4 Brain Tumors

PCV

	Alkylating agent (breakage of chromatids, inhibits mitosis)	Procarbazine (Matulane)	60mg/m^2 PO on d8-21, rep cyc q6-8wk
plus	Alkylating agent (inter- and intrastrand DNA crosslinks)	Lomustine (CCNU, CeeNU)	160mg/m^2 PO on d1, rep cyc q6-8wk
plus	Spindle poison (inhibits intracellular tubulin function/mitosis)	Vincristine (Oncovin, Vincasar, Gens)	1.4mg/m^2 (max 2mg) IV on d8, d29, rep cyc q6-8wk

Monotherapy

	Alkylating agent (breakage of chromatids, inhibits mitosis)	Procarbazine (Matulane)	200 mg/m^2 IV on d1, rep cyc q6-8wk
or	Alkylating agent (inter-, and intrastrand DNA crosslinks)	Carmustine (BiCNU, BCNU)	200mg/m^2 IV on d1, rep cyc q6-8wk
or	Alkylating agent (DNA breaks)	Temozolomide (Temodar)	200mg/m^2 PO qd on d1-5, rep cyc from d28

15.5 Breast Cancer

Adjuvant hormone Tx in "tumor-free" patient for relapse prophylaxis

	Antiestrogen (blockade of peripheral estrogen receptors)	Tamoxifen (Nolvadex)	20-40mg PO qd
or	Gestagen (antiestrogenic, antigonadotropic)	Medroxyprogesterone acetate (Amen, Provera, Gens)	500mg PO qd

Additive Hormone Therapy

	LH-RH-Agonist (down-regulation of pituitary receptors ⇒ sex hormones ↓↓)	Goserelin (Zoladex)	3.6mg SC q4wk

	Aromatase inhibitor (inhibitor of adrenal steroid and extra-adrenal estrogen synthesis)	**Aminoglutethimide** (Cytadren)	*250-500mg PO q6h*
plus	**Glucocorticoid**	**Hydrocortisone** (Gens)	*15mg PO bid*
or	**Aromatase inhibitor** (inhibitor of adrenal steroid and extra-adrenal estrogen synthesis)	**Letrozole** (Femara)	*2.5mg PO qd*
or		**Anastrozole** (Arimidex)	*1mg PO qd*
or	**Selective estrogen receptor antagonist**	**Fulvestrant** (Faslodex)	*250mg IM in buttock monthly*

250. Kaufmann et al. 1989

CMF IV

	Alkylating agent (cross-linking of DNA)	**Cyclophosphamide** (Cytoxan, Neosar, Gens)	*600mg/m² IV on d1 rep cyc from d22*
plus	**Antimetabolite** (folate antagonist)	**Methotrexate** (Folex, Mexate, Trexall, Gens)	*40mg/m² IV on d1 rep cyc from d22*
plus	**Pyrimidine antagonist** (inhibition of thymidine nucleotide synthesis)	**Fluorouracil** (Adrucil, Gens)	*600mg/m² IV on d1 rep cyc from d22*

251. Bonadonna G, et al. Adjuvant cyclophosphamide, methotrexate and fluorouracil in node-positive breast cancer: the results of 20 years of follow-up. N Engl J Med. 1995;332:901-906.

FAC

	Pyrimidine antagonist (inhibition of thymidine nucleotide synthesis)	**Fluorouracil** (Adrucil, Gens)	*500mg/m² IV on d1, d8 rep cyc from d22*
plus	**Cytostatic antibiotic** (binds to DNA, impairs nucleic acid synthesis)	**Doxorubicin** (Adriamycin, Rubex, Gens)	*50mg/m² IV on d8 rep cyc from d22*
plus	**Alkylating agent** (cross-linking of DNA)	**Cyclophosphamide** (Cytoxan, Neosar, Gens)	*500mg/m² IV on d1 rep cyc from d22*

AC

	Cytostatic antibiotic (binds to DNA, impairs nucleic acid synthesis)	**Doxorubicin** (Adriamycin, Rubex, Gens)	*60mg/m² IV bolus on d1 q3wk*
plus	**Alkylating agent** (cross-linking of DNA)	**Cyclophosphamide** (Cytoxan, Neosar, Gens)	*600mg/m² IV on d1 q3wk*

AC→T

	Cytostatic antibiotic (binds to DNA, impairs nucleic acid synthesis)	**Doxorubicin** (Adriamycin, Rubex, Gens)	*60mg/m² IV bolus on d1 q3wk x 4 cyc*
plus	**Alkylating agent** (cross-linking of DNA)	**Cyclophosphamide** (Cytoxan, Neosar, Gens)	*600mg/m² IV on d1 q3wk x 4 cyc*
then	**Spindle poison** (microtubule inhibitor, tubulin polymerization, mitosis inhibition)	**Paclitaxel** (Taxol, Gens)	*175mg/m² IV q3wk x 4 cyc*

HEC

	Cytostatic antibiotic (anthracycline derivative of doxorubicin, mitosis inhibitor)	**Epirubicin** (Ellence)	*100mg/m² IV bolus on d1, rep q3wk up to 6 cyc*
plus	**Alkylating agent** (cross-linking of DNA)	**Cyclophosphamide** (Cytoxan, Neosar, Gens)	*830mg/m² IV bolus on d1, rep q3wk up to 6 cyc*

252. Piccart 2001

	Monoclonal antibody (anti HER-2)	**Herceptin** (Trastuzumab)	*4mg/kg loading dose, then 2mg/kg over 30min qwk*
plus	**Spindle poison** (microtubule inhibitor, tubulin polymerization, mitosis inhibition)	**Paclitaxel** (Taxol, Gens)	*175mg/m² IV inf over 3h, rep q3wk up to 6 cyc*

15.6 Cholangiocarcinoma, Gallbladder Carcinoma

In cholangiocarcinoma palliative Tx, indication with restraint, example:

	Pyrimidine antagonist (inhibition of thymidine nucleotide synthesis)	**Fluorouracil** (Adrucil, Gens)	*500mg/m^2 bolus IV on d1-5 rep cyc from d36*
OR	**Pyrimidine antagonist** (inhibition of thymidine nucleotide synthesis)	**Fluorouracil** (Adrucil, Gens)	*600mg/m^2 IV on d1, d8, d29, d36 rep cyc from d57*
plus	**Cytostatic antibiotic** (binds to DNA, impairs nucleic acid synthesis)	**Doxorubicin** (Adriamycin, Rubex, Gens)	*30mg/m^2 IV on d1, d29 rep cyc from d57*
plus	**Cytostatic antibiotic** (bifunctional alkylating)	**Mitomycin C** (Mutamycin, Mytozytrex, Gens)	*10mg/m^2 IV on d1 rep cyc from d57*

253. Moertel 1984

Cisplatin and Gemcitabine

OR	**Antimetabolite** (cytidine analog, inhibits ribonucleotide reductase)	**Gemcitabine** (Gemzar)	*1000mg/m^2 IV on d1, d8 rep cyc every 3wks*
plus	**Alkylating agent** (intrastrand cross-linking of DNA)	**Cisplatin** (Platinol, Platinol AQ, Gens)	*75mg7m2 IV on d1 rep cyc every 3wks*

15.7 Choriocarcinoma

EMA-CO (Etoposide, Methotrexate + Dactinomycin +Cyclophosaphamide + Vincristine)

	Spindle poison (inhibits DNA-/protein synthesis, mitosis)	**Etoposide** (Etopophos, Toposar, Vepesid)	*100mg/m^2 IV on d1, d2*
plus	**Antimetabolite** (folate antagonist)	**Methotrexate** (Folex, Mexate, Trexall, Gens)	*100mg/kg IV bolus, then 200mg/m^2 IV over 12h on d1*
plus	**Folic acid derivative**	**Folinic acid** (Leucovorin, Gens)	*15mg IV/PO q12h x 4,* **start 24h after MTX**

plus	**Cytostatic antibiotic** (doub.strand DNA breaks)	**Dactinomycin** (Cosmegen)	*0.5mg IV bolus on d1, d2*
plus	**Alkylating agent** (cross-linking of DNA)	**Cyclophosphamide** (Cytoxan, Neosar, Gens)	*600mg/m² IV on d8*
plus	**Spindle poison** (inhibits intracellular tubulin function/mitosis)	**Vincristine** (Oncovin, Vincasar, Gens)	*1mg/m² (max 2mg) on d8*

254. Lurain 1985

PEB (Cisplatin + Etoposide + Bleomycin)

	Alkylating agent (intrastrand cross-linking of DNA)	**Cisplatin** (Platinol, Platinol AQ, Gens)	*20mg/m² IV on d1-5 rep cyc from d22*
plus	**Spindle poison** (inhibits DNA-/protein synthesis, mitosis)	**Etoposide** (Etopophos, Toposar, Vepesid)	*100mg/m² IV over 1h on d1-5 rep cyc from d22*
plus	**Cytostatic antibiotic** (single strand breaks, DNA synthesis ↓)	**Bleomycin** (Blenoxane, Gens)	*30mg IV, on d1, d8, d15 rep cyc from d22*

255. Williams 1991

15.8 Colorectal Carcinoma
15.8.1 Adjuvant Therapy

Mayo Clinic Protocol

	Biomodulator (folinic acid = 5-formyl-tetrahydrofolic acid = citrovorum factor, effectiveness of 5-FU↑)	**Folinic acid** (Leucovorin, Gens)	*20mg/m² IV on d1-5 rep cyc from d29 for 6mo*
plus	**Pyrimidine antagonist** (inhibition of thymidine nucleotide synthesis)	**Fluorouracil** (Adrucil, Gens)	*425mg/m² IV, on d1- d5 rep cyc from d29 for 6mo*

Roswell Park Regimen

	Biomodulator (folinic acid = 5-formyl-tetrahydrofolic acid = citrovorum factor, effectiveness of 5-FU↑)	**Folinic acid** (Leucovorin, Gens)	*500mg/m² IV on d1, d8, d15, d22, d29 + d36 rep cyc if effective after 2wk pause*
plus	**Pyrimidine antagonist** (inhibition of thymidine nucleotide synthesis)	**Fluorouracil** (Adrucil, Gens)	*500mg/m² IV, on d1, d8, d15, d22, d29, d36 rep cyc if effective after 2wk pause*

FOLFOX-4 (for adjuvante and metastatic disease therapy)

	Alkylating agent (third generation platinum, intrastrand cross-linking of DNA)	**Oxaliplatin** (Eloxatin)	*85mg/m2 IV PB over 2h on d1 q2wk*
plus	**Biomodulator** (folinic acid = 5-formyl-tetrahydrofolic acid = citrovorum factor, improves effectiveness of 5-FU)	**Folinic acid** (Leucovorin, Gens)	*200mg/m² IVPB over 2h on d1 and d2 q2wk*
plus	**Pyrimidine antagonist** (inhibition of thymidine nucleotide synthesis)	**Fluorouracil** (Adrucil, Gens)	*400mg/m² IVP mid Folinic acid on d1 and d2 q2wk*
plus	**Pyrimidine antagonist**	**Fluorouracil** (Adrucil, Gens)	*600mg/m² CI over 22h on d1 and d2 q2wk*

15.8.2   Metastatic Disease

Saltz Regimen

	Topoisomerase I inhibitor (double strand DNA breaks)	**Irinotecan** (Camptosar)	*125mg/m² IV over 90min qwk x 4wk rep cyc q6wk*
plus	**Biomodulator** (folinic acid = 5-formyl-tetrahydrofolic acid = citrovorum factor, effectiveness of 5-FU↑)	**Folinic acid** (Leucovorin, Gens)	*20mg/m² IV qwk x 4wk rep cyc q6wk*

plus	Pyrimidine antagonist (inhibition of thymidine nucleotide synthesis)	Fluorouracil (Adrucil, Gens)	*500mg/m² IV qwk x 4wk*

256. Saltz 2000

Or Mayo Clinic Protocol

	Biomodulator (folinic acid = 5-formyl-tetrahydrofolic acid = citrovorum factor, effectiveness of 5-FU↑)	Folinic acid (Leucovorin, Gens)	*20mg/m² IV d1-5 rep q4wk*
plus	Pyrimidine antagonist (inhibition of thymidine nucleotide synthesis)	Fluorouracil (Adrucil, Gens)	*425mg/m² IV d1-5 rep q4wk*

FOLFOX-4 (for adjuvante and metastatic disease therapy)

	Alkylating agent (third generation platinum, intrastrand cross-linking of DNA)	Oxaliplatin (Eloxatin)	*85mg/m² IV PB over 2h on d1 rep q2wk*
plus	Biomodulator (folinic acid = 5-formyl-tetrahydrofolic acid = citrovorum factor, improves effectiveness of 5-FU)	Folinic acid (Leucovorin, Gens)	*200mg/m² IVPB over 2h on d1 and d2 rep q2wk*
plus	Pyrimidine antagonist (inhibition of thymidine nucleotide synthesis)	Fluorouracil (Adrucil, Gens)	*400mg/m² IVP mid Folinic acid on d1 and d2 rep q2wk*
plus	Pyrimidine antagonist	Fluorouracil (Adrucil, Gens)	*600mg/m² CI over 22h on d1 and d2; rep q2wk*

XELOX (CAPOX)

	Alkylating agent (third generation platinum, intrastrand cross-linking of DNA)	Oxaliplatin (Eloxatin)	*130mg/m² IV PB over 2h on d1 rep q3wk*
plus	Pyrimidine antagonist (oral prodrug of 5-Fluorouracil)	Capecitabine (Xeloda)	*1000mg/m² PO bid x 14s, then 1wk rest, rep cyc from d29*

FOLFIRI

	Topoisomerase I inhibitor (double strand DNA breaks)	**Irinotecan** (Camptosar)	180mg/m^2 over 90min d1 only
plus	**Biomodulator** (folinic acid = 5-formyl-tetrahydrofolic acid = citrovorum factor, improves effectiveness of 5-FU)	**Folinic acid** (Leucovorin, Gens)	400mg/m^2 IV over 2h on d1 rep q2wk
plus	**Pyrimidine antagonist** (inhibition of thymidine nucleotide synthesis)	**Fluorouracil** (Adrucil, Gens)	600mg/m^2 IVP mid folinic acid rep q2wk
plus	**Pyrimidine antagonist** (inhibition of thymidine nucleotide synthesis)	**Fluorouracil** (Adrucil, Gens)	2,400mg/m^2 CI over 46h rep q2wk

Bevacizumab-based regimens

IFL plus	**Antiangiogenesis** (Anti-vascular endothelial growth factor VEGF)	**Bevacizumab** (Avastin)	5mg/kg IVPB q2wk (monitor blood pressure and proteinurea)
or	**Antiangiogenesis** (Anti-vascular endothelial growth factor VEGF)	**Bevacizumab** (Avastin)	5mg/kg IVPB q2wk (monitor blood pressure and proteinurea)
plus	**Biomodulator** (folinic acid = 5-formyl-tetrahydrofolic acid = citrovorum factor, improves effectiveness of 5-FU)	**Folinic acid** (Leucovorin, Gens)	500mg/m^2 IV on d1, d8, d15, d22, d29 + d36 rep cyc if effective after 2wk pause
plus	**Pyrimidine antagonist** (inhibition of thymidine nucleotide synthesis)	**Fluorouracil** (Adrucil, Gens)	500mg/m^2 IV on d1, d8, d15, d22, d29 + d36 rep cyc if effective after 2wk pause

Or Irinotecan			
	Topoisomerase I inhibitor (double strand DNA breaks)	**Irinotecan** (Camptosar)	*350mg/m² IV over 30min on d1 rep from d22 (-d29) until progression*

Caution: in diarrhea aggressive interaction with loperamide PO.

Or Capecitabine			
	Pyrimidine antagonist (oral prodrug of 5-Fluorouracil)	**Capecitabine** (Xeloda)	*2500mg/m² PO qd (div bid) x 14d, then 1wk rest, rep cyc from d29*

15.8.3 Relapsed/Refractory Metastatic Colon Cancer

Prior Irinotecan Therapy and EGFR + Tumors			
	Topoisomerase I inhibitor (double strand DNA breaks)	**Irinotecan** (Camptosar)	*Same dose of prior Irinotecan therapy. Either 125 mg/m² weekly x 4 every 6wk or 180mg/m² every 2wk or 350 mg/m² every 3wk*
plus	**Epidermal growth factor receptor (EGFR) inhibitor** (monoklonal antibody, inhibits EGFR-tyrokinase ⇒ cell growth↓)	**Cetuximab** (Erbitux)	*400mg/m² over 2h in wk1, then 259mg/m² weekly. Premedicate with Diphenhydramine 50mg IV*
or alone	**Epidermal growth factor receptor (EGFR) inhibitor** (monoklonal antibody, inhibits EGFR-tyrokinase ⇒ cell growth↓)	**Cetuximab** (Erbitux)	*400mg/m² over 2h in wk1, then 259mg/m2 weekly. Premedicate with Diphenhydramine 50mg IV*

15.9   Esophageal Carcinoma

Cisplatin+ 5 FU and Radiation

	Alkylating agent (intrastrand cross-linking of DNA)	**Cisplatin** (Platinol, Platinol AQ, Gens)	*75mg/m² IV on d1 q4wk*
plus	**Pyrimidine antagonist** (inhibition of thymidine nucleotide synthesis)	**Fluorouracil** (Adrucil, Gens)	*1000mg/m² IV over 24h x 4d q4wk*

Metastatic Disease

	Alkylating agent (intrastrand cross-linking of DNA)	**Cisplatin** (Platinol, Platinol AQ, Gens)	*100mg/m² IV on d1 q4wk*
plus	**Pyrimidine antagonist** (inhibition of thymidine nucleotide synthesis)	**Fluorouracil** (Adrucil, Gens)	*1000mg/m² IV over 24h x 4d q4wk*
or	**Spindle poison** (tubulin polymerization, microtubule stabilization, mitosis inhibitor)	**Docetaxel** (Taxotere)	*75mg/m² IV on d1, rep q3wk*
plus	**Alkylating agent** (intrastrand cross-linking of DNA	**Cisplatin** (Platinol, Platinol AQ, Gens)	*75mg/m² IV on d1, rep q3wk*
OR	**Spindle poison** (microtubule inhibitor, tubulin polymerization, mitosis inhibition)	**Paclitaxel** (Taxol, Gens)	*175-225mg/m2 IV inf over 3h on d1, rep cyc q3wk*
plus	**Alkylating agent** (intrastrand cross-linking of DNA)	**Carboplatin** (Paraplatin)	*AUC 6 IV on d1, rep q3wk*

Gastric Carcinoma 319

15.10 Gastric Carcinoma

EAP (Etoposide + Adriamycin + Cisplatin)

	Spindle poison (inhibits DNA-/protein synthesis, mitosis)	Etoposide (Etopophos, Toposar, Vepesid)	100-120mg/m² IV on d4-6; pat <60yr: 100mg; rep cyc from d22-29
plus	Cytostatic antibiotic (binds to DNA, impairs nucleic acid synthesis)	Doxorubicin (Adriamycin, Rubex, Gens)	20mg/m² IV on d1, d7, rep cyc from d22-29
plus	Alkylating agent (intrastrand cross-linking of DNA)	Cisplatin (Platinol, Platinol AQ, Gens)	40mg/m² IV on d2, d8, rep cyc from d22-29

257. Preusser 1985

ELF (Etoposide + Leucovorin + Fluorouracil)

	Spindle poison (inhibits DNA-/protein synthesis, mitosis)	Etoposide (Etopophos, Toposar, Vepesid)	100-120mg/m² IV on d1-3 rep cyc from d22-29
plus	Biomodulator (folinic acid = 5-formyl-tetrahydrofolic acid = citrovorum factor, effectiveness of 5-FU↑)	Folinic acid (Leucovorin, Gens)	300mg/m² IV on d1-3 rep cyc from d22-29
plus	Pyrimidine antagonist (inhibition of thymidine nucleotide synthesis)	Fluorouracil (Adrucil, Gens)	500mg/m² bolus IV on d1-3 rep cyc from d22-29

258. Wilke 1990

FAM

	Pyrimidine antagonist (inhibition of thymidine nucleotide synthesis)	Fluorouracil (Adrucil, Gens)	600mg/m² IV on d1, d8, d29, d36 rep q8wk
plus	Cytostatic antibiotic (binds to DNA, impairs nucleic acid synthesis)	Doxorubicin (Adriamycin, Rubex, Gens)	30mg/m² on d1, d29 rep q8wk
plus	Cytostatic antibiotic (bifunctional alkylating)	Mitomycin C (Mutamycin, Mytozytrex, Gens)	10mg/m² on d1 rep q8wk

PDA Version on www.media4u.com

FAMTX

	Pyrimidine antagonist (inhibition of thymidine nucleotide synthesis)	**Fluorouracil** (Adrucil, Gens)	*1500mg/m² IV on d1 q28d*
plus	**Biomodulator** (folinic acid = 5-formyltetrahydrofolic acid = citrovorum factor, effectiveness of 5-FU↑)	**Folinic acid** (Leucovorin, Gens)	*15mg/m² PO q6h x 12 doses*
plus	**Cytostatic antibiotic** (binds to DNA, impairs nucleic acid synthesis)	**Doxorubicin** (Adriamycin, Rubex, Gens)	*30mg/m² on d15*
plus	**Antimetabolite** (folate antagonist)	**Methotrexate** (Folex, Mexate, Trexall, Gens)	*1.5g/m² IV on d1*

15.11 Hepatocellular Carcinoma

	Cytostatic antibiotic (binds to DNA, impairs nucleic acid synthesis)	**Doxorubicin** (Adriamycin, Rubex, Gens)	*60mg/m² IV, bolus on d1 rep cyc if effective after 2wk*
OR	**Pyrimidine antagonist** (inhibition of thymidine nucleotide synthesis)	**Fluorouracil** (Adrucil, Gens)	*500mg/m² IV on d1- d5 rep cyc from d36*
OR	**Pyrimidine antagonist** (inhibition of thymidine nucleotide synthesis)	**Fluorouracil** (Adrucil, Gens)	*600mg/m² IV on d1, d8, d29, d36 rep cyc from d57*
plus	**Cytostatic antibiotic** (binds to DNA, impairs nucleic acid synthesis)	**Doxorubicin** (Adriamycin, Rubex, Gens)	*30mg/m² IV on d1, d29 rep cyc from d57*
plus	**Cytostatic antibiotic** (bifunctional alkylating)	**Mitomycin C** (Mutamycin, Mytozytrex, Gens)	*10mg/m² IV on d1 rep cyc from d57*

15.12 Hodgkin's Disease

See Hematology →79

15.13 Insulinoma

	Pyrimidine antagonist (inhibition of thymidine nucleotide synthesis)	**Fluorouracil** (Adrucil, Gens)	*400mg/m² IV on d1-5, rep cyc from d43*
plus	**Alkylating agent** (nitrosourea analog, Inhibits DNA synthesis)	**Streptozocin** (Zanosar)	*500mg/m² IV on d1-5, rep cyc from d43*
plus	**Cytostatic antibiotic** (binds to DNA, impairs nucleic acid synthesis)	**Doxorubicin** (Adriamycin, Rubex, Gens)	*50mg/m² IV on d1, d21, rep cyc from d43*

15.14 Leukemia
15.14.1 Acute Leukemia

See Hematology →70

15.14.2 Chronic Myeloid Leukemia

See Hematology →67

15.14.3 Chronic Lymphocytic Leukemia

See Hematology →77

15.15 Lung Cancer
15.15.1 Small-cell

Limited Disease Stage (chemotherapy + radiation, then consolodation with 2 cycles PE)

	Radiation	*Concurrent chemo-Tx with radiation of 61Gy*	
plus	**Alkylating agent** (intrastrand cross-linking of DNA)	**Cisplatin** (Platinol, Platinol AQ, Gens)	*50mg/m² IV on d1, d8 2 cycs q4wk with radiation*
plus	**Spindle poison** (mitosis inhibitor, DNA-/protein synthesis inhibitor)	**Etoposide** (Etopophos, Toposar, Vepesid)	*50mg/m² IV on d1-5 2 cycs q4wk with radiation*

Extensive Disease Stage

ACO II (extensive disease; Adriamycin + Cyclophosphamide + Oncovin)

	Cytostatic antibiotic (binds to DNA, impairs nucleic acid synthesis)	**Doxorubicin** (Adriamycin, Rubex, Gens)	$40mg/m^2$ IV short inf on d1; 4-6 cycs q3wk
plus	**Alkylating agent** (cross-linking of DNA)	**Cyclophosphamide** (Cytoxan, Neosar, Gens)	$1000mg/m^2$ IV on d1 4-6 cycs q3wk
plus	**Spindle poison** (inhibits intracellular tubulin function/mitosis)	**Vincristine** (Oncovin, Vincasar, Gens)	$1mg/m^2$ (max 2mg) IV, on d1; 4-6 cycs q3wk

259. ACO II Roth 1992

ACE (Adriamycin + Cyclophosphamide + Etoposide)

	Cytostatic antibiotic (binds to DNA, impairs nucleic acid synthesis)	**Doxorubicin** (Adriamycin, Rubex, Gens)	$45mg/m^2$ IV on d1 4-6 cycs q3wk
plus	**Alkylating agent** (cross-linking of DNA)	**Cyclophosphamide** (Cytoxan, Neosar, Gens)	$1000mg/m^2$ IV on d1 4-6 cycs q3wk
plus	**Spindle poison** (mitosis inhibitor, DNA-/protein synthesis inhibitor)	**Etoposide** (Etopophos, Toposar, Vepesid)	$50mg/m^2$ IV on d1-5 4-6 cycs q3wk

260. Aisner 1984

PE

	Alkylating agent (intrastrand cross-linking of DNA)	**Cisplatin** (Platinol, Platinol AQ, Gens)	75-100mg/m^2 IV Inf over 2h on d1, rep q3-4wk
plus	**Spindle poison** (mitosis inhibitor, DNA-/protein synthesis inhibitor)	**Etoposide** (Etopophos, Toposar, Vepesid)	80-120mg/m^2 IV on d1-3, rep q3-4wk

Topotecan (single-agent regimen)

Topoisomerase I inhibitor (double strand DNA breaks)	**Topotecan** (Hycamtin)	1-1.5mg/m^2 IV over 30min qd on d1-5, rep cyc from d22(29) for 4-6 cyc

15.15.2 Non Small Cell Cancer

Adjuvant Therapy (resected stage IB and III)

Carboplatin/Paclitaxel

	Spindle poison (microtubule inhibitor, tubulin polymerization, mitosis inhibition)	Paclitaxel (Taxol, Gens)	175-225mg/m² IV inf over 3h on d1 q3wk x 4 cycles
plus	Alkylating agent (intrastrand cross-linking of DNA)	Carboplatin (Paraplatin)	AUC 6 IV on d1 q3wk x 4 cycles

To calculate the dosage of carboplatin with the AUC-method (AUC=area under the curve of plasma concentration), use formula by A. Calvert:
Dosage of carboplatin (mg) = AUC 6 (mg/ml x min) * [GFR (ml/min) + 25]

Or Cisplatin based regimen

	Alkylating agent (intrastrand cross-linking of DNA)	Cisplatin (Platinol, Platinol AQ, Gens)	75-100mg/m² IV on d1
plus	Any agents approved in lung cancer and used with cisplatin	Navelbine, Etoposide, etc.	

Combination chemotherapy stage IV

Carboplatin/Paclitaxel (+ or -) Avastin

	Spindle poison (microtubule inhibitor, tubulin polymerization, mitosis inhibition)	Paclitaxel (Taxol, Gens)	175-225mg/m² IV over 3h on d1, rep q3wk
plus	Alkylating agent (intrastrand cross-linking of DNA)	Carboplatin (Paraplatin)	AUC 6 IV on d1 rep q3wk
plus	Antiangiogenesis (anti-vascular endothelial growth factor)	Bevacizumab (Avastin)	15mg/kg IVBP d1; rep q3wk (non-squamous cell cancer, no CNS met or hemoptysis)

To calculate the dosage of carboplatin with the AUC-method (AUC=area under the curve of plasma concentration), use formula by A. Calvert:
Dosage of carboplatin (mg) = AUC 6 (mg/ml x min) * [GFR (ml/min) + 25]

Or Cisplatin/Paclitaxel

	Spindle poison (microtubule inhibitor, tubulin polymerization, mitosis inhibition)	Paclitaxel (Taxol, Gens)	*135mg/m² IV over 24h on d1, rep q3wk*
plus	Alkylating agent (intrastrand cross-linking of DNA)	Cisplatin (Platinol, Platinol AQ, Gens)	*75mg/m² IV on d2, rep q3wk*

Or Cisplatin/Gemcitabine

	Antimetabolite (cytidine analog, inhibits ribonucleotide reductase)	Gemcitabine (Gemzar)	*1000mg/m² IV on d1, d8, d15; rep q3-4wk delete d15 in the 3week regimen*
plus	Alkylating agent (intrastrand cross-linking of DNA)	Cisplatin (Platinol, Platinol AQ, Gens)	*100mg/m² IV on d1, rep q3-4wk (use 75mg/m² for the 3week regimen)*

Or Cisplatin/Docetaxel

	Spindle poison (tubulin polymerization, microtubule stabilization, mitosis inhibitor)	Docetaxel (Taxotere)	*75mg/m² IV on d1, rep q3wk*
plus	Alkylating agent (intrastrand cross-linking of DNA)	Cisplatin (Platinol, Platinol AQ, Gens)	*75mg/m² IV on d1, rep q3wk*

261. Schiller 2002

Second or third line

	Multitargeted antifolate	Pemetrexed (Alimta)	*500mg/m² IVP over 15min. Premedicate with Vit. B12 1000mcg IM every 9wk and folic acid 400-1000mcg PO qd. Start vitamins 1-2wks before first cycles.*

| or | **Epidermal growth factor receptor (EGFR) inhibitor** (inhibits EGFR-tyrokinase ⇒ cell growth↓) | **Gefitinib** (Iressa) | *250mg PO qd* |
| or | | **Erlotinib** (Tarceva) | *150mg PO qd* |

15.16 Malignant Melanoma

15.16.1 Adjuvant Therapy

| | **Interferon** (immunostimulation, immunomodulation) | **IFN alpha-2b** (Intron A) | *Ini 20 M IU/m^2 IV 5d/wk for 4 wk, maint 10 M IU/ m^2 tiw for 48wk* |

15.16.2 Advanced and Metastatic

DTIC

| | **Alkylating agent** (depolymerization of DNA, DNA synthesis ↓) | **Dacarbazine** (DTIC-Dome, Gens) | *850-1000mg/m^2 IV on d1, rep cyc from d22-36* |

262. Chapman PB, et al. Phase III multicenter randomized trial of the Dartmouth regimen versus dacarbazine in patients with metastatic melanoma. J Clin Oncol 1999; 17(9): 2745-2751

15.16.3 Combined Therapy

CVD

	Alkylating agent (depolymerization of DNA, DNA synthesis ↓)	**Dacarbazine** (DTIC-Dome, Gens)	*800mg/m^2 IV on d1, rep cyc from d22-d29*
plus	**Alkylating agent** (intrastrand cross-linking of DNA)	**Cisplatin** (Platinol, Platinol AQ, Gens)	*20mg/m^2 IV on d1-5, rep cyc from d22-d29*
plus	**Spindle poison** (inhibits microtubule formation, mitosis ↓)	**Vinblastine** (Velban, Gens)	*1.6mg/m^2 IV on d1-5, rep cyc from d22-d29*

263. Legha SS. Current therapy for malignant melanoma. Semin Oncol. 1989;16(1 suppl 1):34-44

CDBT (Dartmouth Regimen)

	Alkylating agent (intrastrand cross-linking of DNA)	**Cisplatin** (Platinol, Platinol AQ, Gens)	*25mg/m² IV on d1-3, d22-24, rep cyc from d22*
plus	**Alkylating agent** (depolymerization of DNA, DNA synthesis ↓)	**Dacarbazine** (DTIC-Dome, Gens)	*220mg/m² IV on d1-3, d22-24, rep cyc from d22*
plus	**Alkylating agent** (inter-, and intrastrand DNA crosslinks)	**Carmustine** (BiCNU, BCNU)	*150mg/m² IV on d1, rep cyc from d22*
plus	**Antiestrogen** (blockade of peripheral estrogen receptors)	**Tamoxifen** (Nolvadex)	*10mg PO bid on d4, rep cyc from d22*

264. Chapman PB, et al. Phase III multicenter randomized trial of the Dartmouth regimen versus dacarbazine in patients with metastatic melanoma. J Clin Oncol 1999; 17(9): 2745-2751

Temozolomide

	Alkylating agent (DNA breaks)	**Temozolomide** (Temodar)	*150mg/m² d1-5 q28d; if well tolerated incr to 200mg/m²*

IL-2

	Interleukin 2 (IL-2) (growth factor and activator of T cells)	**Aldesleukin** (Proleukin)	*100,000 IU/kg IV qd on d1-5, d15-19, q28d*

15.17 Mesothelioma

	Alkylating agent (intrastrand cross-linking of DNA)	**Cisplatin** (Platinol, Platinol AQ, Gens)	*75mg/m² IV on d1, rep q3wk*
plus	**Multitargeted antifolate**	**Pemetrexed** (Alimta)	*500mg/m² IVP over 15min. Premedicate with Vit. B12 1000mcg IM every 9wk and folic acid 400-1000mcg PO qd. Start vitamins 1-2wks before first cycles.*

265. Vogelzang NJ 2003

Or			
	Alkylating agent (intrastrand cross-linking of DNA)	**Cisplatin** (Platinol, Platinol AQ, Gens)	*75-100mg/m² IV on d1, rep q4wk*
plus	**Antimetabolite** (cytidine analog, inhibits ribonucleotide reductase)	**Gemcitabine** (Gemzar)	*1000mg/m² IV on d1, d8, d15, rep q4wk*

266. Nowak AK, 2002

15.18 Multiple Myeloma

MP (Alexanian I: Melphalan + Prednisolone)			
	Alkylating agent (cross-linking DNA strands, inhibits mitosis)	**Melphalan** (Alkeran)	*9mg/m² PO on d1-4, rep cyc from d43*
plus	**Glucocorticoid** (immunosuppressive, anti-inflammatory)	**Prednisone** (Deltasone, Meticorten, Prednisone Intensol, Gens)	*60mg/m² PO on d1-4, rep cyc from d43*

VAD (Vincristine + Adriamycin + Dexamethasone)			
	Spindle poison (inhibits intracellular tubulin function/mitosis)	**Vincristine** (Oncovin, Vincasar, Gens)	*0.4mg/d IV over 24h d1-4, rep cycle from d29*
plus	**Cytostatic antibiotic** (binds to DNA, impairs nucleic acid synthesis)	**Doxorubicin** (Adriamycin, Rubex, Gens)	*9mg/m² IV over 24h d1-4, rep cycle from d29*
plus	**Glucocorticoid** (anti-inflammatory, immunosuppressive)	**Dexamethasone** (Decadron, Hexadrol, Mymethasone, Gens)	*40mg PO on d1-4, d9-12, d17-20, rep cycle from d29*

Thal-Dex			
Or	**Immunomodulatory** (TNF-alpha production ↓)	**Thalidomide** (Thalomid)	*100-800mg PO qd*
plus	**Glucocorticoid** (anti-inflammatory, immunosuppressive)	**Dexamethasone** (Decadron, Hexadrol, Mymethasone, Gens)	*40mg PO on d1-4, d9-12, d17-20, rep cycle from d29*

15.19 Non–Hodgkin Lymphoma

CHOP

	Alkylating agent (cross-linking of DNA)	**Cyclophosphamide** (Cytoxan, Neosar, Gens)	*750mg/m² IV on d1, rep cyc from d22*
plus	**Cytostatic antibiotic** (binds to DNA, impairs nucleic acid synthesis)	**Doxorubicin** (Adriamycin, Rubex, Gens)	*50mg/m² IV on d1, rep cyc from d22*
plus	**Spindle poison** (inhibits intracellular tubulin function/mitosis)	**Vincristine** (Oncovin, Vincasar, Gens)	*1.5-2mg/m² IV (not to exceed 2mg) on d1, rep cyc from d22*
plus	**Glucocorticoid** (immunosuppressive, anti-inflammatory)	**Prednisone** (Deltasone, Meticorten, Prednisone Intensol, Gens)	*100mg/m² PO on d1-5, rep cyc from d22*

CHOP + Rituximab

	Alkylating agent (cross-linking of DNA)	**Cyclophosphamide** (Cytoxan, Neosar, Gens)	*750mg/m² IV on d1, rep cyc from d22*
plus	**Cytostatic antibiotic** (binds to DNA, impairs nucleic acid synthesis)	**Doxorubicin** (Adriamycin, Rubex, Gens)	*50mg/m² IV on d1, rep cyc from d22*
plus	**Spindle poison** (inhibits intracellular tubulin function/mitosis)	**Vincristine** (Oncovin, Vincasar, Gens)	*1.4mg/m² IV (not to exceed 2mg) on d1, rep cyc from d22*
plus	**Glucocorticoid** (immunosuppressive, anti-inflammatory)	**Prednisone** (Deltasone, Meticorten, Prednisone Intensol, Gens)	*100mg/m² PO on d1-5, rep cyc from d22*
plus	**Monoclonal antibody** (anti CD20)	**Rituximab** (Rituxan)	*375mg/m² on d1 (before chemo-Tx)*

ICE in relapses and primary refractory NHL

	Alkylating agent (DNA cross-linking, DNA and protein synthesis ↓)	**Ifosfamide** (Ifex, Gens)	*1000mg/m² IV over 1h on d1-2, rep cyc q28d*
plus	**Uroprotective agent** (inhibits hemorrhagic cystitis induced by ifosfamide)	**Mesna** (Mesnex, Gens)	*300mg IV before/4h + 8h after Ifosfamide, rep cyc q28d*

plus	**Alkylating agent** (intrastrand cross-linking of DNA)	Carboplatin (Paraplatin)	*200mg/m² on d1-2, rep cyc q28d*
plus	**Spindle poison** (mitosis inhibitor, DNA-/protein synthesis inhibitor)	Etoposide (Etopophos, Toposar, Vepesid)	*150mg/m² IV on d1-2, rep cyc q28d*

COP

	Alkylating agent (cross-linking of DNA)	Cyclophosphamide (Cytoxan, Neosar, Gens)	*800mg/m² IV on d1, rep cyc from d22*
plus	**Spindle poison** (inhibits intracellular tubulin function/mitosis)	Vincristine (Oncovin, Vincasar, Gens)	*1.4mg/m² IV (not to exceed 2mg) on d1, rep cyc from d22*
plus	**Glucocorticoid** (immunosuppressive, anti-inflammatory)	Prednisone (Deltasone, Meticorten, Prednisone Intensol, Gens)	*60mg/m² PO on d1-5, rep cyc from d22*

CP

	Alkylating agent (mitosis inhibitor, lymphosuppression)	Chlorambucil (Leukeran)	*30mg/m² PO on d1, rep cyc q28d*
plus	**Glucocorticoid** (immunosuppressive, anti-inflammatory)	Prednisone (Deltasone, Meticorten, Prednisone Intensol, Gens)	*80mg PO on d1-5, rep cyc q28d*

15.20 Ovarian Carcinoma

Paclitaxel and Carboplatin

	Spindle poison (microtubule inhibitor, tubulin polymerization, mitosis inhibition)	Paclitaxel (Taxol, Gens)	*175mg/m² IV on d1, rep cyc from d22*
plus	**Alkylating agent** (intrastrand cross-linking of DNA)	Carboplatin (Paraplatin)	*AUC 5-7.5 IV on d1, rep cyc from d22*

To calculate the dosage of carboplatin with the AUC-method (AUC=area under the curve of plasma concentration), use formula by A. Calvert:
Dosage of carboplatin (mg) = AUC 7.5 (mg/ml x min) x [GFR (ml/min) + 25]

Paclitaxel and Cisplatin

Or	**Alkylating agent** (intrast. cross-link.ofDNA)	**Cisplatin** (Platinol, Platinol AQ, Gens)	*75mg/m² IV on d2, rep cyc from d22*
plus	**Spindle poison** (microtubule inhibitor, tubulin polymerization, mitosis inhibition)	**Paclitaxel** (Taxol, Gens)	*135mg/m² IV over 24h on d1, rep cyc from d22*

Docetaxel

Or	**Spindle poison** (tubulin polymerization, microtubule stabilization, mitosis inhibitor)	**Docetaxel** (Taxotere)	*75mg/m² IV over 24h on d1, rep cyc from d22*

CAP

	Alkylating agent (cross-linking of DNA)	**Cyclophosphamide** (Cytoxan, Neosar, Gens)	*1000mg/m² IV on d1, rep cyc from d22*
plus	**Alkylating agent** (intra. cross-link. of DNA)	**Cisplatin** (Platinol, Platinol AQ, Gens)	*100mg/m² IV on d1, rep cyc from d22*
plus	**Cytostatic antibiotic** (binds to DNA, impairs nucleic acid synthesis)	**Doxorubicin** (Adriamycin, Rubex, Gens)	*50mg/m² IV on d1, rep cyc from d22*
Or	**Topoisomerase I inhibitor** (doublestrand DNA break)	**Topotecan** (Hycamtin)	*1-1.5 mg/m² IV qd on d1-5, rep cyc from d22(29)*

15.21 Pancreatic Cancer

Gemcitabine and Tarceva

	Antimetabolite (cytidine analog, inhibits ribonucleotide reductase)	**Gemcitabine** (Gemzar)	*1000mg/m² over 30min IV qwk x 7wk, then 1wk rest, then qwk x 3wk with 1wk rest*
Plus	**Epidermal growth factor receptor (EGFR) inhibitor** (inhibits EGFR-tyrosine kinase⇒inhib cell growth	**Erlotinib** (Tarceva)	*100mg PO qd*

Moore 2005

plus	**Cytostatic antibiotic** (binds to DNA, impairs nucleic acid synthesis)	**Doxorubicin** (Adriamycin, Rubex, Gens)	*30mg/m^2 IV on d1, d29, rep cyc from d57*
plus	**Cytostatic antibiotic** (bifunctional alkylating)	**Mitomycin C** (Mutamycin, Mytozytrex, Gens)	*10mg/m^2 IV on d1, rep cyc from d57*
Or	**Antimetabolite** (cytidine analog, inhibits ribonucleotide reductase)	**Gemcitabine** (Gemzar)	*1000mg/m^2 over 30min IV qwk x 7wk, then 1wk rest, then qwk x 3wk with 1wk rest*
Or	**Cytostatic antibiotic** (anthracycline derivative of doxorubicin, mitosis inhibitor)	**Epirubicin** (Ellence)	*90mg/m^2 IV on 1d, rep cyc from d29*

15.22 Prostate Carcinoma

Primary Therapy

	Gonadotropin-RH analog (down-regulation of pituitary receptors ⇒ sex hormones ↓)	**Goserelin** (Zoladex)	*3.6mg SC q4wk or 10.8mg SC q12wk*
		Leuprolide (Eligard, Lupron, Viadur, Gens)	*7.5mg SC q4wk or 22.5mg SC q12wk*
or	**Antiandrogen** (cytosol androgen receptor binding, androgen activity ↓)	**Bicalutamide** (Casodex)	*50mg PO qd*
		Cyproterone acetate (Androcur-Canada; not available in the US)	*100mg PO bid*
		Flutamide (Eulexin)	*250mg PO tid*
		Nilutamide (Nilandron)	*300mg PO qd for 30d, then 150mg PO qd*

Secondary Therapy

| | **Spindle poison** (tubulin polymerization, microtubule stabilization, mitosis inhibitor) | **Docetaxel** (Taxotere) | *60-70mg/m^2 IV on d1, rep q3wk* |

plus	**Alkylating agent** (cytostatic + estrogenic effects)	**Estramustine** (Emcyt)	*280mg PO qdx5 q21days*
Or	**Spindle poison** (tubulin polymerization, microtubule stabilization, mitosis inhibitor)	**Docetaxel** (Taxotere)	*75mg/m² IV on d1, rep q3wk*
plus	**Glucocorticoid** (immunosuppressive, anti-inflammatory)	**Prednisone** (Deltasone, Meticorten, Prednisone Intensol, Gens)	*5mg PO bid*
Or	**Topoisomerase II inhibitor** (DNA intercalation, mitosis inhibitor)	**Mitoxantrone** (Novantrone)	*12mg/m² IV on d1 q3wk*
plus	**Glucocorticoid** (immunosuppressive, anti-inflammatory)	**Prednisone** (Deltasone, Meticorten, Prednisone Intensol, Gens)	*5mg PO bid*
Or	**Pyrimidine antagonist** (inhibition of thymidine nucleotide synthesis)	**Fluorouracil** (Adrucil, Gens)	*500mg/m² IV qwk*
or	**Spindle poison** (microtubule inhibitor, tubulin polymerization, mitosis inhibition)	**Paclitaxel** (Taxol, Gens)	*80mg/m² IV on d1, d8, d15, rep cyc from d28*

15.23 Renal Cell Carcinoma

IL-2 + INF Combination Therapy

	Interleukin 2 (IL-2) (growth factor and activator of T cells)	**Aldesleukin** (Proleukin)	*18 x 10⁶ IU/m² IV CI d1-5 x 2, seperated by 6d break, then 18 x 10⁶ CI d1-5 q3wk x 4 cyc*
plus	**Interferon** (immunostimulating, immunomodulatory)	**IFN alpha-2a** (Roferon A)	*6 M IU/m² SC tiw in combination with IL-2*
		IFN alpha-2b (Intron A)	

267. Negrier S, et al: Recombinant human interleukin-2, recombinant human interferon alfa-2a, or both in metastatic renal-cell carcinoma. Groupe Francais d'Immunotherapie. N Engl J Med 1998 Apr 30; 338(18): 1272-8

High dose IL-2 Therapy		
Interleukin 2 (IL-2) (growth factor and activator of T cells)	**Aldesleukin** (Proleukin)	*600,000-720,000 IU/kg IV over 15min q8h until toxicity or 14 doses; give 2 courses separated by 5-9d, rep 2-course-cyc q6-12 wk*

15.24 Testicular Cancer

PEB (Cisplatin + Etoposide + Bleomycin)

	Alkylating agent (intrastrand cross-linking of DNA)	**Cisplatin** (Platinol, Platinol AQ, Gens)	*20mg/m² IV on d1-5 over 30min, rep cyc from d22*
plus	**Spindle poison** (mitosis ↓, DNA-/protein synthesis inhibitor)	**Etoposide** (Etopophos, Toposar, Vepesid)	*100mg/m² IV over 1h on d1-5, rep cyc from d22*
plus	**Cytostatic antibiotic** (single strand breaks, DNA synthesis ↓)	**Bleomycin** (Blenoxane, Gens)	*30mg IV on d1, d8, d15, rep cyc from d22*

268. Williams SD, Birch R, Einhorn LH, et al: Treatment of disseminated germ-cell tumors with cisplatin, bleomycin, and either vinblastine or etoposide. NEJM 1987; 316: 1435-14

VIP (Etoposide + Ifosfamide + Cisplatin)

	Spindle poison (mitosis inhibitor, DNA-/protein synthesis inhibitor)	**Etoposide** (Etopophos, Toposar, Vepesid)	*75mg/m² IV on d1-5 over 1h, rep cyc from d22*
plus	**Alkylating agent** (DNA cross-linking, DNA and protein synthesis ↓)	**Ifosfamide** (Ifex, Gens)	*1200mg/m² IV on d1- d5 over >1h, rep cyc from d22*
plus	**Uroprotective agent** (inhibits hemorrhagic cystitis induced by ifosfamide)	**Mesna** (Mesnex, Gens)	*400mg IV bolus, then 1200mg/m² IV on d1-5 (rep cyc from d22)*
plus	**Alkylating agent** (DNA double str. linkage)	**Cisplatin** (Platinol AQ, CDDP)	*20mg/m² IV on d1-5 over 30min, rep cyc from d22*

269. Harstrick 1991

16. Toxicology

Susan Smolinske
Managing Director
Regional Poison Control Center
Children's Hospital of Michigan
Wayne State University
Detroit, MI

16.1 Important Notes

16.1.1 General Measures

The primary removal of poisons (gastric lavage, induced vomiting etc.) is not a routine measure. Like pharmacologic therapy of poisonings, the necessity for these measures must be clearly tested and the measure must be clearly indicated. The administration of activated charcoal can replace these measures in many cases. Poison control centers can help with indications.

16.1.2 Pharmacologic Therapy

Drugs or antidotes can have severe adverse effects (deferoxamine, atropine, physostigmine etc.). All the same, it is often impossible to manage without their administration. Because of this, the indication for pharmacologic therapy must be carefully considered for every single case. The indication not only depends on the kind of poison, but also on the amount ingested, the time course of the poisoning, the physical condition of the patient and on other parameters. Benefits and disadvantages for the patient must be carefully considered on an individual basis.

16.1.3 Dosage

Absolute dosages are for adult patients. Dosages for children are specially marked. The specification mg/kg means "mg per kilogram body weight" and can usually be used for adults and children.

270. AACT (1997) Clin Toxicol 35:699-763
271. AACT (1999) Clin Toxicol 37:731-775
272. AACT (2004) Clin Toxicol 42:843-854

16.2 General Measures

16.2.1 Primary Gastric Decontamination

poss.	**Adsorbent** (binding of poison ⇒ resorption ↓ ⇒ poison elimination ↑)	**Activated charcoal** (Actidose, CharcoAid, Insta-Char, Liqui-Char)	*0.5-1g/kg or 10 times the amount of poison ingested PO or NG*
poss.	**Emetic** (induced vomiting ⇒ poison elimination; very rarely indicated)	**Syrup of ipecac** (Gens)	*Adults: 30ml; Ped 6-12m: 5-10ml; Ped 1-12y: 15ml, then 4-8oz H_2O; rep in 30min if no effect*
poss.	**Osmotic cathartic** (laxation ⇒ GI transit ↑)	**Sorbitol** (Gens)	*1-2ml/kg of 70%; Ped 4.3ml/kg of 35%*
poss.	**Gastric lavage** (⇒ poison elimination)	**Wide bore orogastric tube Adults: 36-49 French CH: 24-28 French**	*200-300ml aliquots warm fluid, 0.9% NaCl or water; Ped 10ml/kg warm 0.9% NaCl*
poss.	**Whole bowel irrigation** (⇒ poison elimination)	**PEG electrolyte solution** (Golytely, Colyte)	*2l/h PO or NG until rectal effluent clear; Ped 35ml/kg/h*

16.2.2 Secondary Poison Elimination

poss.	**Multiple dose activated charcoal** (may disrupt entero-hepatic circulation or adsorb drug resorbed from the intestine; "gut dialysis")	**Activated charcoal** (Actidose, CharcoAid, Insta-Char, Liqui-Char)	*0.25-0.5g/kg PO or NG every 2-4h, sorbitol repeated only qd-bid*
poss.	**Extracorporeal measures:** Hemodialysis, hemoperfusion, hemodiafiltration etc. should only be undertaken after consultation with poison control centers or in special poison treatment centers.		

16.3 Specific Management

16.3.1 Acetaminophen

Antidote (detoxification of toxic metabolites, antioxidant)	**Acetylcysteine** (Mucomyst, Mucosil, Acetadote, Gens)	*140mg/kg PO diluted to 5%, then 70mg/kg q4h PO for 17 doses (number of doses can be truncated in many situations)* **or IV** *(if intractable vomiting, ileus or GI bleeding)* *150mg/kg in 200ml D5W over 1h, then 50mg/kg in 500ml D5W over 4h, then 100mg/kg in 1000ml D5W over 16h;* **Peds:** *decrease total volume if < 40kg* **Pregnancy:** *140mg/kg over 1h, then 70mg/kg q4h for 17 doses* **Note:** *use IBW for obese patients*

273. Rumack (2002) Clin Toxicol 40:3–20

16.3.2 Amantadine

Benzodiazepine (anticonvulsant)	**Diazepam** (Valium, Gens)	*0.1–0.2mg/kg IV; may rep q1–4h prn*

16.3.3 Amphetamines

For seizures, agitation, hyperthermia

	Benzodiazepine (anticonvulsant, muscle relaxant ↓, hyperthermia)	**Diazepam** (Valium, Gens)	*0.1–0.2mg/kg IV; may rep q1–4h prn*
	Barbiturate (anticonvulsant)	**Phenobarbital** (Luminal, Gens)	*10–20mg/kg slowly IV*
poss.	**Muscle relaxant** (hyperthermia ↓)	**Dantrolene** (Dantrium)	*2.5mg/kg IV q6h*

For tachycardia

Adenosine (terminates AV nodal reentry-related dysrhythmias)	**Adenosine** (Adenocard, Adenoscan)	*3-6mg IV bolus; may rep 6-12mg q1-2min for 3 doses*
Beta- 1-selective Block. ($CO\downarrow$, neg. chronotropic, neg. inotropic, renin secretion↓, central sympathetic act.↓)	**Esmolol** (Brevibloc)	*50-100µg/kg/min IV inf*

For ventricular fibrillation

Antiarrhythmic Class Ib	**Lidocaine** (Gens)	*Ini 100mg IV, then 2-4mg/min*

274. White (2002) Semin Resp Crit Care Med 23:27-36

16.3.4 Antihistamines

For QRS prolongation (diphenhydramine)

Buffer (Tx of acidosis, Na^+ channel receptor binding↓, QRS↓)	**Sodium bicarbonate 8.4%** (50ml = 50mEq HCO_3^-)	*1-2mEq/kg IV (pH to 7.45-7.55)*

For seizures

Benzodiazepine (anticonvulsant)	**Diazepam** (Valium, Gens)	*0.1-0.2mg/kg IV; may rep q1-4h prn*

For hypotension

Alpha- and Beta-sympathomimetic, D1 receptor agonist (pos. inotropic)	**Dopamine** (Intropin, Gens)	*5-15 µg/kg/min IV*

275. Clark (1992) Ann Emerg Med 21:318-321

16.3.5 Arsenic

Arsenic salts, arsenic acid, arsenite, and arsenate with high As urine levels, not for arsine

Chelator	Succimer (Chemet)	10mg/kg PO tid for 5d, then 10mg/kg bid for 14d (may rep after 2wk interval, depending on arsenic excretion)
Chelator (for severe cases)	Dimercaprol (BAL)	3-5mg/kg IM q4-6h
	DMPS, Unithiol, Dimival (compounding pharmacy)	3-5mg/kg q4h slow IV over 20min; once stable, then 4-8mg/kg q6-8h PO

276. Cullen (1995) Am J Emerg Med 13: 432-435

16.3.6 Aspirin

Sodium bicarbonate (therapy of acidosis, urine alkalinization)	Sodium bicarbonate 8.4% (50ml = 50mEq HCO_3^-)	100-150mEq/l in D5W 3-4ml/kg/h with K^+ 20-40mEq/l (titrate to urine pH >7.5)
poss. Benzodiazepine (anticonvulsant)	Diazepam (Valium, Gens)	0.1-0.2mg/kg IV; may rep q1-4h prn

277. Prescott (1982) Br Med J 285:1383-1386.

16.3.7 Atropine

For severe anticholinergic syndrome (delirium, unstable tachycardia, coma with hypoventilation)

poss. Indirect para-sympatholytic, (cholinesterase inhibition ⇒ anticholinergic and adrenergic effects↓)	Physostigmine (Antilirium)	1-2mg slowly IV, may rep, although usually single dose as diagnostic; Ped 0.02-0.04mg/kg slowly IV
Benzodiazepine (anticonvuls.,antianxiety)	Diazepam (Valium, Gens)	0.1-0.2mg/kg IV; may rep q1-4h prn

278. Burns (2000) Ann Emerg Med 35:374-381

16.3.8	Baclofen		
	Dir. parasympatholytic (cholinergic effects ↓)	**Atropine** (Atropen, Gens)	*0.5-1mg IV; Ped 0.02mg/kg IV*

279. Cohen (1986) Am J Emerg Med 4: 552-553

16.3.9	Barbiturates		
	Buffer (urine alkalization, poison elimination ↑)	**Sodium bicarbonate 8.4%** (50ml = 50mEq HCO₃-)	*100-150mEq/l in D5W 3-4ml/kg/h with K⁺ 20-40mEq/l (titrate to urine pH >7.5; Phenobarbital only)*

280. Frenia (1996) Clin Toxicol 34:169-175

16.3.10	Benzodiazepines		
	Benzodiazepine antagonist (benzodiazepine effects ↑)	**Flumazenil** (Romazicon)	*0.2-0.6mg IV (short EHL, only in vital indication); Ped 0.01-0.02mg/kg q1min to max of 1mg or 0.05mg/kg*

281. Shalansky (1993) Clin Pharm 12:483-487

16.3.11	Betablockers		
	Alpha- and Beta-sympathomimetic, D1 receptor agonist (pos. inotropic)	**Dopamine** (Intropin, Gens)	*5-20 µg/kg/min*
	Beta- (>Alpha-) sympathomimetic (pos. ino-, chrono-, bathmotropic in hypotension, bronchodilatation)	**Epinephrine** (Adrenalin, Epipen, Sus-phrine, Gens)	*0.001-0.01mg/kg IV as single dose, then depending on effects*
	Inotropic agent (CO ↑, HR ↑ in bradycardia)	**Glucagon** (Glucagen, Gens)	*5-10mg IV bolus, then 1-5mg/h;Ped 0.15mg/kg, then: 0.05-0.1mg/kg/h over 24h IV*

poss.	Inotropic agent (BP↑)	**Insulin** (Insulin regular) **Glucose** (Gens)	*0.5-1 IU/kg/h with dextrose 1g/kg/h titrate to euglycemia*
	Buffer (QRS↓)	**Sodium bicarbonate 8.4%** (100ml = 100mEq HCO₃.)	*1-2Eq/kg IV (pH to 7.45-7.55)*
poss.	Calcium (reverses myocardial depression)	**Calcium chloride 10%** (Gens)	*0.1-0.2ml/kg IV q5-10min for 3-4doses, or 20-50mg/kg/h*

282. Kerns (1994) Emerg Med Clin North Am 12:365-390

16.3.12 Black Widow Spider Envenomation

	Antivenin (complexation with venom)	**Latrodectus antivenin**	*1 vial IV, diluted to 10-50ml in saline over 30min*

16.3.13 Botulism

	Specific antidote (poison effects↓)	**Botulinin Antitoxin (ABE)** (CDC)	*1-2 vials IV q4h for 4-5 doses, duration depends on response (not indicated in infants)*

16.3.14 Caffeine

For severe tachycardia or hypotension

	Betablocker (CO↓, neg. chronotropic, neg. inotropic, central sympathetic activity↓)	**Propranolol** (Inderal, Gens)	*1mg q2-5min up to 5mg total IV;* **Ped** *0.1mg/kg IV up to 1mg*
	Betablocker (CO↓, neg. chronotropic, neg. inotropic, central sympathetic activity↓)	**Esmolol** (Brevibloc)	*500µg/kg over 5min, then 50µg/kg/min for 4min; adj prn*

For ventricular fibrillation

	Antiarrhythmic Class Ib	**Lidocaine** (Gens)	*ini 1mg/kg IV bolus, maint 1-4mg/min*

For seizures

	Benzodiazepine (anticonvulsant)	**Diazepam** (Valium, Gens)	*0.1-0.2mg/kg IV; may rep q1-4h prn*

16.3.15 Calcium Channel Blockers

	Calcium (reverses myocardial depression)	**Calcium chloride 10%** (Gens)	*0.1-0.2ml/kg IV q5-10min for 3-4 doses, or 20-50mg/kg/h*
		Calcium gluconate 10% (Gens)	*0.3-0.4ml/kg IV q5-10min for 3-4 doses*
	Direct Parasympatholytic (cholinergic effects ↓)	**Atropine** (Atropen, Gens)	*0.5-1mg q5min to max 0.04mg/kg IV; **Ped** 0.02mg/kg q5min; max dose 0.5mg*
	Alpha- and Beta-sympathomimetic (BP↑, HR↑, pos. inotropic, vasoconstrict., renal vasodilation, natriuresis)	**Epinephrine** (Adrenalin, Epipen, Sus-phrine, Gens)	*0.001-0.01mg/kg IV as single dose, then depending on effects*
	Inotropic agent (CO↑, HR↑ in bradycardia)	**Glucagon** (Glucagen, Gens)	*5-10mg IV bolus, then 1-5mg/h; **Ped** 0.15mg/kg, then 0.05-0.1mg/kg/h over 24h IV*
poss.	Inotropic agent (BP↑)	**Insulin** (Insulin Regular) / **Glucose** (Gens)	*0.5 IU/kg/h with dextrose 1g/kg/h (titrate to euglycemia)*

283. Kerns (1994) Emerg Med Clin North Am 12:365-390
284. Yuan (1999) Clin Toxicol 37:463-474

16.3.16 Carbamate Insecticides

	Direct parasympatholytic (cholinergic effects ↓)	**Atropine** (Atropen, Gens)	*1-5mg IV, poss. rep q5-10min until atropinized (dry pulmonary secretions, reversal bronchospasm) with 5-10mg; **Ped** ini 0.02mg/kg*

16.3.17 Cardiac Glycosides

Specific antidote (glycoside effects↓)	Digitalis Immune Fab (Digibind, Digifab)	#vials =serum dig level (ng/ml) x body weight (kg)/100, over 30min IV. One vial binds 0.5mg dig (total dig levels after antidote falsely high)

16.3.18 Chloral Hydrate

Betablocker (PVCs↓)	Propranolol (Inderal, Gens)	1mg q2-5min up to 5mg total IV; **Ped** 0.1mg/kg IV up to 1mg
Betablocker (PVCs↓)	Esmolol (Brevibloc)	500μg/kg over 5min, then 50μg/kg/min for 4min; adj prn
Antiarrhythmic Class Ib	Lidocaine (Gens)	1mg/kg IV bolus, then 1-4mg/min

285. Pershad (1999) Pediatr Emerg Care 15:432-435

16.3.19 Chloroquine

Buffer (QRS↓)	Sodium bicarbonate 8.4% (50ml = 50mEq HCO₃-)	1-2mEq/kg IV (pH to 7.45-7.55)
Benzodiazepine (prophylaxis of arrhythmias, seizures)	Diazepam (Valium, Gens)	Ini 1-2mg/kg IV (after intubation), then 0.1-0.4mg/kg/h
Beta- (>Alpha-) sympathomimetic (pos. ino-, chrono-, bathmotropic in hypotension, bronchodilatation)	Epinephrine (Adrenalin, Epipen, Sus-phrine, Gens)	0.001-0.01mg/kg IV as single dose, then depending on effects

16.3.20 Clonidine

In bradycardia

Direct parasympatholytic (cholinergic effects ↓)	**Atropine** (Atropen, Gens)	0.5-1mg IV, **Ped** 0.02mg/kg IV

For hypotension

Alpha- and Beta-sympathomimetic, D1 receptor agonist (pos. inotropic)	**Dopamine** (Intropin, Gens)	5-10µg/kg/min

For respiratory depression

Opioid antagonist (opioid effects ↓)	**Naloxone** (Narcan, Gens)	0.4-2mg IV

286. Bamshad (1990) Vet Hum Toxicol 32:220-223

16.3.21 Cocaine

Benzodiazepine (anticonvulsant)	**Diazepam** (Valium, Gens)	0.1-0.2mg/kg IV; may rep q1-4h prn
Barbiturate (anticonvulsant)	**Phenobarbital** (Luminal, Gens)	10-20mg/kg slowly IV (for persistent seizures relaxation)

16.3.22 Copper Salts

Chelator (poison elimination ↑)	**Penicillamine** (Cuprimine, Depen)	1-1.5g PO qd, given q6-12h; **Ped** 10-30mg/kg/d, given q8-12h

16.3.23 Coral Snake Envenomation

Antivenin (complexation with venom)	**Antivenin Micrurus fulvius**	3-5 vials IV, diluted in 50-200ml saline over 15-30min per vial; may rep for continued neurologic symptoms

16.3.24 Crotalinae Envenomation

	Antivenin (complexation with venom)	Antivenin Crotalidae polyvalent (Wyeth)	*Ini 5-10vials IV in 250-500ml saline over 60-90min; rep if progressive edema*
	Antivenin (complexation with venom)	Crotalidae antivenin immune Fab (CroFab)	*Ini 4-6 vials IV in 250ml saline over 60-90min; maint Tx: 2 vials q6h for 3 doses after ini control; rep for recurrent edema or coagulopathy prn*

16.3.25 Cyanide

	Met-Hb-producer (cyanide binding to Met-Hb)	Cyanide antidote kit (amyl nitrite) (Taylor)	*Crush 1-2 ampules and place under nose for 30sec, rep x1 (produces approx 5% Met-Hb)*
then	Met-Hb-producer (cyanide binding to Met-Hb)	Cyanide antidote kit (sodium nitrite) (Taylor)	*300mg (10ml of 3%) IV over 3-5min; Ped 0.15-0.33ml/kg up to 10ml; adj based on Hb conc, can rep ½ dose (⇒ ca. 30% Met-Hb)*
then	Cyanide binding (form Met-Hb ⇒ change into thiocyanate ⇒ cyanide elimination)	Cyanide antidote kit (sodium thiosulfate) (Taylor)	*12.5g (50ml of 25%) IV at 2.5-5ml/min; Ped 400mg/kg (1.6ml/kg of 25%) IV up to 50ml, can rep ½ dose*

16.3.26 Cyclic Antidepressants

For arrhythmias

	Buffer (Tx of acidosis, binding of Na channel rec.↓, QRS↓)	Sodium bicarbonate 8.4% (50ml = 50mEq HCO_3^-)	*1-2mEq/kg IV (pH to 7.45-7.55)*
	Antiarrhythmic Class Ib	Lidocaine (Gens)	*1mg/kg slowly IV*

In hypotension

Alpha- and Beta-Sympathomimetic, D1 receptor agonist (pos. inotropic)	Dopamine (Intropin, Gens)	10-15µg/kg/min IV (do not use beta agonists)
Alpha-Sympathomimetic (periph. resist.↑, BP↑)	Norepinephrine (Levophed)	Ini 0.1µg/kg/min

287. Mackway-Jones (1999) J Accid Emerg Med 16:139-140

16.3.27 Ergot Derivatives

Direct vasodilator (antihypertensive therapy)	Sodium Nitroprusside (Nipride, Nitropress)	0.3µg/kg/min, titrate to effect, usual range 0.5 to 10µg/kg/min IV (only in very severe cases)

16.3.28 Ethylene Glycol

Alcohol Dehydrogenase blocker (competitive inhibition of alcohol dehydrogenase ⇒ metabolization↓)	Fomepizole (Antizol)	Ini 15mg/kg IV over 30min, then: 10mg/kg q12h for 4 doses, then incr to 15mg/kg q12h until ethylene glycol levels are <20mg/dl
Alcohol Dehydrogenase blocker (competitive inhibition of alcohol dehydrogenase ⇒ metabolization↓)	Ethanol	Ini 7.5ml/kg IV of 10% in dextrose 5% or 2ml/kg PO of 50%, then: 1-2ml/kg/h IV inf. or 0.2-0.4ml/kg/h PO maint. doses (aim for ethanol conc. 100mg/dl)
Metabolism cofactor (improve glyoxylic acid elimination)	Pyridoxine (=Vit. B6; Gens)	50mg IV q6h
	Thiamine (=Vit. B1; Gens)	100mg IV q6h

288. Brent. (2000) Drugs 61:979-988

16.3.29 Heparin

Specific antidote (reversal of heparin effects)	Protamine (Gens)	*1-1.5mg slowly IV per 100 IU heparin if immediately after heparin dose, ½ if 30-60min, ¼ if >2h (monitor PTT)*

16.3.30 Iron

Chelator (iron elimination ↑)	Deferoxamine (Desferal)	*15mg/kg/h IV, max: 6g q24h (avoid inf >24h) up to 50mg/kg/h and 16g/d in severe intoxication*
Whole bowel irrigation (⇒ poison elimination)	PEG electrolyte solution	*Adults: 2 l/h PO or NG until rectal effluent clear* **Ped** *35ml/kg/h*

289. Tenenbein (1996) Clin Toxicol 34:485-489
290. Howland (1996) Clin Toxicol 34:491-497

16.3.31 Lead

Chelator (poison elimination ↑)	Dimercaprol (BAL)	*3-5mg/kg IM q4-6h*
Chelator (poison elimination ↑)	Ethylendiamintetra-acetic acid (Ca-disodium EDTA)	*1000-1500mg/m²/d, as continuous inf. of 2-4mg/ml in D5W or NS for 5d (begin 4h after BAL if combined Tx)*
Chelator (poison elimination ↑)	Succimer (Chemet)	*10mg/kg PO tid for 5d, then 10mg/kg bid for 14d*

291. Campbell (2000) Curr Opin Pediatr 12:428-437

16.3.32 Levothyroxine

Betablocker (CO↓, neg. chronotropic, neg. inotropic, central sympathetic activity ↓)	Propranolol (Inderal, Gens)	*40mg PO tid*

16.3.33 Lithium

Saline hydration (Replace fluid/electrolyte deficits ⇒ poison elimination)	Saline 0.45–0.9%	*Ini 1-2l 0.9% IV; Ped 10-20ml/kg; then 0.45% at normal maintenance*
Whole bowel irrigation (⇒ poison elimination)	PEG electrolyte solution (Golytely, Colyte)	*Adults: 2 l/h PO or NG until rectal effluent clear; Ped 35ml/kg/h*

16.3.34 MAO Inhibitors

	Serotonin antagonist	Cyproheptadine (Periactin, Gens)	*4mg PO q1h up to 3 doses*
poss.	Muscle relaxant (hyperthermia ↓)	Dantrolene (Dantrium)	*2.5mg/kg IV q6h*
	Alphablocker (BP↓)	Phentolamine (Regitine, Rogitine, Gens)	*1-5mg IV bolus, rep q5-10min (to diastolic <100mmHg); Ped 0.02-0.2mg/kg*

16.3.35 Mercury

Depending on whole blood or 24 hour urine mercury concentration

Chelator (poison elimination↑)	Succimer (Chemet)	*10mg/kg PO tid for 5d, then 10mg/kg bid for 14d*
Chelator (for severe inorganic HG)	DMPS, Unithiol, Dimival (compounding pharmacy)	*3-5mg/kg q4h slow IV over 20min, once stable, then 4-8mg/kg q6-8h PO*

16.3.36 Metformin

Insulin/Dextrose (therapy of acidosis)	**Insulin** (regular) **/Dextrose 5%**	*10-20 IU IV q4h with dextrose 5-12.5g IV q4h*
Glucose (for hypoglycemia)	**Glucose 50%, then Glucose 5%**	*Depending on BS*
Buffer (therapy of acidosis)	**Sodium bicarbonate 8.4%** (50ml = 50 mEo HCO$_3^-$)	*1-2mEq/kg IV*

292. Misbin (1998) N Engl J Med 338:265-266

16.3.37 Methanol

Alcohol Dehydrogenase blocker (competitive inhibition of alcohol dehydrogenase ⇒ inhibition of metabolization)	**Fomepizole** (Antizol)	*Ini 15mg/kg IV over 30min, then: 10mg/kg q12h for 4 doses, then incr to 15mg/kg q12 until methanol levels are <20mg/dl*
Alcohol Dehydrogenase blocker (competitive inhibition of alcohol dehydrogenase ⇒ inhibition of metabolization)	**Ethanol**	*Ini 7.5ml/kg IV of 10% in dextrose 5% or 2ml/kg PO of 50%, t then: 1-2ml/kg/h IV inf. or 0.2-0.4ml/kg/h PO maint. doses (aim for ethanol conc. of 100mg/dl)*
To improve formic acid elimination	**Folic acid** (Folicet, Folvite, Gens) **Leucovorin Calcium** (Wellcovorin, Gens)	*Leucovorin 1mg/kg (up to 50 mg) IV q4h for 2 doses, then folic acid PO 1mg/kg q4-6h*

293. Brent (2001) N Engl J Med 344:424-429

16.3.38 Methaemoglobin Causing Agents

Reduction of Met-Hb (poison effects ↓)	**Methylene blue** (Gens)	*1-2mg/kg IV, may rep in 30-60min for 2 doses, max 15mg/kg. Maint (if needed) 1-2mg/kg q6-8h*

16.3.39 Methotrexate

Specific antidote (poison effects↓)	**Leucovorin Calcium** (Wellcovorin, Gens)	*Same dose as MTX or 75mg IV then 12mg q12h for 4 doses (give within 1h of MTX); rep doses if 24h MTX level >0.1μM to total 12 doses*
Enhance elimination (investigational)	**Carboxypeptidase G2** (Voraxaze)	*50U/kg IV*

16.3.40 Mushrooms (Cyclopeptide)

Adsorbent (interrupt enterohepatic recirculation)	**Activated charcoal** (Actidose, CharcoAid, Insta-Char, Liqui-Char)	*0.5g/kg q4h*
Antidote (Antioxidant)	**Acetylcysteine** (Mucomyst, Mucosil, Acetadote, Gens)	*140mg/kg PO diluted to 5%, then 70mg/kg q4h PO for 17 doses (number of doses can be truncated in many sit.); or IV (if intractable vomiting, ileus or GI bleeding) 150mg/kg in 200ml D5W over 1h, then 50mg/kg in 500ml D5W over 4h, then 100mg/kg in 1000ml D5W over 16h; Peds: decrease total volume if < 40kg; Pregnancy: 140mg/kg over 1h, then 70mg/kg q4h for 17 doses; Note: use IBW for obese patients*

294. Floersheim (1987) Med Toxicol 2:1-9
295. Enjalbert (2002) Clin Toxicol 40:715-757

16.3.41 Neuroleptics/Antipsychotics

For ventricular arrhythmias

Buffer (QRS↓)	Sodium bicarbonate 8.4% (50ml = 50mEq HCO₃-)	1-2mEq/kg IV (pH to 7.45-7.55)
Antiarrhythmic Class Ib	Lidocaine (Gens)	1mg/kg IV bolus, then 1-4mg/min

For hypotension

Alpha- and Beta-sympathomimetic, D1 receptor agonist (pos. inotropic)	Dopamine (Intropin, Gens)	5-10µg/kg/min
Alpha-sympatho-mimetic (periph. resist.↑, BP↑)	Norepinephrine (Levophed)	Ini 0.1µg/kg/min
Dopamine agonist (adjunct in NMS)	Bromocriptine (Parlodel)	2.5-10mg PO or NG 2-6 times daily

16.3.42 Opiates

Opioid antagonist (opioid effects↓)	Naloxone (Narcan)	0.4-2mg IV q2-3min continuous inf 0.4-0.8mg/h in 0.9% Na⁺Cl⁻ or D5W (long-acting opioids)
Opioid antagonist (opioid effects↓)	Nalmefene (Revex)	0.25-0.5mg q2-5min IV until respiration restored May require rep doses

296. Clarke (2002) Emerg Med J 19:249-250

16.3.43 Organophosphates

Direct parasympatholytic (cholinergic effects ↓)	Atropine (Atropen, Gens)	1-5mg IV, poss. rep q5-10min until atropinized (dry pulm secretions, reversal bronchospasm) with 5-10mg; Ped ini 0.02mg/kg

Cholinesterase activator (antidote)	Pralidoxime (2-PAM, Protopam)	*Ini-2g IV over 5-10min; maint. 200-500mg/h as 1% solution;* **Ped** *25-50mg/kg; maint. 5-10mg/kg/h*

16.3.44 Quinine

Membrane stabilizing effects

Buffer (QRS↓)	Sodium bicarbonate 8.4% (50ml = 50mEq HCO₃-)	*1-2mEq/kg IV (pH to 7.45-7.55)*
Benzodiazepine (anticonvulsant, antianxiety)	Diazepam (Valium, Gens)	*0.1-0.2mg/kg IV; may rep q1-4h prn*

16.3.45 Serotonin Reuptake Inhibitors

Serotonin antagonist	Cyproheptadine (Periactin, Gens)	*4mg PO q1h up to 3 doses*

297. Mills (1997) Med Toxicol 13:763-783

16.3.46 Sulfonylureas

Antidote (insulin release↓)	Octreotide (Sandostatin)	*50-100µg SC or IV q4-12h, up to 125µg/h* **Ped** *4-5µg/kg per dose given q6-12h*

298. McLaughlin (2000) Ann Emerg Med 36:133-138

16.3.47 Theophylline

Barbiturate (seizure treatment/ prophylaxis)	Phenobarbital (Luminal, Gens)	*2mg/kg slow IV, rep q15min up to 10-20mg/kg IV*
Benzodiazepine (seizure treatment/ prophylaxis)	Diazepam (Valium, Gens)	*0.1-0.2mg/kg IV; may rep q1-4h prn*

Betablocker (HR↓, BP↑)	Propranolol (Inderal, Gens)	1mg q2-5 in up to 5mg total IV; Ped 0.1mg/kg IV up to 1mg
Betablocker (HR↓, BP↑)	Esmolol (Brevibloc)	500µg/kg over 5min, then 50µg/kg/min for 4min; adj prn

16.3.48 Valproic Acid

For encephalopathy with hyperammonemia

Antidote (serum ammonia↓)	L-carnitine (Carnitor)	150-500mg/kg IV up to 3g/d

299. Raskind (2000) Ann Pharmacother 34:630-638

16.3.49 Warfarin/Superwarfarins

Vitamin K (Vit-K antagonism↓)	Phytonadione (Aquamephyton, Vitamin K1, Gens)	10-25mg PO qd (50-200mg/d may be required), 0.6mg/kg IV; Ped 5-10mg PO qd (in long-acting anticoagulant rodenticides poss. over months)

16.3.50 Zinc

Chelator (poison elimination↑)	Ethylendiamintetra-acetic acid (Ca-disodium EDTA)	1000-1500mg/m²/d, as cont. Inf of 2-4mg/ml in D5W or NS for 5d (ini 4h after BAL if combined Tx)
Chelator (poison elimination↑)	Dimercaprol (BAL)	3-5mg/kg IM q4-6h

Poison Control Centers

The American Association of Poison Control Centers (AAPCC) has launched a nationwide number for access to the 62 US poison control centers. The number, **1-800-222-1222**, is routed to the local poison center serving the caller, based on the area code and exchange of the caller. The number is functional 24-hours a day in the 50 states, the District of Columbia, the US Virgin Islands, and Puerto Rico.

ALABAMA

Alabama Poison Center
408-A Paul Bryant Drive
Tuscaloosa, AL 35401
Phone: (800) 462-0800 [AL only]; (205) 345-0600
Regional Poison Control Center
The Children's Hospital of Alabama,
1600 - 7th Avenue South
Birmingham, AL 35233-1711
Phone: (205) 939-9201; (800) 222-1222

ALASKA

Anchorage Poison Control Center
Providence Hospital Pharmacy
PO Box 196604
Anchorage, AK 95516-6604
Phone: (800) 222-1222
(907) 261-3193

ARIZONA

Arizona Poison and Drug Information Center
Arizona Health Sciences Center
1501 N. Campbell Avenue,
Rm #1156,
Tucson, AZ 85724
Phone: (800) 222-1222;
(520) 626-6016
Samaritan Regional Poison Center
1111 E. McDowell Road,
Ancillary - 1,
Phoenix, AZ 85006
Phone: (602) 253-3334;
(800) 222-1222

ARKANSAS

Arkansas Poison and Drug Information Center
University of Arkansas for
Medical Sciences
4301 West Markham-Slot 522
Little Rock, AR 72205
Phone: (800) 222-1222

CALIFORNIA

California Poison Control System, Central Office
University of California,
San Francisco
School of Pharmacy, Box
1262San Francisco, CA 94143
Phone: (800) 222-1222

COLORADO

Rocky Mountain Poison and Drug Center
8802 E. 9th Avenue
Denver, CO 80220-6800
Phone: (303) 629-1123
(800) 222-1222

CONNECTICUT

Connecticut Poison Control Center
University of Connecticut
Health Center
263 Farmington Avenue
Farmington, CT 06030
Phone: (800) 222-1222

DELAWARE

The Poison Control Center
3600 Sciences Center, Ste. 220
Philadelphia, PA 19104-2641
Phone: (215) 386-2100;
(800) 222-1222

DISTRICT OF COLUMBIA

National Capital Poison Center
3201 New Mexico Avenue, N.W.,
Suite 310
Washington, DC 20016
Phone: (800) 222-1222
(202) 625-3333;
(202) 362-8563 [TTY]

FLORIDA

Florida Poison Information Center
University Medical Center
University of Florida Health
Science Center
655 West 8th Street
Jacksonville, FL 32209
Emergency Numbers: (904) 549-4465; (800) 222-1222

Florida Poison Information Center
University of Miami/Jackson Memorial Hospital
1611 NW 12th Avenue
Urgent Care Center Bldg., Rm. 219, Miami, FL 33136
Phone: (800) 222-1222
The Florida Poison Information and Toxicology Resource Center
Tampa General Hospital
PO Box 1289
Tampa, FL 33601
Phone: (813) 256-4444 [Tampa only];
(800) 222-1222

GEORGIA
Georgia Poison Center
Hughes Spalding Children's Hospital
Grady Health Systems
80 Butler Street, S.E.
PO Box 26066
Atlanta, GA 30335-3801
Phone: (800) 222-1222
(404) 616-9000 [GA only]

HAWAII
Hawaii Poison Center
1500 S. Beretania Street, Rm. #113
Honolulu, HI 96826
Phone: (808) 941-4411
(800) 222-1222

IDAHO
Idaho Poison Center
3092 Elder Street
Boise, ID 83720-0036
Phone: (208) 334-4570;
(800) 222-1222

ILLINOIS
Illinois Poison Center
222 South Riverside Plaza, Suite 1900
Chicago, IL 60606
Phone: (800) 222-1222

INDIANA
Indiana Poison Center
Methodist Hospital of Indiana
I-65 and 21st St.
PO Box 1367
Indianapolis, IN 46206-1367
Phone: (800) 222-1222
(317) 929-2323

IOWA
St. Luke's Poison Center
St. Luke's Regional Medical Center
2720 Stone Park Boulevard
Sioux City, IA 51104
Phone: (712) 277-2222;
(800) 222-1222
Mid-Iowa Poison and Drug Information Center
Variety Club Poison and Drug Information Center
Iowa Methodist Medical Center
1200 Pleasant Street
Des Moines, IA 50309
Phone: (515) 241-6254;
(800) 222-1222
Poison Control Center
The University of Iowa Hospitals and Clinics
Pharmacy Department
200 Hawkins Drive
Iowa City, IA 52242
Phone: (800) 222-1222

KANSAS
Mid-America Poison Control Center
University of Kansas Medical Center
3901 Rainbow Blvd., Room B-400
Kansas City, KS 66160-7231
Phone: (913) 588-6633;
(800) 222-1222

KENTUCKY
Kentucky Regional Poison Center of Kosair Children's Hospital
Medical Towers South, Suite 572
PO Box 35070
Louisville, KY 40232-5070
Phone: (502) 589-8222;
(800) 222-1222

LOUISIANA
Louisiana Drug and Poison Information Center
Northeast Louisiana University
Sugar Hall
Monroe, LA 71209-6430
Phone: (800) 222-1222
(318) 362-5393

MAINE
Maine Poison Control Center
Maine Medical Center
Department of Emergency Medicine
22 Bramhall Street
Portland, ME 04102
Phone: (207) 871-2950;
(800) 222-1222

MARYLAND
Maryland Poison Center
University of Maryland School
of Pharmacy
20 N. Pine Street
Baltimore, MD 21201
Phone: (410) 528-7701;
(800) 222-1222

MASSACHUSETTS
**Massachusetts Poison Control
System**
300 Longwood Avenue
Boston, MA 02115
Phone: (617) 232-2120;
(800) 222-1222

MICHIGAN
**Blodgett Regional Poison
Center**
1840 Wealthy S.E.
Grand Rapids, MI 49506-2968
Phone: (800) POISON1;
(800) 222-1222
Poison Control Center
Children's Hospital of Michigan
Harper Professional Office Bldg.
4160 John R., Suite 425
Detroit, MI 48201
Phone: (313) 745-5711;
(800) 222-1222
Marquette General Hospital
420 W. Magnetic Street
Marquette, MI 49855
Phone: (906) 225-3497;
(800) 222-1222

MINNESOTA
**Hennepin Regional Poison
Center**
Hennepin County Medical
Center
701 Park Avenue
Minneapolis, MN 55415
Phone: (612) 347-3141;
(612) 337-7387 [Petline];
(800) 222-1222
**Minnesota Regional Poison
Center**
8100 34th Avenue S.
P.O. Box 1309
Minneapolis, MN 55440-1309
Phone: (612) 221-2113
(800) 222-1222

MISSISSIPPI
**Mississippi Regional Poison
Control Center**
University of Mississippi Medical
Center
2500 North State Street
Jackson, MS 39216-4505
Phone: (601) 354-7660
(800) 222-1222

MISSOURI
**Cardinal Glennon Children's
Hospital Regional Poison
Center**
1465 S. Grand Blvd.
St. Louis, MO 63104
Phone: (314) 772-5200;
(800) 222-1222
Children's Mercy Hospital
2401 Gillham Road
Kansas City, MO 64108
Phone: (816) 234-3430
(800) 222-1222

MONTANA
**Rocky Mountain Poison and
Drug Center**
8802 E. 9th Avenue
Denver, CO 80220-6800
Phone: (303) 629-1123
(800) 222-1222

NEBRASKA
The Poison Center
8301 Dodge Street.
Omaha, NE 68114
Phone: (402) 390-5555
[Omaha];
(800) 222-1222

NEVADA
**Rocky Mountain Poison and
Drug Center**
8802 E. 9th Avenue
Denver, CO 80220-6800
Phone: (303) 629-1123;
(303) 739-1127 [TTY]
(800) 222-1222

NEW HAMPSHIRE
**New Hampshire Poison
Information Center**
Dartmouth-Hitchcock Medical
Center
One Medical Center Drive
Lebanon, NH 03756
Phone: (603) 650-8000;
(603) 650-5000 [11pm-8am];
(800) 222-1222

NEW JERSEY
**New Jersey Poison
Information and Education
System**
201 Lyons Avenue
Newark, NJ 07112
Phone: (800) 222-1222

NEW MEXICO
New Mexico Poison and Drug Information Center
University of New Mexico
Health Sciences Library,
Room 125
Albuquerque, NM 87131-1076
Phone: (505) 843-2551;
(800) 222-1222

NEW YORK
Central New York Poison Control Center
SUNY Health Science Center
750 E. Adams Street
Syracuse, NY 13210
Phone: (315) 476-4766;
(800) 222-1222
Finger Lakes Regional Poison Center
Box 777
University of Rochester Medical Center
601 Elmwood Avenue, Box 321,
Rm. G-3275
Rochester, NY 14642
Phone: (716) 275-5151;
(800) 222-1222
Hudson Valley Regional Poison Center
Phelps Memorial Hospital Center
701 North Broadway
North Tarrytown, NY 10591
Phone: (800) 222-1222
(914) 366-3030
Long Island Regional Poison Control Center
Winthrop University Hospital
259 First Street
Mineola, NY 11501
Phone: (516) 542-2323
(800) 222-1222

New York City Poison Control Center
N.Y.C. Department of Health
455 First Avenue, Room 123
New York, NY 10016
Phone: (212) 340-4494;
(212) 689-9014 [TDD]
(800) 222-1222
Western New York Regional Poison Control Center
Children's Hospital of Buffalo
219 Bryant Street
Buffalo, NY 14222
Phone: (716) 878-7654;
Also Extensions: 7655, 7856,
7857 (800) 222-1222

NORTH CAROLINA
Carolinas Poison Center
1000 Blythe Boulevard
P.O. Box 32861
Charlotte, NC 28232-2861
Phone: (704) 355-4000;
(800) 222-1222
Catawba Memorial Hospital Poison Control Center
Pharmacy Department
810 Fairgrove Church Road
Hickory, NC 28602
Phone: (704) 322-6649
(800) 222-1222
Duke Poison Control Center
North Carolina Regional Center,
Duke University
Box 3007
Durham, NC 27710
Phone: (919) 684-8111;
(800) 222-1222
Triad Poison Center
1200 N. Elm Street
Greensboro, NC 27401-1020
Phone: (910) 574-8105;
(800) 222-1222

NORTH DAKOTA
North Dakota Poison Information Center
MeritCare Medical Center
720 4th Street North
Fargo, ND 58122
Phone: (701) 234-5575;
(800) 222-1222

OHIO
Akron Regional Poison Center
1 Perkins Square
Akron, OH 44308
Phone: (216) 379-8562;
(800) 222-1222
(216) 379-8446 [TTY]
Bethesda Poison Control Center
2951 Maple Avenue
Zanesville, OH 43701
Phone: (614) 454-4221
(800) 222-1222
Central Ohio Poison Center
700 Children's Drive
Columbus, OH 43205-2696
Phone: (614) 228-1323;
(800) 222-1222
(614) 228-2272 [TTY]
(614) 461-2012
Cincinnati Drug & Poison Information and Regional Poison Control System
P.O. Box 670144
Cincinnati, OH 45267-0144
Phone: (513) 558-5111;
(800) 222-1222
(800) 253-7955 [TTY]
Greater Cleveland Poison Control Center
11100 Euclid Avenue
Cleveland, OH 44106
Phone: (216) 231-4455
(800) 222-1222

Medical College of Ohio
Poison and Drug Information Center
3000 Arlington Avenue
Toledo, OH 43614
Phone: (419) 381-3897;
(800) 222-1222
Northeast Ohio Poison Education/Information Center
1320 Timken Mercy Drive N.W.
Canton, OH 44708
Phone: (800) 222-1222

OKLAHOMA
Oklahoma Poison Control Center
940 N.E. 13th Street, Rm. 3N118
Oklahoma, OK 73104
Phone: (405) 271-5454;
(800) 222-1222

OREGON
Oregon Poison Center
Oregon Health Sciences University
3181 S.W. Sam Jackson Park Road, CB550
Portland, OR 97201
Phone: (503) 494-8968;
(800) 222-1222

PENNSYLVANIA
Central Pennsylvania Poison Center
University Hospital
Milton S. Hershey Medical Center
Hershey, PA 17033-0850
Phone: (800) 222-1222
(717) 531-6111

Lehigh Valley Hospital Poison Prevention Program
17th & Chew Streets
P.O. Box 7017
Allentown, PA 18105-7017
The Poison Control Center
3600 Sciences Center, Suite 220
Philadelphia, PA 19104-2641
Phone: (215) 386-2100
(800) 222-1222
Pittsburgh Poison Center
3705 Fifth Avenue
Pittsburgh, PA 15213
Phone: (412) 681-6669;
(800) 222-1222
Regional Poison Prevention Education Center
Mercy Regional Health System
2500 Seventh Avenue
Altoona, PA 16602
Phone: (800) 222-1222

RHODE ISLAND
Rhode Island Poison Center
593 Eddy Street
Providence, RI 02903
Phone: (401) 444-5727
(800) 222-1222

SOUTH CAROLINA
Palmetto Poison Center
College of Pharmacy
University of South Carolina
Columbia, SC 29208
Phone: (803) 765-7359;
(800) 222-1222;
(706) 724-5050;
(803) 777-1117

SOUTH DAKOTA
McKennan Poison Control Center
Box 5045
800 E. 21st Street
Sioux Falls, SD 57117-5045
Phone: (605) 336-3894;
(800) 222-1222

TENNESSEE
Middle Tennessee Poison Center
The Center for Clinical Toxicology
Vanderbilt University Medical Center
1161 21st Avenue South
501 Oxford House
Nashville, TN 37232-4632
Phone: (615) 936-2034 [local];
(800) 222-1222
Southern Poison Center, Inc.
847 Monroe Avenue, Suite 230
Memphis, TN 38163
Phone: (901) 528-6048;
(800) 222-1222

TEXAS
Central Texas Poison Center
Scott & White Memorial Clinic & Hospital
2401 S. 31st Street
Temple TX 76508
Phone: (817) 774-2005;
(800) 222-1222
North Texas Poison Center
Texas Poison Center Network at Parkland Memorial Hospital
5201 Harry Hines Blvd.
Dallas, TX 75235
Phone: (800) 222-1222

South Texas Poison Center
7703 Floyd Curl Drive
San Antonio, TX 78284-7834
Phone: (800) 222-1222

Texas Poison Control Network
PO Box 1110, 1501 S. Coulter
Amarillo, TX 79175
Phone: (800) 222-1222

Texas Poison Control Network
Southeast Texas Poison Center
The University of Texas Medical
Branch
301 University Avenue
Galveston, TX 77555-1175
Phone: (409)-765-1420
[Galveston];
(713) 654-1701 [Houston];
(800) 222-1222

**West Texas Regional Poison
Center**
4815 Alameda Avenue
El Paso, TX 79905
Phone: (800) 222-1222

UTAH
Utah Poison Control Center
410 Chipeta Way, Suite 230
Salt Lake City, UT 84108
Phone: (801) 581-2151;
(800) 222-1222

VERMONT
Vermont Poison Center
Fletcher Allen Health Care
111 Colchester Avenue
Burlington, VT 05401
Phone: (802) 658-3456
(800) 222-1222

VIRGINIA
Blue Ridge Poison Center
University of Virginia
Blue Ridge Hospital
Charlottesville, VA 22901
Phone: (804) 924-5543;
(800) 222-1222

Virginia Poison Center
401 N. 12th Street
Virginia Commonwealth
University
Richmond, VA 23298-0522
Phone: (804) 828-9123
[Richmond];
(800) 222-1222

WASHINGTON
Washington Poison Center
155 N.E. 100th Street,
Suite #400
Seattle, WA 98125
Phone: (206) 526-2121;
(800) 222-1222
(206) 517-2394 [TDD];
(206) 517-2394 [TDD; WA only]

WEST VIRGINIA
West Virginia Poison Center
3110 MacCorkle Avenue, S.E.
Charleston, WV 25304
Phone: (800) 222-1222
(304) 348-4211

WISCONSIN
**Poison Center of Eastern
Wisconsin**
Children's Hospital of Wisconsin
P.O. Box 1997
Milwaukee, WI 53201
Phone: (414) 266-2222;
(800) 222-1222

**University of Wisconsin
Hospital Regional Poison
Center**
E5/238 CSC
600 Highland Avenue
Madison, WI 53792
Phone: (608) 262-3702;
(800) 222-1222

WYOMING
The Poison Center
8301 Dodge Street
Omaha, NE 68114
Phone: (402) 390-5555
[Omaha]; (800) 222-1222

Numerics

5-azacytidine 69
5-AZC 69

A

A-200 299
Abacavir 191
Abbokinase 44
Abilify 231, 234, 235, 236
Abscess 285
- eyelids 243
Acamprosate 232
Acarbose 116
Accolate 83
Accupril 157, 158
Accutane 287
ACE inhibitors 17, 18, 22, 24, 26, 28, 33, 157, 158
Acephen 190, 195, 196, 278, 282
Acetadote 336, 349
Acetaminophen 89, 96, 105, 146, 161, 190, 195, 196, 207, 210, 255, 278, 282
Acetaminophen intoxication 336
Acetasol 280
Acetazolamide 59, 264, 271–272
Acetic acid 281
Acetic acid sol 280
Acetic acid derivatives 109, 110
Acetylcysteine 159, 336, 349
Achalasia 141
Achromycin 242, 248, 286, 288, 295, 301–303
ACI 230, 231
Acidosis 56
- lactic 57
- metabolic 56

Acids
- fibric 118, 119
- folic 63
- valproic 235
Acinetobacter species 169
Acitretin 296, 297, 301
Acne vulgaris
- comedonal 285
- nodulocystic 287
- papulopustular 285
Acromegaly 137
Actidose 335, 349
Actigall 148, 150
Actinomyces species 169
Actiq/PO 206
Activase I.V. 212, 213
Activated charcoal 335, 349
Actos 116
Acular 256
- *PF* 160
- *preservative free* 256
Acute
- agitation 228
- alcohol withdrawal 229, 232
- catatonia 237
- coronary syndrome 23
- excitement 228
- fear 238
- high anion gap acidosis 57
- intermittent porphyria 121
- leukemia 321
- lymphocytic leukemia 71, 72
- mania 235
- myelogenous leukemia (AML) 70
- non-anion gap acidosis 56
- panic attack 238
- post-streptococcal glomerulonephritis 155
- promyelocytic leukemia 74
- prostatitis 164
- renal failure 152
- suicidality 229

- tubulointerstitial nephritis 158
- urinary tract infection 161
- urticaria 304
- visual loss 263
Acyclovir 190, 194, 196, 244, 253, 260, 282, 295, 296
Acylaminopenicillins 146, 150, 169, 184
Adalat 16, 104, 141, 305
Adalat cc 16, 104
Adalimumab 107
Adapalene 285, 298, 301, 305
Addison crisis 132
Addison disease 131
Additive hormone therapy 309
Adefovir dipivoxil 147
Adenocard 37, 337
Adenoscan 337
Adenosine 37, 337
Adjuvant hormone therapy 309
Adoxa 286, 288, 295, 298, 302, 303
Adrenal insufficiency 131
Adrenalin 339, 341, 342
Adrenergic agonists, topical 269
Adriamycin 138, 308, 310–312, 319–322, 327–331
- *PFS* 73, 77– 80
- *RDF* 73, 77–80
Adrucil 138, 307, 310–321, 332
Adsorbents 335, 349
Advil 96, 105, 205, 210, 256, 257, 266, 281
- *Children's* 106, 280
- *Migraine* 210
Aerobid 82, 83, 84
Aerolate 19
Afrin 20, 275
Agenerase 191
Aggrenox 213, 214
Agitation 228
Agoraphobia 239

B

Bacillus anthracis 170
Bacitracin 243
- oint 241–244, 248, 253, 255
Baclofen 208, 212
Baclofen intoxication 339
Bacterial conjunctivitis 248
Bacteroides fragilis 171
Bactocill 40, 245, 285, 296
Bactrim 102, 113, 158, 161, 162, 163, 164, 170–173, 181, 183, 185, 188, 189, 192, 193, 282, 302
Bactroban 296
BAL 338, 346, 352
Barbiturate intoxication 339
Bayer Aspirin 20–24, 27, 35, 40, 43, 46, 104, 205, 213, 214, 263, 265, 278
BCNU 309, 326
Bebulin VH 61
Beclomethasone 82, 83, 84, 276, 277
Beconase 276, 277
Beepen VK 155, 169, 171, 186, 187
Benadryl 247, 292, 304
Benazepril 157, 158
BeneFix 61
Benlyin 279
Benzac 286
Benzaclin 286
Benzamycin 286
Benzathine Penicillin 39, 40, 278, 302
Benzimidazole derivates 197
Benzodiazepines 24, 128, 175, 208, 217, 218, 226, 228, 229, 232, 235, 237–239, 283, 306
- antagonists 339
Benzodiazepin intoxication 339
Benzoyl peroxide 286

Benztropine 222, 223
Benztropine mesylate 237
Benzylpenicillins 40, 41, 97, 169–175, 180–183, 186–188, 278–280, 302
Bepanthen 113
Beta-adrenergic agonists 38
Beta-adrenergic blockers 33
Beta-blockers 16–28, 33–35, 38, 39, 46, 121, 127, 128, 132, 133, 149, 175, 211, 237, 339
- beta-1-selective 16
- topical 260, 261, 262, 264, 266, 268, 270, 272, 273
Betadine 294, 295
Betagan 264, 268, 272, 273
Beta-hemolytic streptococci 187
Beta-interferons 225
Beta-lactamase inhibitors 95, 146, 162, 169, 243, 244, 246, 251, 275, 276, 278, 282, 283
Betamethasone 293
Betapace 36, 37, 38
Betapace AF 36, 37, 38
Betapen VK 39, 155, 169, 171, 186, 187
Betaseron 225
Beta-sympathomimetics 82, 83, 84, 85, 86, 87, 102
Beta-thalassemia major 63
Betatrex 293
Betaval 293
Betaxolol 269
Betimol 260, 262, 264, 266, 268, 272, 273
Betoptic S 269
Bevacizumab 316
Biaxin 88, 89, 143, 163, 171, 173, 174, 176, 180–183, 186, 194, 277–280, 293, 294
Biaxin XL 88, 89
Bicalutamide 331

Bicillin L-A 39, 40, 278, 302
BiCNU 309, 326
Biguanides 116
Bile acid sequestrants 118, 146, 148
Biliary cirrhosis 148
Biliary colic 150
Biltricide 200, 201
Bimatoprost 269
Biocef 285, 293, 295, 297
Bioclate 60
Biomodulators 313–316, 319, 320
Bion Tears 241, 247, 253, 255
Biperiden 237
Biphasic insulins 114, 117
Bisacodyl 151
Bisoprolol 16, 21, 28, 33
Bisphosphonates 55, 81, 122, 125, 133
Black widow spider envenomation 340
b-Lactamase inhibitors 162
Bladder cancer 307
Blenoxane 79, 305, 313, 333
Bleomycin 79, 305, 313
Bleph-10 248
Blepharitis anterior 241
Blepharitis posterior 242
Blocadren 211
Bordetella pertussis 171
Borrelia burgdorferi 171
Borrelia recurrentis 172
Borreliosis 298
Bosentan 100, 112
Botox 141
Botulinin Antitoxin (ABE) 175, 340
Botulinum toxin 141
Botulism 175, 340
Bradycard arrhythmias 39
Bradycardia 26
Brain tumors 309

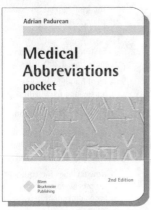

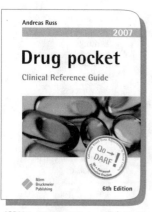

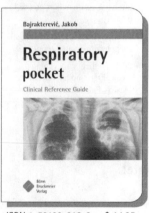

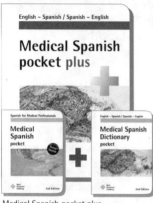
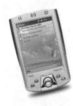

Börm Bruckmeier Publishing
PO Box 388
Ashland, OH 44805

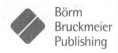

Börm
Bruckmeier
Publishing

Phone: 888-322-6657
Fax: 419-281-6883

Name		E-mail	
Address			
City		State	Zip

	Subtotal	
Sales Tax, add only for: CA 8%; OH 6.25%	**+ Sales Tax**	
Shipping & Handling for US address: UPS Standard: 10% of subtotal with a minimum of $5.00 UPS 2nd Day Air: 20% of subtotal with a minimum of $8.00	**+ S & H**	
	= Total	

Credit Card: ☐ Visa ☐ Mastercard ☐ Amex ☐ Discover
Card Number

Exp. Date   Signature

**For foreign orders,
quantity rebate, optional
shipping and payment
please inquire:
service@media4u.com**

Books and Pocketcards also available at ...   www.media4u.com

Börm Bruckmeier Products

	COPIES		PRICE/COPIES		PRICE
pockets					
Anatomy pocket		x	US $ 16.95	=	
Canadian Drug pocket 2006–2007		x	US $ 14.95	=	
Differential Diagnosis pocket		x	US $ 14.95	=	
Drug pocket 2007		x	US $ 12.95	=	
Drug pocket plus 2007		x	US $ 24.95	=	
Drug Therapy pocket 2006–2007		x	US $ 16.95	=	
ECG pocket		x	US $ 16.95	=	
ECG Cases pocket		x	US $ 16.95	=	
EMS pocket		x	US $ 14.95	=	
Homeopathy pocket		x	US $ 14.95	=	
Medical Abbreviations pocket		x	US $ 16.95	=	
Medical Classifications pocket		x	US $ 16.95	=	
Medical Spanish pocket		x	US $ 16.95	=	
Medical Spanish Dictionary pocket		x	US $ 16.95	=	
Medical Spanish pocket plus		x	US $ 22.95	=	
Normal Values pocket		x	US $ 12.95	=	
Respiratory pocket		x	US $ 16.95	=	
pocketcards					
Alcohol Withdrawal pocketcard		x	US $ 3.95	=	
Antibiotics pocketcard 2007		x	US $ 3.95	=	
Antifungals pocketcard		x	US $ 3.95	=	
ECG pocketcard		x	US $ 3.95	=	
ECG Evaluation pocketcard		x	US $ 3.95	=	
ECG Ruler pocketcard		x	US $ 3.95	=	
ECG pocketcard Set (3)		x	US $ 9.95	=	
Echocardiography pocketcard Set (2)		x	US $ 6.95	=	
Epilepsy pocketcard Set (2)		x	US $ 6.95	=	
Geriatrics pocketcard Set (3)		x	US $ 9.95	=	
History & Physical Exam pocketcard		x	US $ 3.95	=	
Medical Abbreviations pocketcard Set (2)		x	US $ 6.95	=	
Medical Spanish pocketcard		x	US $ 3.95	=	
Medical Spanish pocketcard Set (2)		x	US $ 6.95	=	
Neurology pocketcard Set (2)		x	US $ 6.95	=	
Normal Values pocketcard		x	US $ 3.95	=	
Periodic Table pocketcard		x	US $ 3.95	=	
Psychiatry pocketcard Set (2)		x	US $ 6.95	=	
Vision pocketcard		x	US $ 3.95	=	

Books and Pocketcards also available at …   www.media4u.com